BIOCHEMICAL PHARMACOLOGY AS AN APPROACH TO GASTROINTESTINAL DISORDERS

IUPHAR GI PHARMACOLOGY SYMPOSIUM

BIOCHEMICAL PHARMACOLOGY AS AN APPROACH TO GASTROINTESTINAL DISORDERS

Basic Science to Clinical Perspectives (1996)

Editors:

Timothy S. Gaginella

School of Pharmacy, University of Wisconsin, Madison, WI, USA

Gyula Mózsik

First Department of Medicine, University Medical School of Pécs, Pécs, Hungary

K.D. Rainsford

Department of Biomedical Sciences, Sheffield Hallam University, Sheffield, UK

SPRINGER-SCIENCE+BUSINESS MEDIA, B.V.

Library of Congress Cataloging-in-Publication Data is available.

ISBN 978-94-010-6267-1 ISBN 978-94-011-5390-4 (eBook)
DOI 10.1007/978-94-011-5390-4

Printed on acid-free paper

CONTENTS

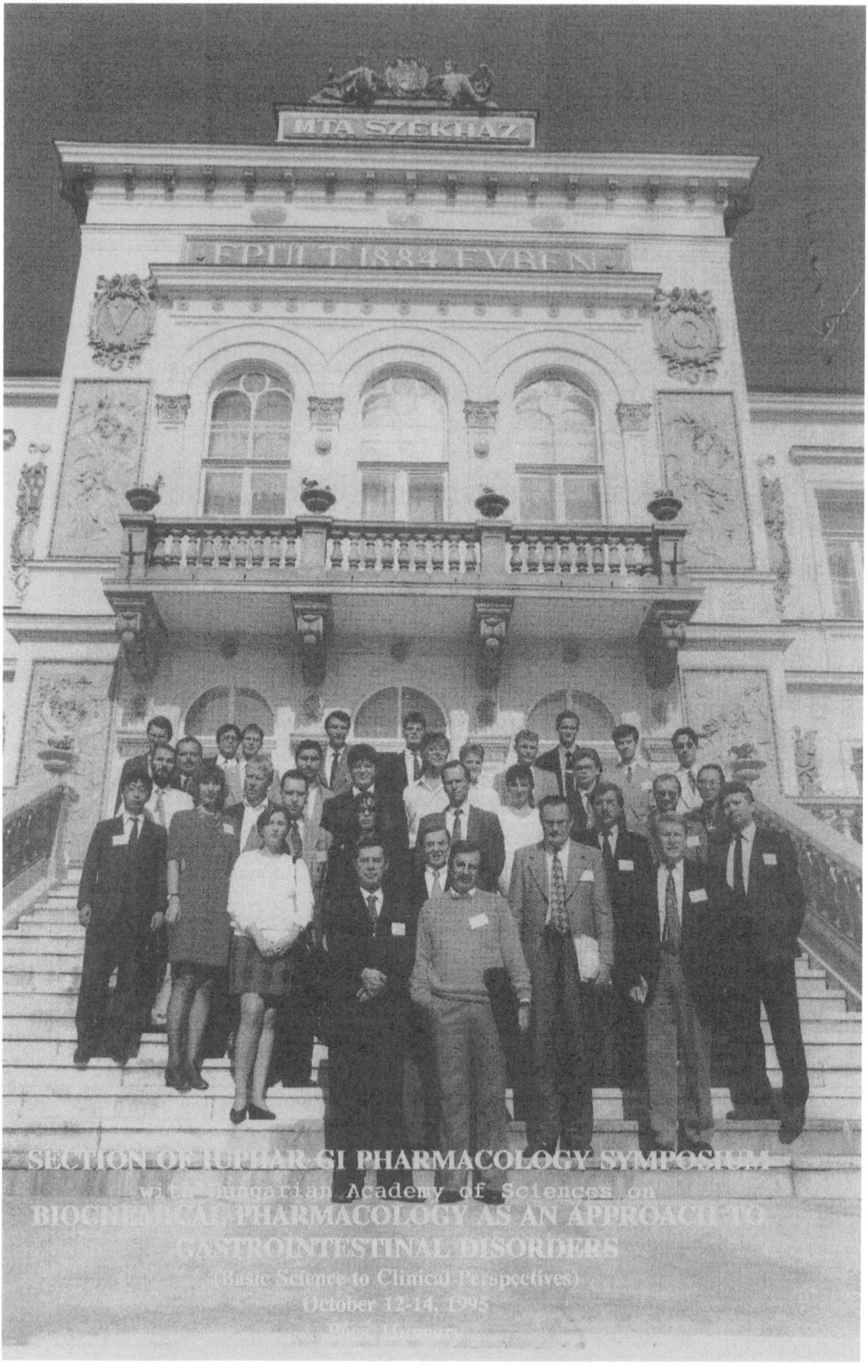
MTA SZÉKHÁZ
ÉPÜLT 1884 ÉVBEN
SECTION OF IUPHAR GI PHARMACOLOGY SYMPOSIUM
with Hungarian Academy of Sciences on
BIOCHEMICAL PHARMACOLOGY AS AN APPROACH TO
GASTROINTESTINAL DISORDERS
(Basic Science to Clinical Perspectives)
October 12-14, 1995

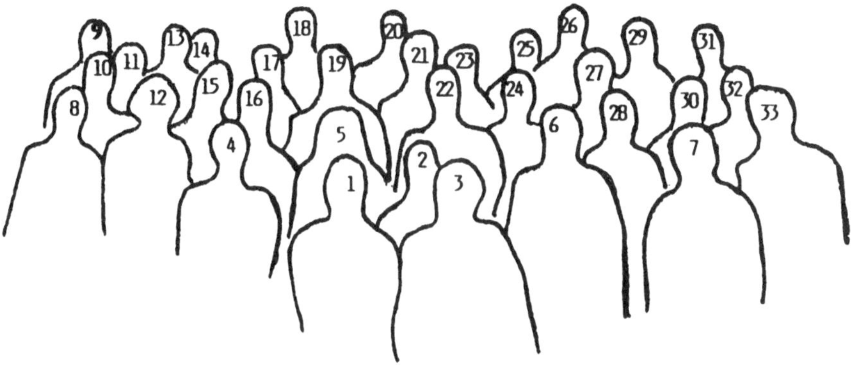

PARTICIPANTS

1. P. Sikiric (Zagreb, Croatia)
2. T. S. Gaginella (Madison, USA)
3. V. Calderaro (Naples, Italy)
4. L. Jurina (Zagreb, Croatia)
5. S. Giljanovic (Zagreb, Croatia)
6. Gy. Mózsik (Pécs, Hungary)
7. M. Palkovits (Budapest, Hungary; Bethesda, USA)
8. M. Nakamura (Tokyo, Japan)
9. L. Barthó (Pécs, Hungary)
10. J. Blazsek (Budapest, Hungary)
11. G. Varga (Budapest, Hungary)
12. M. Veljaca (Zagreb, Croatia)
13. K. Takeuchi (Kyoto, Japan)
14. O. Karádi (Pécs, Hungary)
15. G. Flemström (Uppsala, Sweden)
16. V. Simicevic (Zagreb, Croatia)
17. O.M.E. Abdel-Salem (Pécs, Hungary)
18. S. Evangelista (Firenze, Italy)
19. G. Sütő (Pécs, Hungary)
20. Gy. Rumi (Pécs, Hungary)
21. B. Hunyadi (Bethesda MD, USA)
22. Á. Vincze (Long Beach, USA)
23. K. Kalmár (Pécs, Hungary)
24. B. Bódis (Pécs, Hungary)
25. K. Kovács (Pécs, Hungary)
26. P. Csere (Pécs, Hungary)
27. I. Szabó (Pécs, Hungary)
28. E. Beubler (Graz, Austria)
29. A. Debreceni (Pécs, Hungary)
30. M. Diener (Zürich, Switzerland)
31. G. Várbíró (Pécs, Hungary)
32. D. Chen (Lund, Sweden)
33. Z.K. Krowicki (New Orleans, USA)

SECTION OF IUPHAR GI PHARMACOLOGY SYMPOSIUM
with Hungarian Academy of Sciences
on
BIOCHEMICAL PHARMACOLOGY AS AN APPROACH TO GASTROINTESTINAL DISORDERS
(Basic Science to Clinical Perspectives)

October 12–14, 1995
Pécs, Hungary

PREFACE

The Gastrointestinal Section of International Union of Pharmacology (IUPHAR) was established in 1994 in Montreal, Canada. The establishment of the GI Section recognizes the international progress of gastrointestinal pharmacology, including basic and human studies.

The Gastrointestinal Section will actively participate in the main congress (IUPHAR). Smaller symposia will be organized for times between the main IUPHAR congresses.

The Gastrointestinal Section of IUPHAR had organized the first symposium as 'Biochemical Pharmacology as an Approach to Gastrointestinal Diseases: from Basic Science to Clinical Perspectives' in October 10–12, 1995, Pécs, Hungary.

The main topics were 1) Gastrointestinal secretory and excretory functions, 2) Gastrointestinal motility, 3) Biochemical-pharmacological mechanisms in neural and hormonal actions involved in GI functions, 4) Main normal and pathological biochemical mechanisms in GI functions, 5) GI mucosal injury and protection, 6) Molecular mechanisms of premalignant and malignant diseases in GI tract, 7) Use of isolated cells and cell cultures in biochemical-pharmacological studies to approach GI diseases.

The presented papers are published in this book.

The abstracts of this meeting were published in *Digestive Diseases and Sciences*, and we record appreciation of the Editor of that journal for their publication.

Some of the papers published here have appeared in *Inflammopharmacology* 1996;4:261–305, 1996;4:399–413 and 1997;5:21–103.

Timothy S. Gaginella, PhD
School of Pharmacy, University of Wisconsin, Madison, WI, USA
Gyula Mózsik, *MD, ScD (med)*
First Department of Medicine, University Medical School of Pécs, Pécs, Hungary
KD Rainsford, *PhD, FRCPath, FRSC, FIBiol*
Department of Biomedical Sciences, Sheffield Hallam University, Sheffield, UK

TS Gaginella et al. (eds.), Biochemical Pharmacology as an Approach to Gastrointestinal Disorders, 1–3.

INTRODUCTION: ADVANCES IN THE BIOCHEMICAL PHARMACOLOGY OF GASTROINTESTINAL (GI) FUNCTIONS AS AN APPROACH TO UNDERSTANDING GI DISORDERS

K.D. RAINSFORD
Department of Biomedical Sciences, Sheffield Hallam University, Sheffield, UK

This book contains the proceedings of the first international meeting of the IUPHAR Section on Gastroenterology. It is recognition of how gastrointestinal pharmacology has now progressed to be a discipline in its own right. The past three decades have seen this subject evolve in a unique manner, especially compared with that of many other fields of pharmacology. In the first place many of the specialist developments have arisen from research in the pharmaceutical industry and physician-scientists as well as from the contributions of academics. We recall that the first Nobel Prize to an industry biomedical scientist was to Sir James Black, who could be described as a biochemical pharmacologist. His work on histamine receptor studies set the stage for the development of the first of the truly specific anti-ulcer drugs, the H_2 receptor antagonists, modelled initially by metiamide but then followed by the highly successful drug cimetidine. The latter drug is now deemed to be so safe and effective that it is now sold over the counter in a number of countries. We should also remember how many of us benefited from the generosity of companies like Smith, Kline and French who in the days when the H_2-receptor field was evolving readily gave samples of drugs like metiamide and cimetidine for experimental studies. Whilst it could be said with hindsight that the company stood to benefit from this, it was much less clear then.

The clinical side of gastroenterology has developed in the past 2–3 decades with recognition of the value of scientific advances. Many notable gastroenterologists have made outstanding contributions to gastrointestinal pharmacology. The basic scientists in universities, independent institutes and industry, driven by curiosity, have evolved a deep understanding of the molecular and cellular processes underlying ulcerogenesis in different regions of the gastrointestinal tract and the actions of new and established anti-ulcer drugs and ulcerogenic compounds. The field has thus evolved on a truly multidisciplinary basis involving a partnership of all – physicians, academic and industrial scientists – whose contributions have been synergistic.

The recognition and establishment of the Gastrointestinal Pharmacology Section of IUPHAR would not have been possible without the hard work and persistent efforts of Dr Tim Gaginella, who has himself worked in both industry and academia, and made significant contributions from both sides. Those who have joined with him to form the GI Pharmacology Section all support the ethos of bringing together basic and clinical GI pharmacology and the multi-disciplinary nature of this field.

The past decade has seen the emergence not only of new drugs with unique anti-ulcer activities (e.g. misoprostol, omeprazole) but also the recognition of the role of

Helicobacter pylori as an aetiological agent in peptic ulcer disease, the role of growth factors in ulcer repair, and the importance of a whole range of inflammatory mediators and cells of the immuno-inflammatory system in the pathogenesis of ulcer diseases in the various regions of the GI tract. Advances in molecular and cell biology have had a powerful influence on our understanding of the mechanisms of ulcer disease. GI research has undoubtedly benefited considerably from advances in other fields (even immunology) and also from the development of biologics by the biotechnology industry.

While some would say that there has been a tendency in some GI pharmacology studies to apply these biologics without much rationality, as always happens in science there have been some remarkable observations, e.g. in the application of growth factors as potential anti-ulcer agents. Among these advances has been the understanding of the control of regenerative/restorative processes in the GI mucosa in response to ulcerogenic agents. Linked with this have been studies of the anti-ulcer/ulcer healing effects of biologics, such as acid-resistant basic fibroblast growth factor following the pioneering observations by Professors Sandor Szabo and Judah Folkunan of Harvard University (see chapters by Vincze et al., Nakamura et al. and Watanabe et al., in these Proceedings). Here is an example of where the new GI biochemical pharmacology is emerging linked to advances in molecular biology.

The tools and techniques provided from advances in molecular biology (growth factors, cytokines), immunology (monoclonal antibodies), cell biology (isolated cell systems, single cell ion monitoring) and the neurosciences (neuroregulatory peptides and specific receptor antagonists/agonists) have all had an enormous impact. Future research in the field of GI functions, drug development and mucosal protection will undoubtedly benefit from other advances in cell and molecular biology to encompass the new GI biochemical pharmacology.

The papers in proceedings cover the field of research ranging from studies on gastrointestinal secretion and excretion, through motility disorders, neural controls, mucosal protection, molecular mechanisms of premalignant and malignant changes in gastrointestinal cancers, to the cellular and molecular targets used in understanding drug actions.

This symposium would not have been possible were it not for the hard work and enthusiasm of the two principal organizers, Dr Tim Gaginella and Professor Gyula Mózsik, whose high standing in the field of gastrointestinal pharmacology is well known. The support of the local and international organizing committee has also been most impressive. This all gives support to what has been a successful start to the development of the Section on Gastrointestinal Pharmacology which has now been established and under which this symposium was organized.

Of course the location of the symposium in Hungary is recognition of the high standing and considerable efforts of the scientists and physicians in Hungary who have made extensive contributions to the science of gastroenterology over the decades. The location of the symposium in Pécs was most appropriate for Professor Mózsik and his colleagues have been among the major contributors to the research in this field. There is also the added benefit that this classical city is a beautiful and relaxing place in which to have a meeting!

The help of Mr Phil Johnstone and editorial staff at Kluwer Academic Publishers in producing this book and the publication in the Journal is most gratefully acknowledged.

Section I

GASTROINTESTINAL SECRETORY AND EXCRETORY FUNCTIONS

TS Gaginella et al. (eds.), Biochemical Pharmacology as an Approach to Gastrointestinal Disorders, 7–23

POSSIBLE COMPENSATION IN EPIDERMAL GROWTH FACTOR PRODUCTION BY SALIVA IN RAT

J. BLAZSEK[1*], K. OFFENMÜLLER[1], B. BURGHARDT[2], I. KISFALVI Jr[2], K. BIRKI[1], M. WENCZL[1], G. VARGA[2] AND T. ZELLES[1]
[1]Department of Oral Biology, Semmelweis Medical University; [2]Institute of Experimental Medicine, Hungarian Academy of Science, Budapest, Hungary
*Correspondence

This paper was first published in: Inflammopharmacology. 1996;4:279–295.

ABSTRACT

In the present work, the authors investigated the effect of both main vegetative transmitters and some regulatory peptides on epidermal growth factor (EGF) secretion into whole saliva. We studied how the salivary and glandular EGF levels depend on the functional activity of salivary glands in rats. Experimental groups comprised: (a) control, (b) bilateral ablation (AB) of submandibular and sublingual salivary glands, (c) 0.5% citric acid in drinking water treatment (Cit), and (d) ablation plus citric acid combination (AB+Cit). On the 7th day under narcosis, pilocarpine-stimulated saliva was collected and the amylase activity was measured along with concentrations of EGF and the protein, both in saliva and in salivary glands. In the first study, in conscious rats adrenergic activation of EGF secretion was observed. During noradrenaline stimulation, the curve showing EGF discharge was parallel to the amylase secretory curve. Salivary amylase secretion was stimulated by adrenergic, cholinergic and VIP-ergic actions. Other regulatory peptides, such as CCK, bombesin and somatostatin, did not seem to be involved in controlling EGF or amylase secretion. In the second study, 7 days after ablation, protein concentration of salivary glands decreased in control animals 30 min after pilocarpine stimulation. There was no significant change in protein concentration after this stimulation in the other groups. EGF concentration increased about 40% in submandibular tissues of the Cit group of animals, and decreased in the parotid tissues in all treated groups. The EGF concentration decreased after pilocarpine stimulation to a great extent in all salivary tissues. Protein concentration in saliva was significantly higher than the initial level in all treated groups (AB: +240%; Cit: +80%; AB+Cit: +350%). EGF concentration of saliva was slightly decreased in the ablation group (–10%), while it increased in the other treated animals (Cit: +20%, AB+Cit: +200%). Changes in the EGF level in saliva were lower than 10% in the control group. In conclusion:

1. EGF secretion is controlled by adrenergic pathways but not by cholinergic mechanisms or by VIP, CCK, bombesin or somatostatin,
2. The EGF level in saliva can be increased by enhanced activity of salivary glands,
3. EGF in saliva is not exclusively produced by one type of salivary glands,
4. Parotid glands can compensate the EGF secretion to saliva when functional activity of the other main gland is lost.

Keywords: ablation, citric acid, functional compensation, epidermal growth factor, gustatoric stimulus, salivary glands, regulatory peptides, VIP, CCK, bombesin, somatostatin

---

This paper was presented at the Section of IUPHAR GI Pharmacology Symposium on 'Biochemical pharmacology as an approach to gastrointestinal disorders (basic science to clinical perspectives)', October 12–14, 1995, Pécs, Hungary.

INTRODUCTION

The intact surface of mucous membrane is very important for normal physiological function of the gastrointestinal (GI) tract. Epidermal growth factor (EGF) plays an important role in vital function, regulation of GI cells, with many favourable effects (trophic, cytoprotective, etc.). This peptide is regarded as an important factor in the regeneration of epithelial cells in normal conditions as well as during inflammation or ulceration in the gastrointestinal tract [1]. EGF is a polypeptide comprising 53 amino acids. It was originally isolated from mouse submandibular glands and from human urine. The role of EGF in cell function is in controlling cAMP adenylate cyclase and protein kinase C activity, inositol-P_3 turnover and mRNA transcription [2]. The peptide stimulates cellular growth and differentiation, inhibits gastric acid secretion and prevents experimentally induced gastric and duodenal ulcers [3,4]. In an established cell line of human oral epithelial cells, these cells exhibit chemotaxis to EGF and maximal chemotactic response occurs within the physiological concentration range for EGF found in human saliva [5].

EGF is localized mainly in salivary and Brunner's glands [6]. In humans, the relative proportions of EGF levels in submandibular gland saliva, parotid saliva and whole saliva are 1:6:4. Consequently, the main area of production and storage is the parotid gland in man [7]. In contrast, submandibular gland produces the majority of EGF and the parotid has only a secondary role [8,9]. EGF immunoreactivity can be found, not only in saliva, but also gastric, duodenal and pancreatic secretions. Chewing of parafilm significantly increased salivary but not gastric or duodenal EGF output in man [6]. Salivary EGF, like other salivary constituents, is secreted in a diurnal pattern, and the rhythm is related to the pattern of food intake. During stimulation, the rate of EGF secretion doubles but the concentration falls by 70% because of dilution of salivary fluid [7,10]. We also found this diurnal rhythm of salivary EGF secretion in mouse. Urinary and serum EGF levels have no obvious diurnal rhythm [11]. Salivary EGF levels are significantly lower in younger than in older people. There were no significant differences between EGF levels in saliva of male and female humans. In mice, however, the EGF concentration in saliva is 10-fold higher in males than in females [12].

In a clinical study, higher EGF levels were found in the saliva of patients suffering from juvenile periodontitis (JP) [13], reflux oesophagitis without columnar metaplasia [1], gastric ulcer, duodenal ulcer and gastrointestinal ulcer [14]. Unfortunately, others have reported the opposite changes: lower EGF concentration in gastritis, and no significant change in Barrett's oesophagus and oesophagitis [15]. Salivary EGF levels were found to be very low in patients with oral inflammation (stomatitis aphthosa or peritonsillar abscess), head and neck tumours (squamous cell carcinoma of the tongue, oral cavity, hypopharynx or larynx) [7] and oropharyngeal carcinoma [16]. The salivary EGF level is also lowered in smokers [16,17] and in alcoholic subjects with liver disease[18]. The contradictory results found in human studies could be due to the lack of standard laboratory conditions, the variability in living conditions of patients, and the influence of intermittent diseases.

Investigations with experimental animals allow better understanding of the role of salivary EGF in normal and pathological conditions. In rats, excision of the submandibular salivary glands, which have high EGF production and accumulation in rodents, led to an increased H^+ ion reflux of mucous membrane [19] and an increase in ulceration of mucous membrane [12] was observed. Treatment of sialoadenectomized male mice with EGF (1 μg/ml in drinking water) restored the rate of wound healing to normal levels [12]. Treatment of rats with exogenous EGF (10 μg/kg ip, twice daily for 3 days) caused an increase in amylase activity in saliva in response to pilocarpine stimulation, and a corresponding decrease in enzyme activity in the parotid gland. Analysis of parotid-gland RNA by reverse transcriptase PCR generated a single predicted amylase-derived cDNA product of 576 bp. The level of mRNA for amylase in EGF-treated parotid total RNA showed a 1.8-fold increase compared with untreated controls [2].

The cell types that produce salivary EGF are not well characterized. In rats, in the submandibular glands, EGF is localized to the cells of the granulated convoluted tubules (GCT cells), which are surrounded by an intense network of adrenergic nerves [20,21]. Indeed, noradrenaline in mice and rats increases the concentration of EGF in plasma and in saliva [22–24], an effect mediated by α-adrenergic receptors [25].

Little is known about the physiological role of gastrointestinal peptides in control of salivary secretion. However, experiments involving nerve stimulation in vivo suggest that a significant neuronal regulation of salivary secretion by non-adrenergic non-cholinergic mechanisms may exist in rats [26]. Among the potential mediators, the bioactivity of VIP (vasoactive intestinal peptide), CCK (cholecystokinin), bombesin and somatostatin in other regions of the gastrointestinal tract has already been well documented [27].

The purposes of the present study were (a) to clarify the peptidergic regulation of salivary EGF and amylase secretion in conscious rats, and (b) to determine the effect of sialoadenectomy and gustatoric stimulation on EGF secretion and storage in salivary glands.

MATERIALS AND METHODS

Experiments with conscious rats

Female 250–300 g Wistar Crl.(Wi)Br rats (Charles River) were used. Surgery was performed under di-ethylether anaesthesia. For infusions, a polyethylene catheter (PE50) was inserted into the right jugular vein. Another polyethylene catheter (PE24O) was introduced into the lower oesophagus through a ruminal incision, secured in place by two ligatures at the level of the cardia and rumen, and conducted through the abdominal wall. The muscle and skin were sutured and the rat was placed in a Bollman cage. Two hours after recovery from anaesthesia, saliva was collected at 30-min fractions in 5-ml graduated tubes. The volume of saliva samples was measured to the nearest 0.1 ml. Amylase and EGF output was evaluated as described in a separate section.

In each study, basal salivary secretion was collected for at least two basal periods before the various treatments. In the first two experiments, noradrenaline and carbachol were infused in successively increasing doses. In subsequent studies, a submaximal dose of carbachol (0.03 mg kg^{-1} h^{-1}) was used as a background infusion to study the effect of peptides. VIP (vasoactive intestinal peptide, Sigma), CCK (cholecystokinin, Research Plus), bombesin (Peninsula) and a long-acting somatostatin analogue (Sandostatin, Sandoz) were infused in increasing doses.

Experiments on increased salivary activity

At the beginning of all experiments, under light sodium pentobarbital (30 mg/kg ip, Serva) anaesthesia, samples of saliva were collected for 15 min from 250–300 g Wistar Crl.(Wi)Br female rats, following pilocarpine stimulation (Pilocarpine-HCl, Serva, 2.5 mg/kg ip). The secreted saliva from the oral cavity was collected in eppendorf tubes. After 15-min saliva collection, bilateral submandibular (SM) and sublingual (SL) sialoadenotomy (ablation) was performed on half the animals through a sagittal neck incision under local subcutaneously injected lidocaine (0.1 ml, 2% solution, EGIS Co.). Intact and ablated animals were divided into groups, receiving either drinking tap water or water containing 0.5% citric acid. Experimental groups were the following: control, ablation (AB), citric acid (Cit) and ablation and citric acid (AB+Cit). These treatments were continued for one week. Food (from LATI Ltd.) and the drinking solutions were provided ad libitum. Food was withdrawn 12–16 h before experiments. On the experimental day, under necrosis, 15-min pilocarpine-stimulated saliva was collected from every second rat. After bleeding, the salivary glands were excised from all animals. The glands were weighed and tissues were homogenized in a blender in 20 mmol/L phosphate-buffered saline, pH 7.4.

Determination of EGF, protein and amylase

EGF level was measured in both saliva samples and in glandular homogenates by radioreceptor assay, using a preparation of human placental syncytiotrophoblast microvilli membranes [28]. Aliquots (100 µl) were added to 100 µl human placental microvillus membranes and ^{125}I-labelled human EGF (100 µl/50 000 cpm). After incubation at room temperature overnight, the membrane solution was diluted in 1000 µl 5% polyethylene glycol, centrifuged for 10 min at 1500*g* and the supernatant was aspirated and discarded. The radiolabel associated with the membrane was determined in a γ-counter. Using this method, the binding is independent of the species of EGF source [29]. Protein concentration was measured by the Bio-Rad Protein Micro Assay based on the method of Bradford [30], with a microplate reader Bio-Rad model 3550, using bovine serum albumin as a standard. The amylase activity was determined by an enzyme activity assay [31] using starch as substrate. One unit (U) of amylase was defined as the activity of amylase that hydrolyses 1 mg starch/min at 37°C.

Statistics

The results are expressed as mean ± standard error of mean (SEM). Statistical significance was calculated by analysis of variance followed by Dunnett test or by Student's *t*-test. Differences were considered significant when $p < 0.05$.

RESULTS

Studies on peptidergic regulation of EGF secretion

Intravenous infusion of noradrenaline (1.5–5.0 mg kg^{-1} h^{-1}) increased the secretion of salivary amylase dose dependently in conscious rats (Figure 1a). Carbachol (0.03–0.3 mg kg^{-1} h^{-1}) infusion also led to an increased amylase output (Figure 2a). Similarly, VIP (0.1, 1.0 and 10.0 nmol kg^{-1} h^{-1}) stimulated the discharge of the enzyme (Figure 3a) when given together with a submaximal carbachol dose (0.03 mg kg^{-1} h^{-1}). CCK (0.25–2.5 nmol kg^{-1} h^{-1}), bombesin (1–10 nmol kg^{-1} h^{-1}) and somatostatin (1.5–15 µg kg^{-1} h^{-1}) did not influence the secretion of salivary amylase over a wide dose range in conscious rats (Figure 4a).

In conscious rats, noradrenaline (1.5–5.0 mg kg^{-1} h^{-1}) induced a substantial increase in EGF secretion into the saliva (Figure 1b). On the other hand, carbachol administration did not affect the discharge of this regulatory peptide (Figure 2b). Neither VIP (Figure 3b) nor CCK, bombesin or somatostatin (Figure 4b) modified EGF output under our experimental conditions.

Studies on adaptive changes in salivary EGF secretion and storage

In a second series of experiments, we studied EGF and protein levels in whole saliva and salivary glands in rats after bilateral submandibular and sublingual gland ablation, citric acid administration, and the combination of the two treatments. Pilocarpine was used to stimulate salivary function. Pilocarpine has a dual action, a main cholinergic and a secondary sympathetic effect. Therefore, it is an optimal stimulus for salivary secretion [32].

Animal body weights over 7 days under our experimental conditions did not change (Table 1). The weight of the parotid glands was elevated in the AB group by 10%, in the Cit group by 30% and in the AB+Cit group by 90%. The weight of the SM glands did not alter over one week of citric-acid treatment (Table 2). Non-significant trends in the protein concentration of parotid tissue were: 25% decrease following AB in non-stimulated animals (and no difference after pilocarpine stimulation), 12% increase in the Cit group and 20% reduction in the AB+Cit group (Figure 5a). In the SM glands, the protein concentration did not change following citric acid treatment (Figure 6a).

The EGF concentrations in the parotid tissues of all three treated groups were decreased by 90–95% compared with controls (Figure 5b). By contrast, the EGF concentration in SM glands was elevated following citric acid treatment by 40%

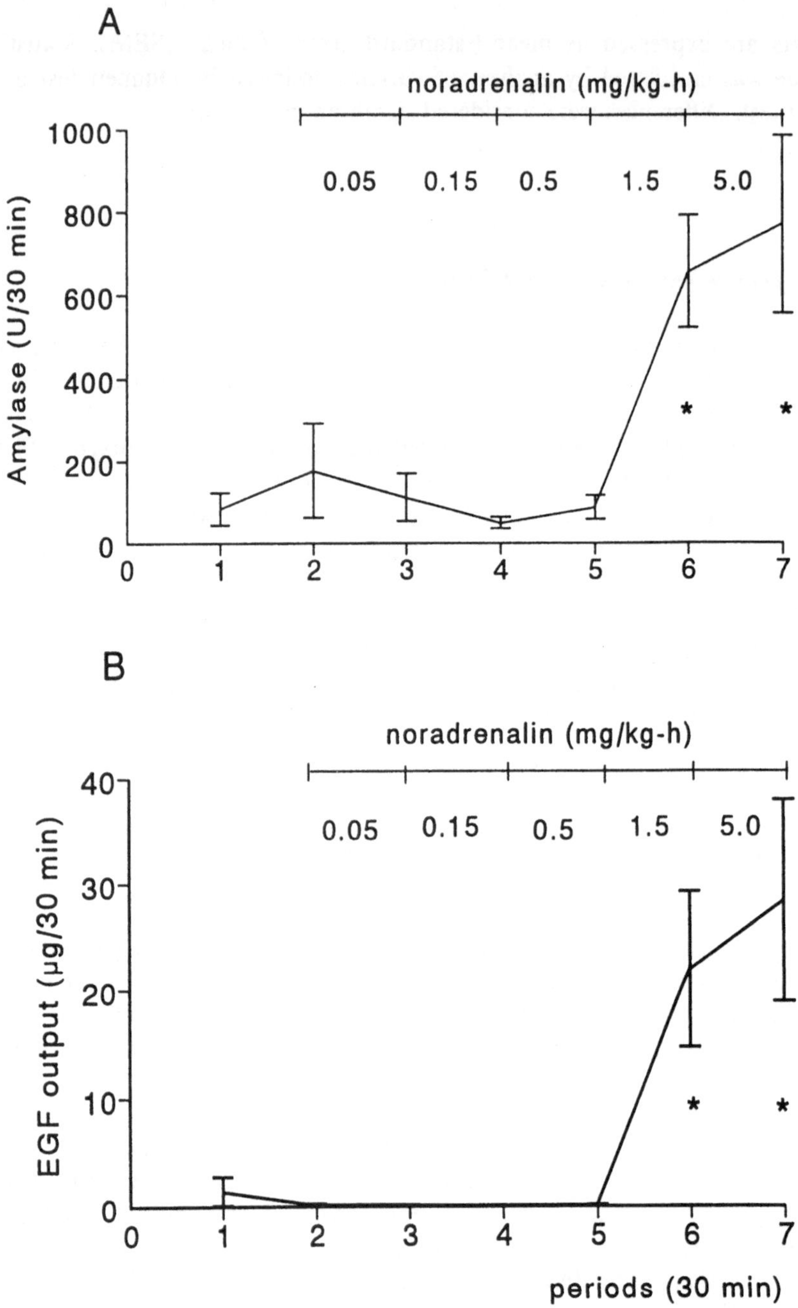

Figure 1. Effect of noradrenaline (0.15–5.0 mg kg^{-1} h^{-1}) on salivary amylase (A) and EGF (B) secretion in conscious rats. Values are mean ± SEM. *$p < 0.05$ vs. basal secretion

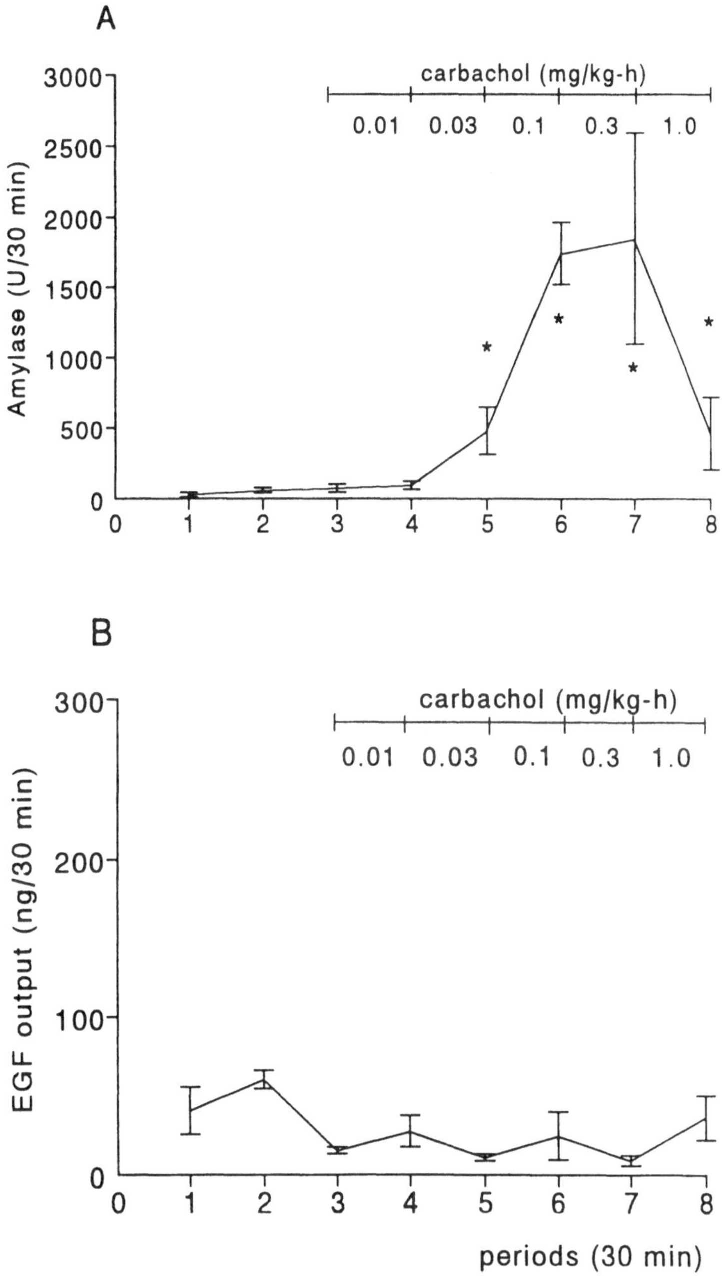

Figure 2. Effect of carbachol (0.03–1.0 mg kg^{-1} h^{-1}) on salivary amylase (A) and EGF (B) secretion in conscious rats. Values are mean ± SEM. $p < 0.05$ vs. basal secretion

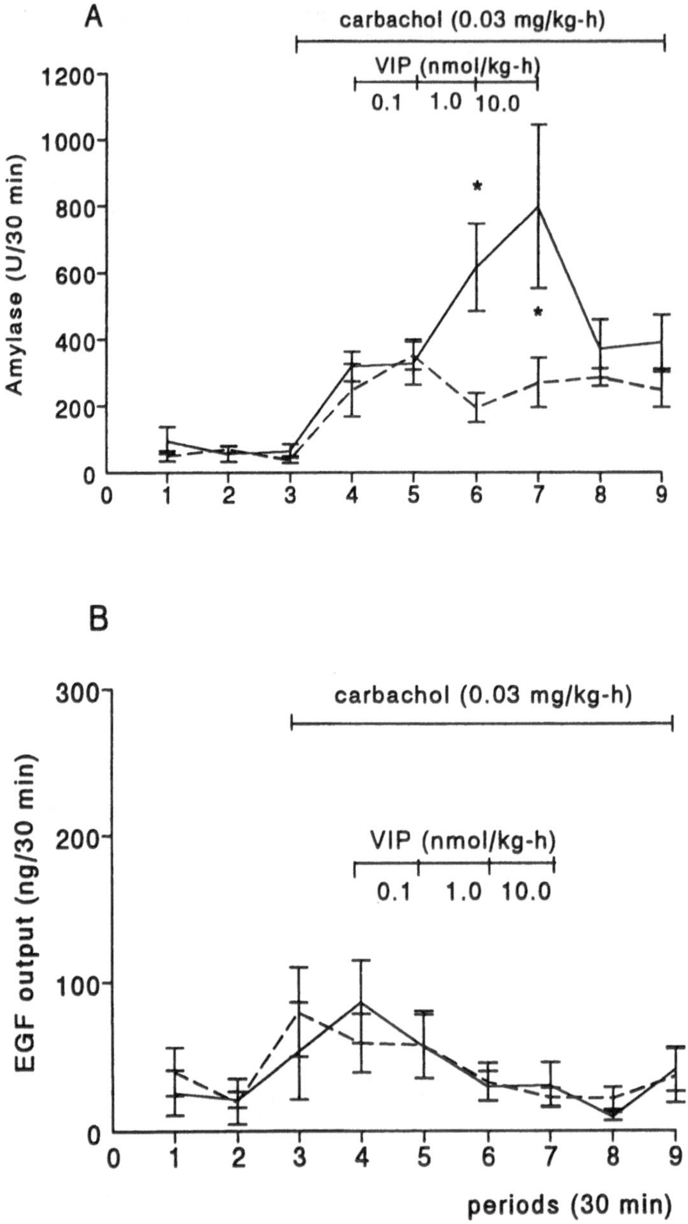

Figure 3. Effect of vehicle (- - -) or VIP (——) (0.1, 1.0, 10.0 nmol kg^{-1} h^{-1}) on amylase (A) and EGF (B) secretion during carbachol (0.03 mg kg^{-1} h^{-1}) background infusion in conscious rats. Values are mean $\pm$ SEM. *$p<0.05$ vs. the 3rd collection period of the same group (the period in which carbachol was given alone)

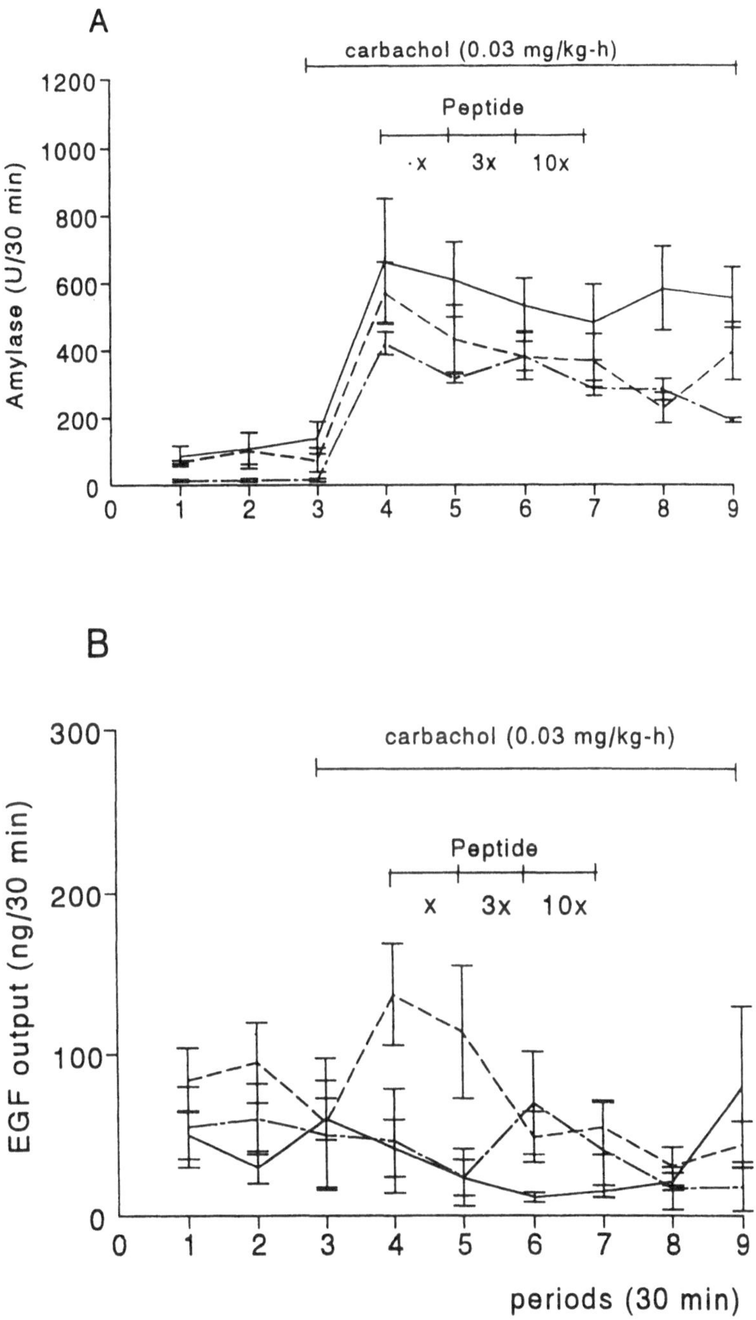

Figure 4. Effect of CCK (——) (0.25, 0.75 and 2.5 nmol kg^{-1} h^{-1}), bombesin (– – –) (1, 3 and 10 nmol kg^{-1} h^{-1}) and somatostatin (- · -) (1.5, 4.5 and 15 μg kg^{-1} h^{-1}) on salivary amylase (A) and EGF (B) secretion during carbachol (0.3 mg kg^{-1} h^{-1}) background infusion in conscious rats. Values are mean ± SEM

TABLE 1

Body weight (g) of rats on day 0 and 7 days after ablation, 0.5% citric acid drinking, and combined treatment (AB+Cit)

	Control		Ablation		Citric acid		AB+Cit	
	day 0	day 7	day 0	day 7	day 0	day 7	day 0	day 7
Mean	271.8	277.8	261.8	268.0	272.0	280.0	272.7	270.8
SEM	9.2	9.9	10.7	9.9	4.7	5.9	10.8	15.5
p	NS		NS		NS		NS	

NS = not significant

TABLE 2

Weight (mg) of the submandibular and parotid glands of fasted non-stimulated (Rest) and pilocarpine-stimulated (Stim) rats

	day 0	Control (day 7)		Ablation (day 7)		Citric acid (day 7)		AB+Cit (day 7)	
	Stim	Rest	Stim	Rest	Stim	Rest	Stim	Rest	Stim
Submandibular gland									
Mean	371.3	407.3	383.3	–	–	402.0	384.7	–	–
SEM	11.8	31.5	10.1	–	–	11.2	17.4	–	–
p						NS			
Parotid gland									
Mean	–	305.0	325.7	332.0	384.0	410.7	374.3	658.3	518.3
SEM	–	16.2	7.4	58.6	16.6	37.2	7.2	63.6	70.5
p				NS	*	**	**	**	**

NS = not significant; $^*p<0.05$; $^{**}p<0.01$ compared with controls

(Figure 6b). In both glands, the EGF concentration decreased following pilocarpine treatment (Figures 5b and 6b). A substantial rise in the protein concentration was observed in saliva samples of all treated groups when compared with controls (AB +240%, Cit +80%, AB+Cit +350%). The change in the salivary protein concentration of the control groups did not exceed 10% (Figure 7a). The EGF concentrations of saliva samples of the AB group were 10% lower than the initial values; these values were significantly elevated in the other groups (Figure 7b). In the saliva on the seventh day, the EGF/protein ratio was lower in all treated groups than in controls (AB group: –80%; Cit group –40%; AB+Cit group: –40%) (Figure 8).

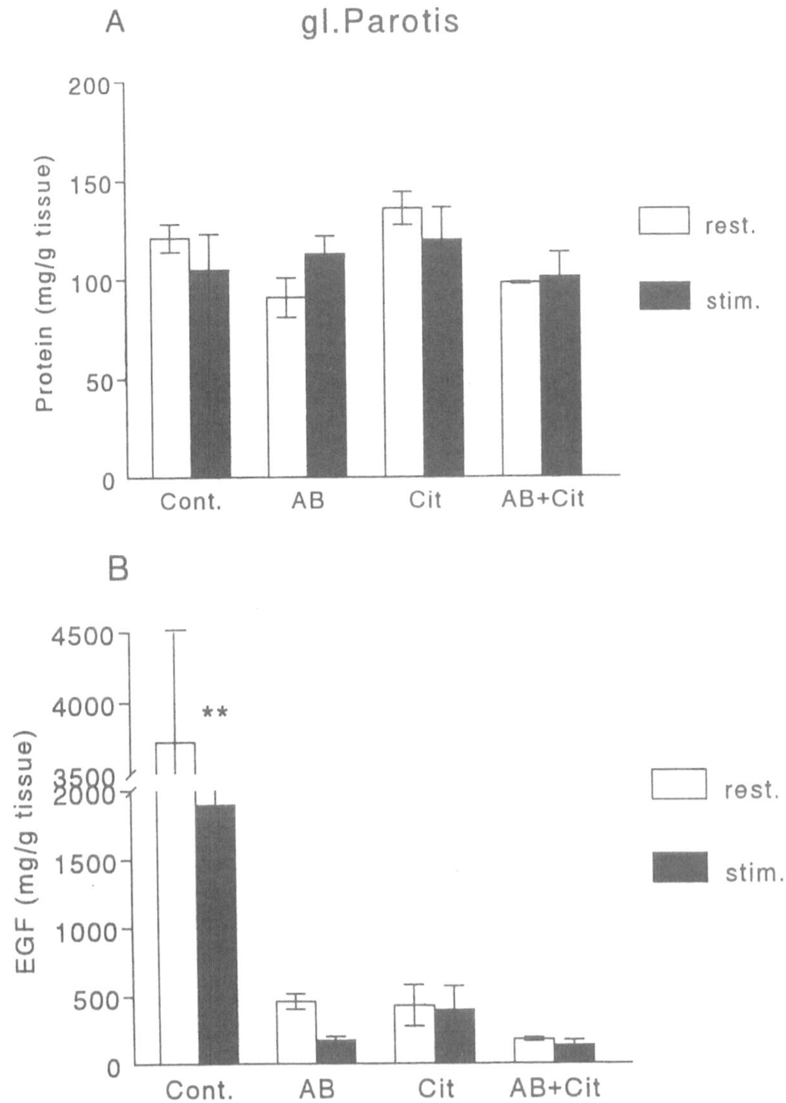

Figure 5. Protein (A) and EGF (B) concentration in parotid glands after 7 days' treatment by ablation (AB), 0.5% citric acid drinking (Cit), and the combination of these (AB+Cit) and control values (Cont), in fasted non-stimulated (rest.), and 2.5 mg/kg pilocarpine-stimulated (stim.) rats. Values are mean ± SEM, $^{**}p < 0.01$ stim. vs. rest

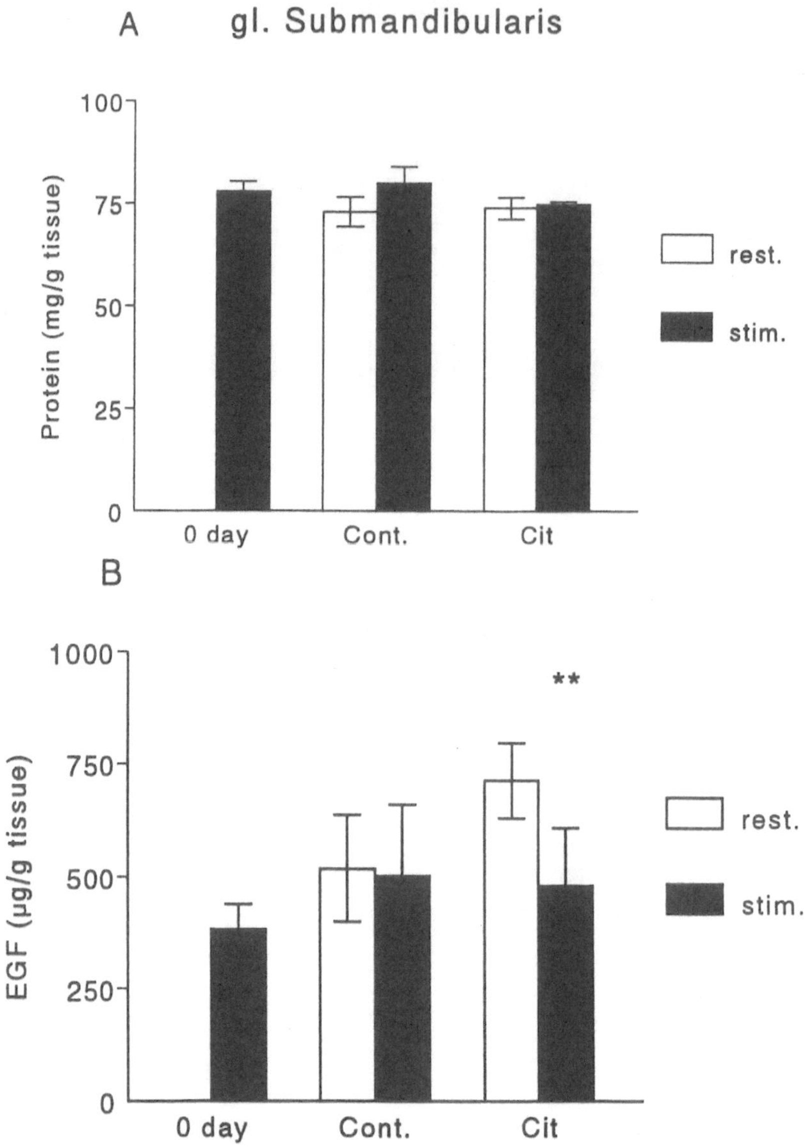

Figure 6. Protein (A) and EGF (B) concentration in submandibular glands on day 0 and after 7 days' treatment by 0.5% citric acid drinking in fasted non-stimulated (rest). and 2.5 mg/kg pilocarpine-stimulated (stim.) rats. Values are mean ± SEM, $^{**}p < 0.01$ stim. vs. rest

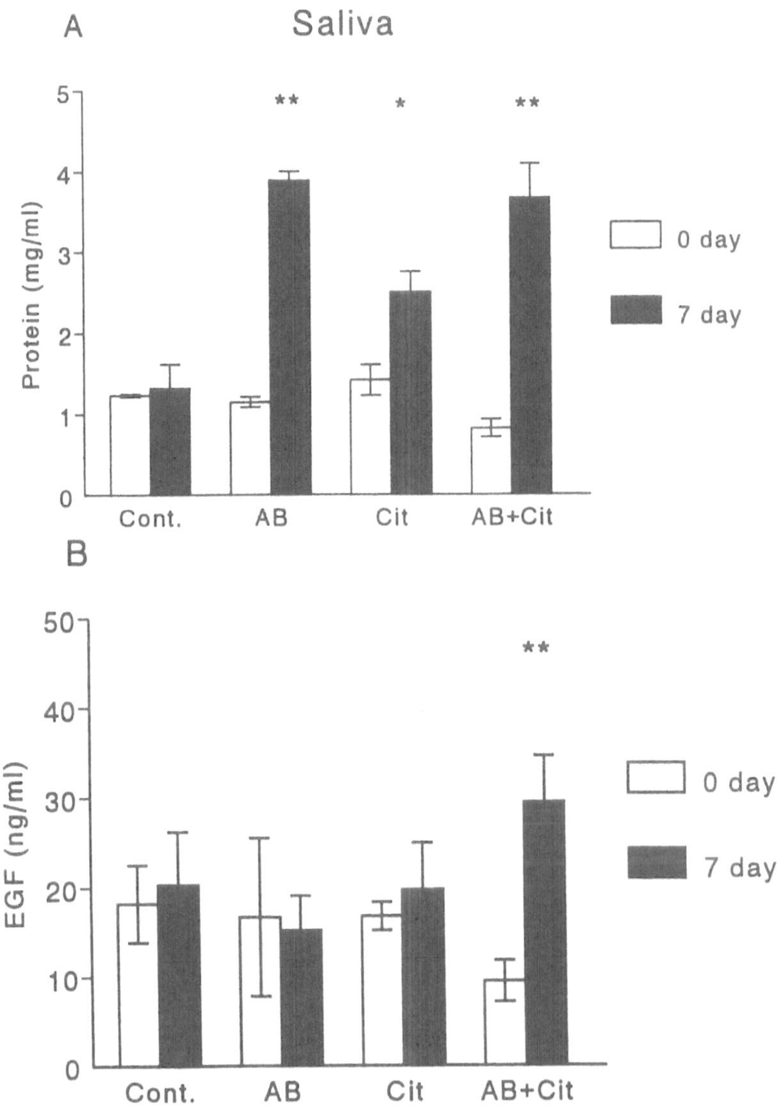

Figure 7. Protein (A) and EGF (B) concentration in whole saliva collected for 15 min after 2.5 mg/kg pilocarpine stimulation on day 0 and after 7 days' treatment by ablation (AB), 0.5% citric acid drinking (Cit), the combination of these (AB+Cit) and control values (Cont). Values are mean ± SEM, $^{*}p<0.05$, $^{**}p<0.01$ stim. vs. rest

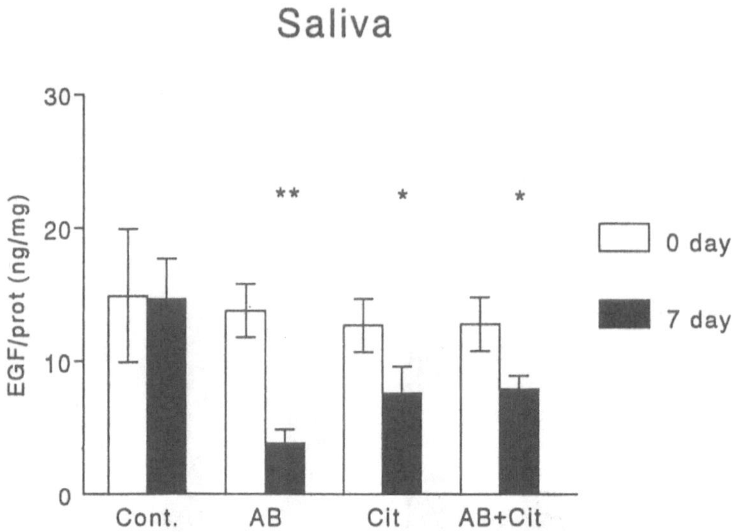

Figure 8. The EGF/protein ratio in 15-min fractions of whole saliva, after 2.5 mg/kg ip pilocarpine stimulus, on day 0 and after 7 days' treatment by ablation (AB), 0.5% citric acid drinking (Cit), the combination of these (AB+Cit) and control values (Cont). Values are mean ± SEM, *$p<0.05$, **$p<0.01$ stim vs. rest

DISCUSSION

The present investigation confirms previous findings that salivary glands secrete a large amount of EGF into the saliva [25]. We have also confirmed that discharge of EGF is under adrenergic control [25]. In addition, we have observed that muscarinic cholinergic stimulation does not affect EGF secretion from salivary glands.

Previous experiments studying the role of regulatory peptides in amylase from salivary glands led to controversial results. The stimulatory effect of VIP on salivary amylase secretion has been reported previously both in vitro [33] and in vivo [34]. CCK immunoreactivity was observed in salivary glands [35] but CCK was found to be ineffective on salivary secretion [36]. Bombesin-like immunoreactivity was also observed in salivary glands [37] but gastrin-releasing peptide, a mammalian form of bombesin, did not stimulate amylase discharge from isolated parotid acini [33]. Immunocytochemical studies revealed the presence of immunoreactive somatostatin in salivary glands without determining the function of this peptide at this location [38]. Our data suggest that VIP, indeed, play a role in the physiological regulation of amylase secretion in the salivary glands. CCK, bombesin and somatostatin are probably not involved in this control since none of them affected salivary secretion in the dose range in which they exert their effects on other organs [27].

The present observations, that VIP, CCK, bombesin and somatostatin do not affect salivary EGF secretion in rats, cannot be compared with other studies since no data are available on peptidergic regulation of salivary EGF secretion in the literature.

Sialoadenotomy and citric acid treatment both induced parotid gland enlargement in our experimental system. Previous studies also showed a compensatory tissue hypertrophy [39] and an increase in amylase mRNA level [2] in parotid glands. The gustatoric stimulatory effect of 0.5% citric acid in drinking water was also reported to increase the functional activity of salivary glands [40]. Ablation resulted in increased activity and slight increase in weight of the parotid glands. The 25% decrease in the tissue protein concentration of the parotid glands can be accounted for, at least in part, by the substantial increase in the protein concentration in saliva.

In our experiments, EGF concentration in saliva decreased by only 10% following submandibular ablation, probably because of the activation of parotid glands and other minor salivary glands. In mice, after ablation of submandibular glands, a dramatic decrease in salivary EGF concentration was observed by Noguchi et al. [12]. The differences between our results and their data may be due to differences in species (rat vs mice), time course and/or types of secretagogues used. In our experiments the compensation effect is indicated by our finding that the tissue EGF level decreased by 90% while EGF in saliva hardly changed. It is also interesting to note that the activity of the parotid glands was further increased by ablation combined with citric acid drinking in our experiment.

Gustatoric stimulation by citric acid induced increases in gland weight and protein concentration in parotid glands. The EGF concentration of the parotid tissue, as in the ablation group, decreased by 90%. On the other hand, a 20% EGF concentration increase was measured in the saliva following citric acid drinking. This slight increase was accompanied by a substantial elevation in protein concentration in salivary juice. The weight and protein concentration of the submandibular glands did not show significant changes in response to citric-acid stimulation. On the other hand, the tissue EGF content was increased by 40%. This increased EGF level in submandibular glands was depleted by pilocarpine stimulation.

Summarizing the results of our experiment:

1. EGF secretion from salivary glands is regulated by nonadrenaline but not by cholinergic pathways, VIP, CCK, bombesin or somatostatin;

2. Ablation of SM and SL glands does not lead to the complete depression of salivary EGF secretion;

3. The EGF in saliva is secreted by more than one type of salivary gland;

4. The EGF level in saliva can be increased by the stimulation of glandular activity;

5. Parotid glands could continuously secrete a significant amount of protein and EGF while the EGF and protein pools in the glands were minimal;

6. In the case of defected or ablated glands, complementary gland(s) may compensate for the depleted function.

ACKNOWLEDGEMENTS

We thank Ms Zs. Horváth and Ms E. Sarkady for their excellent technical assistance. This work was supported by grants ETT T-02 352/93, T-02 149/93 and OTKA T-5429.

REFERENCES

1. Gray MR, Donnelly RJ, Kingsnorth AN. Role of salivary epidermal growth factor in the pathogenesis of Barrett's columnar lined oesophagus. Br J Surg. 1991;78:1461–6.
2. Purushotham KR, Zelles T, Blazsek J et al. Effect of EGF on rat parotid gland secretory function. Comp Biochem Physiol. 1995;110:7–14.
3. Carpenter G, Cohen S. Epidermal growth factor. Annu Rev Biochem. 1979;48:193–216.
4. Kirkegaard P, Skov Olsen P, Poulsen SS, Nexo E. Epidermal growth factor inhibits cysteamine-induced duodenal ulcers. Gastroenterology. 1983;85:1277–83.
5. Royce LS, Baum BJ. Physiologic levels of salivary epidermal growth factor stimulate migration of an oral epithelial cell line. Biochim Biophys Acta. 1991;1092:401–3.
6. Konturek JW, Bielanski W, Konturek SJ, Bogdal J, Oleksy J. Distribution and release of epidermal growth factor in man. Gut. 1989;30:1194–200.
7. Ino M, Ushiro K, Ino C, Yamashita T, Kumazawa T. Kinetics of epidermal growth factor in saliva. Acta Otolaryngol Suppl Stockh. 1993;500:126–30.
8. Cohen S. Isolation of a mouse submaxillary gland protein accelerating incisor eruption and eyelid opening in the new-born animal. J Biol Chem. 1962;237:1555–62.
9. Barka T. Biologically active polypeptides in submandibular glands. J Histochem Cytochem. 1980;28:836–59.
10. McGurk M, Hanford L, Justice S, Metcalfe RA. The secretory characteristics of epidermal growth factor in human saliva. Arch Oral Biol. 1990;35:653–9.
11. Siminoski K, Bernanke J, Murphy RA. Nerve growth factor and epidermal growth factor in mouse submandibular glands: identical diurnal changes and rate of secretagogue-induced synthesis. Endocrinology. 1993;1332:2031–7.
12. Noguchi S, Ohba Y, Oka T. Effect of salivary epidermal growth factor on wound healing of tongue in mice. Am J Physiol. 1991;260:620–5.
13. Hormia M, Thesleff I, Perheentupa J, Pesonen K, Saxen L. Increased rate of salivary epidermal growth factor secretion in patients with juvenile periodontitis. Scand J Dent Res. 1993;101:138–44.
14. Hirasawa Y, Asaki S, Hongo M et al. Salivary epidermal growth factor in patients with peptic ulcer. Nippon Shokakibyo Gakkai Zasshi. 1991;88:1043–50.
15. Maccini DM, Veit BC. Salivary epidermal growth factor in patients with and without acid peptic disease. Am J Gastroenterol. 1990;85:1102–4.
16. Bergler W, Petroianu G, Metzler R. Diminution of epidermal growth factor in saliva of patients with carcinoma of the oropharynx. Acta Otorrinolaringol Esp. 1992;43:173–5.
17. Wang SL, Milles M, Wu-Wang CY et al. Effect of cigarette smoking on salivary epidermal growth factor (EGF) and EGF receptor in human buccal mucosa. Toxicology. 1992;75:145–57.
18. Dutta SK, Orestes M, Vengulekur S, Kwo P. Ethanol and human saliva: effect of chronic alcoholism on flow rate, composition, and epidermal growth factor. Am J Gastroenterol. 1992;87:350–4.
19. Sarosiek J, Feng T, McCallum RW. The interrelationship between salivary epidermal growth factor and the functional integrity of the esophageal mucosal barrier in the rat. Am J Med Sci. 1991;302:359–63.
20. Gresik EW, Van der Noen H, Barka T. Epidermal growth factor-like material in rat submandibular gland. Am J Anat. 1979;156:83–9.
21. Alm P, Bloom GD, Carlsö B. Adrenergic and cholinergic nerves of bovine, guinea-pig and hamster salivary glands. A light and electronmicroscopic study. Z Zellforsch. 1973;138:407–20.
22. Byyny RL, Orth DN, Cohen S, Doyne ES. Epidermal growth factor: effects of androgens and adrenergic agents. Endocrinology. 1974;95:776–82.
23. Murphy RA, Pantazis NJ, Papastavros M. Epidermal growth factor and nerve growth factor in mouse saliva: a comparative study. Dev Biol. 1979;71:356–70.
24. Roberts ML. The in vitro secretion of epidermal growth factor by mouse submandibular salivary gland. Arch Pharmacol. 1977;296:301–5.

25. Olsen PS, Kirkegaard P, Poulsen SS, Nexo E. Adrenergic effects on exocrine secretion of rat submandibular epidermal growth factor. Gut. 1984;25:1234–40.
26. Mansson B, Ekström J. On the non-adrenergic, non-cholinergic contribution to the parasympathetic nerve-evoked secretion of parotid saliva in the rat. Acta Physiol Scand. 1991;251:C175–85.
27. Walsh JH, Dockray GJ. Gut Peptides. New York: Raven Press; 1994.
28. Booth AG, Olaniyan O, Vanderpuye OA. An improved method for the preparation of human placental syncytiotrophoblast microvilli. Placenta. 1980;1:327–36.
29. Simpson RJ, Smith JA, Moritz RL et al. Rat epidermal growth factor: complete amino acid sequence. Homology with the corresponding murine and human protein; isolation of *a* form truncated at both ends with full *in vitro* biological activity. Eur J Biochem. 1985;153:629–37.
30. Bradford MM. A rapid and sensitive method for the quantitation of microgram quantities of protein utilizing the principle of protein-dye binding. Anal Biochem. 1976;72:248–54.
31. Bernfield P. Amylases, alpha and beta. Meth Enzymol. 1955;1:149–58.
32. Schneier CA, Hall HD. Autonomic pathways involved in a sympathetic-like action of pilocarpine on salivary composition. Proc Soc Exp Biol Med. 1966;121:96–101.
33. Goll R, Poulsen JH, Schmidt P, Schjoldager B, Poulsen SS, Holst JJ. Peptide-evoked release of amylase from isolated acini of the rat parotid gland. Regul Peptides. 1994;51:237–54.
34. Tazi-Saad K, Chariot J, Roze C. Control of pepsin secretion by regulatory peptides in the rat stomach: comparison with acid secretion. Peptides. 1992;13:233–9.
35. Ichikawa H. Leucine enkephaline, neurokinin A and cholecystokinin like immunoreactivities in the guinea pig tongue. Arch Oral Biol. 1990;35:181–91.
36. Liddle R. Cholecystokinin. In: Walsh JH, Dockray GJ, eds. Gut Peptides. New York: Raven Press; 1994:175–216.
37. Frazen L, Forsgen S, Gustafsson H, Henriksson R. Irradiation induced effects on the innervation of rat salivary glands, changes in enkephalin and bombesin like immunoreactivity in ganglionic cells and intraglandular nerve fibers. Cell Tissue Res. 1993;271:529–36.
38. Letic-Gavrilovic A, Abe K. Localization of chromogranins, nonneurospecific enolase, and different forms of somatostatin in submandibular salivary glands of mice. J Dent Res. 1990;69:1494–9.
39. Hall HD, Schneier CA. Functional mediation of compensatory enlargement of the parotid gland. Cell Tissue Res. 1977;184:249–54.
40. Zelles T, Blazsek J, Kóbor A, Gelencsér F, Enlargement of the parotid gland induced by gustatory stimulus. Fogorv Szle. 1984;77:315–18.

Manuscript received 3 Nov. 95.
Accepted for publication 8 Nov. 95.

TS Gaginella et al. (eds.), Biochemical Pharmacology as an Approach to Gastrointestinal Disorders, 25–37

REGULATORY MECHANISM OF ACID SECRETION IN RAT STOMACH AFTER DAMAGE – ROLE OF NITRIC OXIDE, HISTAMINE AND SENSORY NEURONS

K. TAKEUCHI AND S. KATO
Department of Pharmacology and Experimental Therapeutics, Kyoto Pharmaceutical University, Misasagi, Yamashina, Kyoto 607, Japan

This paper was first published in: Inflammopharmacology. 1997;5:43–55.

ABSTRACT

The gastric mucosa responds to mucosal damaging agents by significantly decreasing acid secretion. However, the inhibition of nitric oxide (NO) biosynthesis by N^G-nitro-L-arginine methyl ester (L-NAME) turned the acid-secretory response in the damaged stomach from the 'inhibition' into 'stimulation' state. The present study was performed to investigate the mechanism underlying stimulation of acid secretion in the stomach after damage in the presence of L-NAME. Exposure of the chambered rat stomach to 20 mmol/L taurocholate (TC) for 30 min decreased acid secretion with concomitant reduction of transmucosal potential difference (PD). Pretreatment with L-NAME, although it had no effect on basal acid secretion, apparently increased the acid secretion in the stomach after exposure to TC without any change in the PD response. The acid-stimulatory effect of L-NAME in the damaged stomach was reversed by the co-administration of L-arginine but not D-arginine. Such acid-secretory responses in the presence of L-NAME were also inhibited by prior administration of cimetidine, FPL-52694 (a mast cell stabilizer), spantide (a substance P antagonist) or sensory defunctionalization with capsaicin pretreatment. In contrast, mucosal exposure to TC significantly decreased the number of mucosal mast cells and increased histamine output in the lumen, and these responses were significantly inhibited by FPL-52794, spantide or sensory deafferentation. These findings suggest that:

1. Damage in the stomach may activate the acid-stimulatory pathway in addition to the NO-dependent inhibitory pathway, although the latter effect overcomes the former, resulting in a decrease in acid secretion;
2. The stimulatory pathway is dependent on histamine which may be released from mucosal mast cells in association with capsaicin-sensitive sensory nerves; and
3. L-NAME unmasks the acid-stimulatory response by suppressing the inhibitory pathway.

Keywords: stomach, barrier disruption, taurocholate, acid secretion, nitric oxide, histamine, sensory neuron

INTRODUCTION

The application of a mucosal-damaging agent to the stomach has been shown to cause a luminal alkalinization, mainly by the inhibition of acid secretion [1–3]. The inhibition of acid secretion in the damaged stomach is mediated by both endogenous prostaglandins (PGs) and nitric oxide (NO), since this response is attenuated by pretreatment of

This paper was presented at the Section of IUPHAR GI Pharmacology Symposium on 'Biochemical pharmacology as an approach to gastrointestinal disorders (basic science to clinical perspectives)', October 12–14, 1995, Pécs, Hungary.

the animals with either the NO synthase inhibitor, N^G-nitro-L-arginine methyl ester (L-NAME), or the cyclo-oxygenase inhibitor, indomethacin [4,5]. L-NAME completely abolished the decreased acid-secretory response in the stomach after damage by taurocholate (TC) and enhanced the acid secretion over the basal levels [6]. However, the mechanism underlying stimulation by L-NAME of acid secretion in the damaged stomach has not been clearly explained.

It has been shown that histamine is released into gastric venous blood following injury of the gastric mucosa by acetic or salicylic acid [7] and that this substance is important in the increased acid secretion in the damaged stomach [8]. In addition, mast cell degranulation has been shown in the stomach after administration of mucosal-damaging agents [9]. In the gastrointestinal mucosa, mast cells have been shown to be opposed to substance P containing nerve endings, and substance P is known to stimulate release of histamine from mast cells [10,11]. Furthermore, a recent study showed that NO plays a part as a regulatory mediator of mast cell reactivity [12]. Thus, it is possible to speculate that histamine may play an important role in the regulatory mechanism of acid secretion in the damaged stomach, where NO is released.

In the present study, we examined the acid-secretory response in the stomach after damage with TC in the presence or absence of L-NAME and investigated the roles of NO and histamine in the regulatory mechanism of acid secretion in the damaged stomach.

MATERIALS AND METHODS

Male Sprague–Dawley rats (220–250 g; Nihon Charles River, Atsugi, Japan), kept in individual cages with raised mesh bottoms, were deprived of food but allowed free access to tap water for 18 h prior to the experiments. All studies used 4–7 rats per group under urethane anaesthesia (1.25 g/kg ip).

Determination of PD and luminal pH

Gastric transmucosal potential difference (PD) and luminal pH were measured simultaneously as previously described [5,13]. Briefly, the stomachs were obtained, mounted on ex-vivo chambers (the area exposed = 3.14 cm^2), and superperfused at a flow rate of 1 ml/min with saline (154 mmol/L NaCl) that was suffused with 100% O_2 and kept in a reservoir. The pH of the fluid emerging from the chamber was measured using a flow-type pH glass electrode (6901-25T Horiba, Kyoto, Japan) while PD was determined using two agar bridges, one positioned in the chamber and the other in the abdominal cavity. Changes in both PD and pH were monitored simultaneously on a two-pen recorder (U-228, Tokai-irika, Tokyo, Japan). After both PD and pH had stabilized, the perfusion system was interrupted, and the solution in the chamber was withdrawn. The mucosa was then exposed for 30 min to 2 ml of 20 mmol/L sodium taurocholate (TC). After application of TC, the mucosa was rinsed with saline, another

2 ml of saline was instilled and the perfusion resumed. The pH monitoring was interrupted for 30 min while the mucosa was exposed to TC, whereas PD recording was continuously measured throughout the 2-h test period. L-NAME (10 mg/kg) was given iv as a bolus injection 5 min before exposure to TC. L- or D-arginine (200 mg/kg) was given iv 5 min prior to the administration of L-NAME. In some animals, the effects of the following drugs or treatment on the acid secretory response to TC were examined: cimetidine (50 mg/kg; an H_2 antagonist), FPL-52694 (100 mg/kg; a mast cell stabilizer) [14], spantide (100 μg/kg; a substance P antagonist) and chemical ablation of capsaicin-sensitive sensory neurons. Cimetidine and FPL-52694 were given ip 30 min before the administration of L-NAME, while spantide was administered iv 5 min before L-NAME. Sensory deafferentation was performed by three consecutive sc injections of capsaicin (total dose: 100 mg/kg) for 3 days, 2 weeks before the experiment [15].

Determination of gastric acid secretion

The total amount of acid output in the stomach was measured before and after exposure to 20 mmol/L TC by introducing an automatic titrator (Hiranuma Comtite-7, Tokyo, Japan) into the perfusion system [5]. Under these conditions, the titration was performed at luminal pH 7.0 using the pH-stat method and by adding 50 mmol/L NaOH to the reservoir, in which both entry and exit tubes were positioned. In some cases, the recording of pulses of titrants was performed using a Zero Suppression Adaptor (Toha Denpa, C-93611B, Tokyo, Japan) every 5 min. After basal acid secretion had stabilized, the mucosa was exposed for 30 min to TC, and acid secretion was measured for 90 min thereafter. L-NAME (10 mg/kg) was given iv 5 min before injection of L-NAME. In some animals, the effects of cimetidine (50 mg/kg), FPL-52694 (100 mg/kg), spantide (100 μg/kg) and sensory deafferentation were examined on the acid secretory response to TC.

Determination of luminal histamine output

The luminal levels of histamine were determined in the stomach before, during and after exposure for 30 min to 20 mmol/L TC using HPLC. The stomach was mounted on the chamber, rinsed and exposed to 2 ml of saline for 30 min as a control condition. The mucosa was exposed for 30 min to 2 ml of 20 mmol/L TC, followed again by exposure to saline for 30 min. In each case, the gastric samples collected were deproteinized by adding perchloric acid at a final concentration of 3% and then centrifuged at 4°C for 10 min at 10 000*g*. Histamine levels of each sample were determined by using the fluorometer and HPLC-autoanalyser system (Hitachi, Ibaraki, Japan) [16,17]. The experiment was performed in rats without pretreatment of L-NAME (10 mg/kg iv), and the effect of spantide or sensory deafferentation was also examined.

Examination of gastric mucosal mast cells

The method of staining and determining the number of mast cells in the gastric mucosa was similar to that used by Cho et al. [18]. The corpus portion of the stomach, immediately after exposure to 20 mmol/L TC for 30 min, was fixed in freshly prepared 4% (w/v) lead acetate solution. Following a 2-day fixation period, the tissue was dehydrated with alcohol, cleared with xylene, and embedded in paraffin. Sections (7 μm thick) were then made by cutting the paraffin block in a plane vertical to the mucosal surface of the tissue; these were mounted and stained with an aqueous solution of 0.5% (w/v) toluidine blue. The mast cell count was expressed as the number of granulated metachromatically stained mast cells seen in an area immediately below and parallel to the surface epithelium of the mucosa. The experiment was performed in rats with or without pretreatment with L-NAME (10 mg/kg iv), and, in the former, the effect of FPL-52694 or sensory deafferentation was also examined.

Preparation of drugs

Drugs used were urethane (Tokyo Kasei, Tokyo, Japan), taurocholate Na (Difco Lab., Detroit, MI, USA), N^G-nitro-L-arginine methyl ester (L-NAME), L-arginine, D-arginine, cimetidine, capsaicin (Sigma Chemicals, St. Louis, MO, USA), FPL-52694 (Fison/Fujisawa, Osaka, Japan), spantide (Peptide Institute, Kyoto, Japan), and toluidine blue (Merck, Darmstadt, Germany). Cimetidine was suspended in 0.5% carboxymethylcellulose. Capsaicin was dissolved in a solution consisting of 10% ethanol, 10% Tween 80 (Wako, Osaka, Japan) and 80% saline. Other agents were dissolved in saline. Each agent was prepared immediately before use and was given iv in a volume of 0.1 ml/100 g body weight, and ip or sc in a volume of 0.5 ml/100 g body weight.

Statistics

Data are presented as the means $\pm$ SE of values from 4–7 rats per group. Statistical analyses were performed using the two-tailed Dunnett's multiple comparison test for unpaired samples, and $p < 0.05$ was regarded as significant.

RESULTS

Effect of L*-NAME on gastric PD, pH and acid secretory responses induced by taurocholate*

PD and pH

Normal stomachs mounted on the chamber and perfused with saline generated a stable PD of –30–35 mV (mucosa negative) and secreted acid to keep the luminal pH at 3.3–3.8 under anaesthetized conditions. Mucosal exposure to 20 mmol/L TC for 30 min produced a reduction in PD, followed by a marked increase in luminal pH (Figure 1). After removal of TC from the chamber, the pH increased from 3.6 ± 0.1 to the

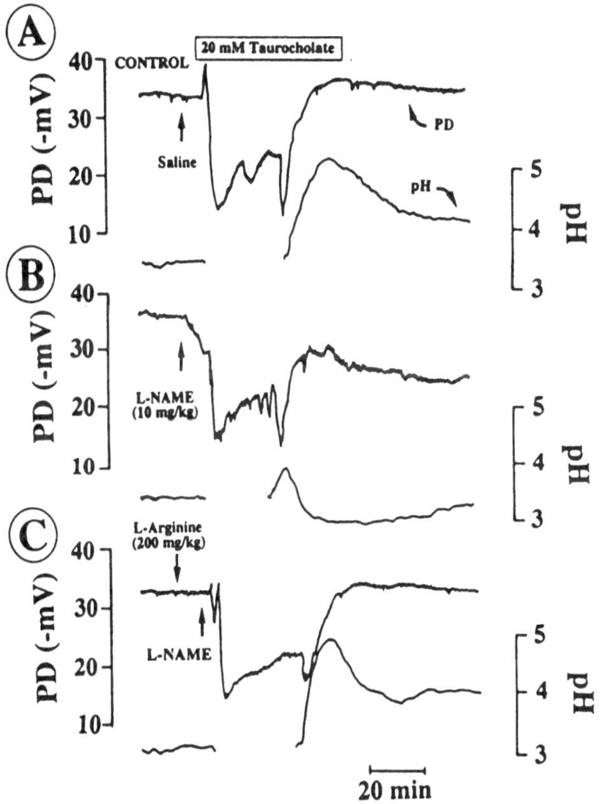

Figure 1. Representative recordings of changes in PD and pH of the stomach before, during and after the exposure to 20 mmol/L TC for 30 min in anaesthetized rats. L-NAME (10 mg/kg) was administered iv as a bolus injection 5 min before TC treatment. L-arginine (200 mg/kg) was administered iv 5 min before the administration of L-NAME. Note that in the animals pretreated with L-NAME (**B**) the luminal pH was decreased below basal levels after the exposure to TC

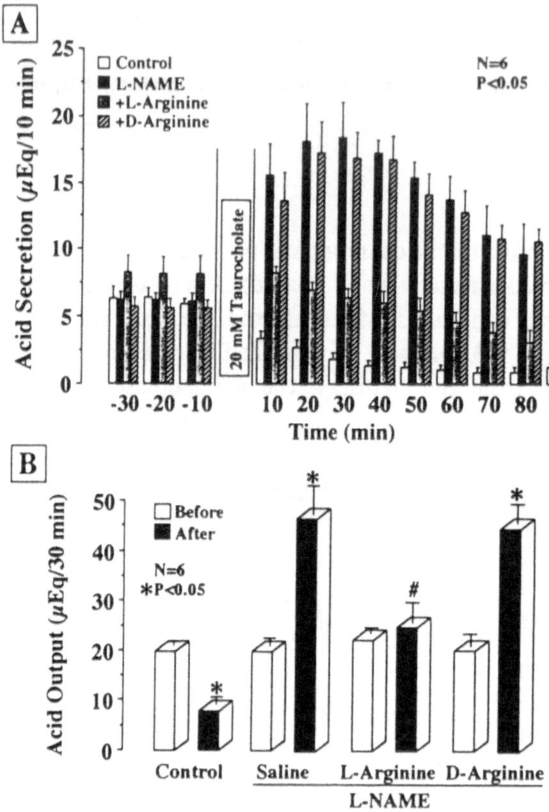

Figure 2. Effect of L-NAME, either alone or in combination with L- or D-arginine, on acid-secretory responses induced by TC in anaesthetized rats. The stomach was exposed for 30 min to 20 mmol/L TC and perfused with saline before and after the exposure. L-NAME (10 mg/kg) was administered iv 5 min before TC treatment, while L- or D-arginine (200 mg/kg) was administered 5 min before L-NAME. Data are presented as the means ± SE of values determined every 10 min from 6 rats. Lower panel (**B**) shows total acid output obtained for 30 min after exposure to TC, and values are presented as the means ± SE of 6 rats. Statistically significant differences at $p<0.05$: *from values in the 'before' group; # from values in the 'after' group with saline (L-NAME alone)

maximal values of 5.4 ± 0.2 (ΔpH 1.8 ± 0.2) within 20 min and remained elevated for over 1 h. Prior administration of L-NAME did not affect the reduction of PD in *response to* TC but completely attenuated the increase of pH after exposure to TC, and the pH decreased below the basal levels within 20 min following exposure to TC; ΔpH at 20 min post-exposure was −0.3 ± 0.1. This effect of L-NAME on the increased pH response caused by TC was apparently antagonized by the subsequent administration of L-arginine but not D-arginine.

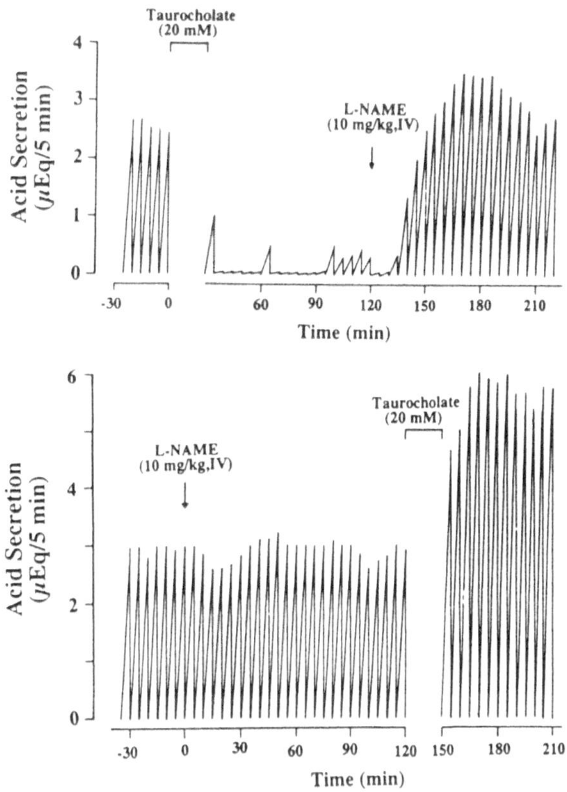

Figure 3. Representative figures showing the effect of L-NAME on gastric acid secretory responses induced by mucosal exposure to 20 mmol/L TC in anaesthetized rats. The stomach was exposed for 30 min to 20 mmol/L TC, and L-NAME (10 mg/kg) was administered iv as a single injection 5 min before TC treatment. The recording of pulses of titrant was performed every 5 min using a Zero Suppression Adapter. Note that the mucosal exposure to TC in the presence of L-NAME apparently increases acid secretion

Acid secretion

The anaesthetized stomachs spontaneously secreted acid at the rate of 4–6 μEq/10 min under normal conditions. Mucosal exposure to 20 mmol/L TC for 30 min caused a decrease in acid secretion from 6.0 ± 0.4 μEq/10 min to the lowest values of 0.8 ± 0.2 μEq/10 min within 1 h; the total acid output for 30 min after TC treatment was 7.6 ± 1.5 μEq/30 min, which is only 37.4% of that obtained in control animals without TC treatment (20.3 ± 2.4 μEq/30 min) (Figure 2). Figure 3 shows typical recordings of acid-secretory responses before and after exposure of the stomach to TC. Mucosal application of TC markedly reduced acid secretion but this decreased acid secretion was restored to above basal levels by the subsequent administration of L-NAME. On the other hand, L-NAME alone did not affect basal acid secretion. However, prior admininstration of L-NAME completely attenuated the decreased acid-secretory response caused by TC, and the acid secretion was enhanced to above basal levels; the acid output obtained after TC treatment was 48.6±8.2 μEq/30 min which is significantly greater than that in control animals given saline. This increased acid response caused by TC in the presence of L-NAME was significantly inhibited by the simultaneous administration of L-arginine but not D-arginine; acid outputs after TC treatment were 23.8±4.8 μEq/30 min and 46.7±5.6 μEq/30 min, respectively.

Effects of cimetidine, FPL-52694, spantide and sensory deafferentation on acid-secretory response caused by taurocholate plus L-NAME

To investigate the characteristics of the enhanced acid secretory response induced by TC in the L-NAME-treated animals, we first examined the effects of cimetidine and FPL-52694 on this phenomenon. In the presence of L-NAME, the mucosal application of 20 mmol/L TC increased acid secretion from 3.2±0.2 μEq/5 min to the maximal values of 9.6±1.4 μEq/5 min, the total acid output for 30 min after TC treatment being 55.2±7.6 μEq/30 min (Figure 4). Prior administration of cimetidine significantly decreased the basal rates of acid secretion and almost totally abolished the enhanced acid-secretory response caused by TC in the L-NAME-treated rats; the acid output remained unchanged before and after TC treatment, the values being 6.8±1.0 μEq/30 min and 8.6±0.8 μEq/30 min, respectively. On the other hand, FPL-52694 did not affect basal rates of acid secretion, yet significantly attenuated the increased acid secretory response following the mucosal application of TC in the presence of L-NAME; the total acid output after TC treatment was 12.4±2.1 μEq/30 min, which is much lower than that obtained in the saline group.

On the other hand, sensory deafferentation did not affect acid secretion before exposure of TC but significantly decreased the enhanced acid-secretory response following the mucosal application of TC; the total acid output was 19.2±3.6 μEq/30 min, which is significantly lower than that of control animals (Figure 4). Likewise, prior administration of spantide significantly reduced the enhancement of acid secretion seen after exposure to TC plus L-NAME, without any effect on the basal acid secretion. All the treatments used here (cimetidine, FPL-52694, spantide, sensory deafferentation) had no influence on PD reduction but significantly antagonized the increased pH response induced by the mucosal application of TC (not shown).

Luminal histamine levels and mucosal mast cell counts

To further investigate the mechanism underlying the enhancement of acid secretion caused by TC plus L-NAME, we measured the luminal histamine levels and mucosal mast cell counts before, during and after exposure of the stomach to TC for 30 min. The amount of histamine which appeared in the gastric lumen was 0.17±0.04 nmol/

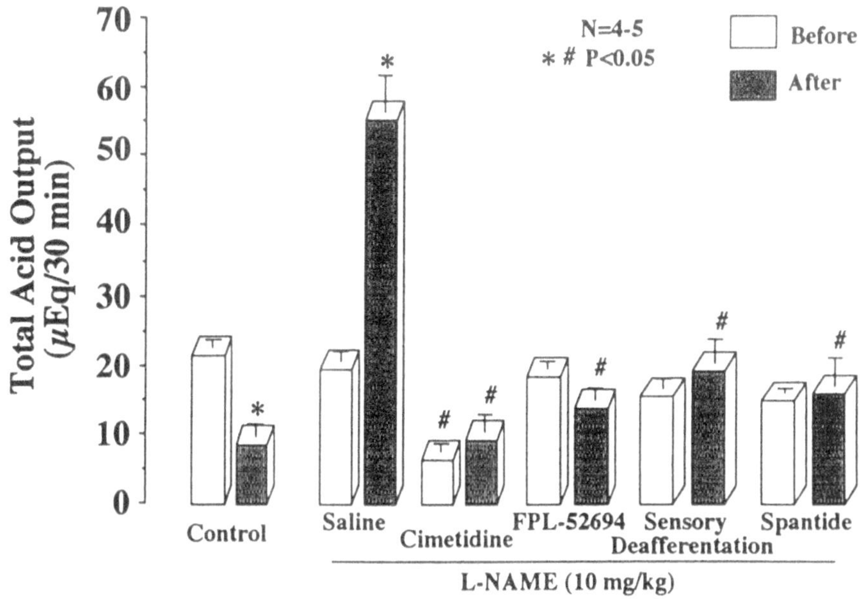

Figure 4. Effects of cimetidine, FPL-52694, spantide and sensory deafferentation on the stimulatory acid-secretory responses induced by TC in the presence of L-NAME in anaesthetized rats. The stomach was exposed for 30 min to 20 mmol/L TC, and L-NAME (10 mg/kg) was administered iv 5 min before TC treatment. Cimetidine (50 mg/kg) or FPL-52694 (200 mg/kg) was given ip 30 min before the exposure of the stomach to TC, while spantide (100 μg/kg) was administered iv 5 min before the injection of L-NAME. Sensory deafferentation was performed by three consecutive injections of capsaicin (total 100 mg/kg) two weeks before the experiment. Values show total acid output obtained for 30 min before and after exposure to TC and are presented as the means ± SE from 5–6 rats. Statistically significant difference at $p < 0.05$; *from values in the 'before' group; # from values in the 'after' group with saline

30 min under basal conditions without TC treatment. The histamine output was increased during exposure to 20 mmol/L TC to levels of about 4 times greater (0.72 ± 0.08 nmol/30 min) than basal values, and remained significantly higher for another 30 min following TC treatment. The increased histamine response to TC was significantly reduced by pretreatment with spantide or sensory deafferentation, the values obtained during TC treatment being 0.38 ± 0.12 nmol/30 min or 0.30 ± 0.15 nmol/30 min, respectively.

On the other hand, the number of mucosal mast cells stained by toluidine blue was significantly reduced in stomachs exposed to 20 mmol/L TC for 30 min. Prior administration of L-NAME slightly but significantly potentiated the degranulation of the mast cells caused by TC (not shown). However, such changes in mast cell counts seen after exposure to TC in the presence of L-NAME were significantly mitigated by either FPL-52694 or sensory deafferentation.

DISCUSSION

The local release of NO is considered to be important in the modulation of various gastric functions affecting mucosal integrity [5,6,19,20]. In a previous study, we showed that NO is involved in the mechanism of luminal alkalinization that occurs in the stomach following the exposure to hypertonic NaCl [5]. The present study demonstrated that L-NAME attenuates the inhibitory acid response induced in the rat stomach by TC, confirming the involvement of NO in this phenomenon, and further suggesting that damage in the stomach may activate the acid-stimulatory pathway in addition to the inhibitory one, and that L-NAME unmasks the acid-stimulatory influence by suppressing the NO-related inhibitory pathway. We also demonstrated that the mechanism of acid-stimulatory response after damage involves histamine release from mast cells, probably through stimulation of capsaicin-sensitive sensory neurons.

First, we confirmed our previous findings that the NO synthase inhibitor, L-NAME, attenuates the increase in luminal pH induced by TC without affecting the PD response [6]. The increase in luminal pH is mainly based on the decrease in acid secretion because this pH response is totally attenuated by pretreatment with L-NAME without any changes in HCO_3^- levels in the lumen [6]. The attenuation by L-NAME of the inhibitory acid response is associated with the inhibition of endogenous NO production since this effect is significantly antagonized by the simultaneous administration of L-arginine but not D-arginine. These results suggest that mucosal irritation by TC may activate NO synthase and increase the local release of NO which in turn inhibits acid secretion. Indeed, we have previously noted an increase in NO generation in the gastric mucosa following exposure to 20 mmol/L TC when determined using the NO-sensitive electrode [21]. On the other hand, the NO involved in this phenomenon may depend on the constitutive type of NO synthase activity because the selective inhibitor of inducible NO synthase aminoguanidine had no effect on the increased pH response in the stomach after damage by TC [6,21].

The most interesting finding in this study is that acid secretion was enhanced in the stomach following exposure to TC in the presence of L-NAME. This is also supported by the pH recordings, and the luminal pH was reduced further below basal levels following TC treatment. Thompson [8] reported an increase in acid output in the canine stomach during irrigation with TC and suggested that acid back diffusion may stimulate acid secretion. Johnson and Overholt [7] demonstrated the release of histamine into gastric venous blood following injury to the gastric mucosa by acetic or salicylic acid. In addition, mast cell degranulation has been shown in the stomach after administration of the mucosal damaging agent [9]. In the present study, the mucosal application of TC increased the luminal histamine levels, suggesting that the increase in acid secretion in the damaged stomach may be mediated by histamine. This contention is supported by the fact that the enhanced acid response was significantly mitigated not only by cimetidine but by FPL-52694 as well.

It is also known that the mast cells in the gastrointestinal mucosa are opposed to substance P-containing sensory neurons [10,11]. Gronbech and Lacy [22] recently reported that stimulation of capsaicin-sensitive sensory neurons activates mucosal

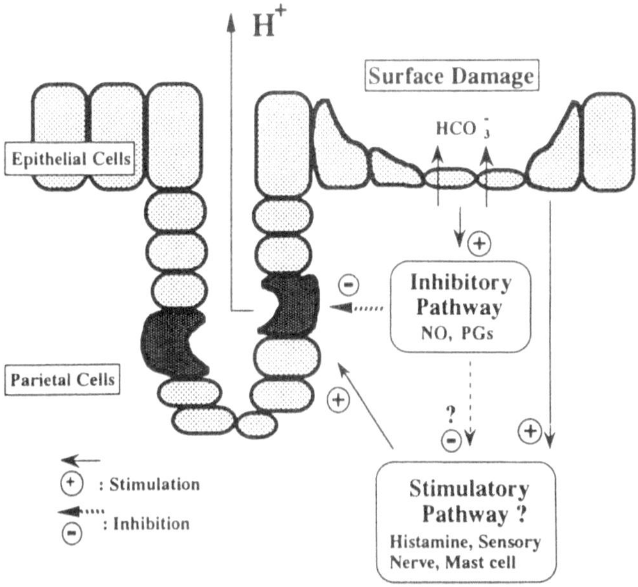

Figure 5. Possible regulatory mechanism of gastric acid secretion in the rat stomach after damage. Irritation of the stomach (surface cell damage) may release NO as well as PGs in the mucosa, both of which in turn inhibit acid secretion locally and unmask luminal alkalinization due to HCO_3^- flux from the damaged portion. Damage in the stomach may also enhance the acid-stimulatory pathway in addition to the inhibitory mechanism, though the latter effect overcomes the former, resulting in a decrease in acid secretion. L-NAME may turn the acid-secretory response in the damaged stomach from the 'inhibitory' into the 'stimulatory' state, mainly by attenuating the inhibitory pathway. The acid-stimulatory pathway may involve histamine released from mucosal mast cells through capsaicin-sensitive sensory neurons

mast cells in the stomach through the release of substance P. As expected, the enhanced acid-secretory response to TC in the presence of L-NAME was significantly mitigated by either sensory deafferentation or the prior administration of the substance P antagonist, spantide. In addition, the luminal appearance of histamine during exposure to TC was also significantly decreased by these treatments. We previously reported that the mucosal application of TC induced gastric hyperaemic response mediated by capsaicin-sensitive sensory neurons, inasmuch as this response was significantly attenuated by sensory deafferentation with capsaicin pretreatment [15]. These results taken together suggest that the acid-stimulatory pathway in the damaged stomach may involve histamine release from the mucosal mast cells.

Recently, Massini et al. [23] reported the potentiation of histamine release by *Escherichia coli* lipopolysaccharide after preincubation of rat serosal mast cells with N^G-monomethyl-L-arginine and suggested that mast cell histamine release can be modulated by an intrinsically generated NO-like factor. The same authors also showed that exogenous NO donors significantly reduced both the release of histamine and the loss of mast cell metachromasia in the heart after ischaemia reperfusion [24]. In agreement with these observations, we found that prior administration of L-NAME significantly enhanced the luminal output of histamine and the loss of mast cell metachromasia during exposure to TC. Certainly, these effects of L-NAME were all significantly mitigated by sensory deafferentation, again supporting the interaction of NO with mucosal mast cells. Thus, it may be assumed that endogenous NO plays a role not only in the acid inhibitory mechanism but also the acid stimulatory pathway in the stomach after damage. NO might suppress the mast cell activation and results in inhibition of histamine release. Certainly, as nitroprusside inhibits histamine-induced acid secretion [5], the direct influence of NO on acid-secreting cells should also be considered.

In conclusion, the present findings suggest that damage in the gastric mucosa may enhance the acid-stimulatory pathway in addition to the NO-mediated inhibitory one, though the latter effect overcomes the former, resulting in a decrease in acid secretion (Figure 5). The acid-stimulatory pathway may involve histamine released from mucosal mast cells through capsaicin-sensitive sensory neurons. It may be assumed that L-NAME turns the acid-secretory response to TC from the 'inhibitory' into the 'stimulatory' state, probably by affecting both the inhibitory and stimulatory pathways of acid secretion operating in the damaged stomach.

REFERENCES

1. Swierczek JS, Konturek SJ. Gastric alkaline response to mucosa-damaging agents: effect of 16,16-dimethyl prostaglandin E_2. Am J Physiol. 1981;241:G509–15.
2. Svanes K, Ito S, Takeuchi K, Silen W. Restitution of the surface epithelium of the in vitro frog gastric mucosa after damage with hyperosmolar sodium chloride: morphologic and physiologic characteristics. Gastroenterology. 1982;82:1409–26.
3. Nobuhara Y, Takeuchi K. Possible role of endogenous prostaglandins in alkaline response in rat gastric mucosa damaged by hypertonic NaCl. Dig Dis Sci. 1984;29:1142–7.
4. Takeuchi K, Ueki S, Tanaka H. Endogenous prostaglandins in gastric alkaline response in the rat stomach after damage. Am J Physiol. 1986;250:G842–9.
5. Takeuchi K. Ohuchi T, Okabe S. Endogenous nitric oxide in gastric alkaline response in the rat stomach after damage. Gastroenterology. 1994;106:367–74.
6. Takeuchi K, Takehara K, Kaneko T, Okabe S. Nitric oxide and prostaglandins in regulation of acid secretory response in rat stomach following injury. J Pharmacol Exp Ther. 1995;272:357–63.
7. Johnson LR, Overholt BF. Release of histamine into gastric venous blood following injury by acetic or salicylic acid. Gastroenterology. 1967;52:505–9.
8. Thompson MR. Studies on the acid secretion that occurs during injury to the gastric mucosa. Gastroenterology. 1976;71:286–90.
9. Beck PL, Morris GP, Wallace JL. Reduction of ethanol-induced gastric damage by sodium cromoglycate and FPL-52694: Role of leukotrienes, prostaglandins, and mast cells in the protective mechanism. Can J Physiol Pharmacol. 1988;67:287–94.
10. Stead RH, Dixon MF, Brammwell NH, Riddel RH, Bienenstock J. Mast cells are closely opposed to nerves in the human gastrointestinal mucosa. Gastroenterology. 1989;97:575–81.
11. Mio M, Izushi K, Tasaka K. Substance P-induced histamine release from rat peritoneal mast cells and its inhibition by antiallergic agents and calmodulin inhibitors. Immunopharmacology. 1991;22:59–66.
12. Salvemini D, Masini E, Pistelli A, Mannaioni PF, Vane JR. Nitric oxide: A regulatory mediator of mast cell reactivity. J Cardiovasc Pharmacol. 1991;17(suppl.3):S258–62.

13. Takeuchi K, Ishihara Y, Okada M, Niida H, Okabe S. A continuous monitoring of mucosal integrity and secretory activity in rat stomach: a preparation using a lucite chamber. Jpn J Pharmacol. 1989;49:235–44.
14. Takeuchi K, Ohtsuki H, Nakagawa S, Okabe S. Characterization of FPL-52694 [5-(2-hydroxypropoxyl)-8-propyl-4-oxo-4H-benzopyran-2-carboxylic acid Na] on histamine release from rat peritoneal mast cells induced by antigen, compound 48/80 and A23187. Agents Actions. 1985;17:10–13.
15. Takeuchi K, Ohuchi T, Narita M, Okabe S. Capsaicin-sensitive sensory nerves in recovery of gastric mucosal integrity after damage by sodium taurocholate in rats. Jpn J Pharmacol. 1993;63:479–86.
16. Yamatodani A, Maeyama K, Watanabe T, Wada T, Kitamura Y. Tissue distribution of histamine in a mutant mouse deficient in mast cells. Biochem Pharmacol. 1983;31:305–9.
17. Takeuchi K, Ohtsuki H, Okabe S. Pathogenesis of compound 48/80-induced gastric lesions in rats. Dig Dis Sci. 1986;31:392–400.
18. Cho CH, Ogle CW, Dai S. Effects of zinc chloride on gastric secretion and ulcer formation in pylorus-occluded rats. Eur J Pharmacol. 1976;38:337–41.
19. Whittle BJR, Lopes-Bermonte J, Moncada S. Regulation of gastric mucosal integrity by endogenous nitric oxide: Interactions with prostaglandins and sensory neuropeptides in the rat. Br J Pharmacol. 1990;99:607–11.
20. Moncada S, Palmer RMJ, Higgs EA. Nitric oxide: Physiology, pathophysiology and pharmacology. Pharmacol Rev. 1991;43:109–42.
21. Takeuchi K, Ohuchi T, Okabe S. Nitric oxide mediates inhibition of gastric acid secretion in the damaged stomach: Interaction with endogenous prostaglandins. Gastroenterology (abstract). 1994;106:A-1692.
22. Gronbech JE, Lacy ER. Substance P attenuates gastric mucosal hyperemia after stimulation of sensory neurons in the rat stomach. Gastroenterology. 1994;106:440–9.
23. Masini E, Bianchi S, Mugnai L et al. The effect of nitric oxide generators on ischemia reperfusion injury and histamine release in isolated perfused guinea-pig heart. Agents Actions. 1991;33:53–6.
24. Masini E, Salvemini D, Pistelli A, Mannaioni PF, Vane JR. Rat mast cells synthesize a nitric oxide like-factor which modulates the release of histamine. Agents Actions. 1991·33:61–3

Manuscript received 14 Oct. 95
Accepted for publication 19 Oct. 95

TS Gaginella et al. (eds.), Biochemical Pharmacology as an Approach to Gastrointestinal Disorders, 39–55

SECRETORY PATHWAYS IN HISTAMINE-CONTAINING ENTEROCHROMAFFIN-LIKE CELLS OF RAT STOMACH

D. CHEN, C.-M. ZHAO, K. ANDERSSON AND R. HÅKANSON*
Department of Pharmacology, University of Lund, S-223 62 Lund, Sweden
*Correspondence

ABSTRACT

Histamine-producing enterochromaffin-like (ECL) cells are numerous in the oxyntic mucosa of the rat stomach. They respond to gastrin by secretory activation, hypertrophy and hyperplasia. They contain cytoplasmic granules and vesicles. The present study addresses the questions of how histamine is stored in the ECL cells and how it is released upon stimulation with gastrin. α-Fluoromethylhistidine (α-FMH) was given to the adult rats to deplete histamine from the ECL cells by inhibiting the histamine-forming enzyme, histidine decarboxylase. Gastrin-17 infusion or omeprazole treatment was used to induce hypergastrinaemia. ECL cell profiles (electron micrographs) were analysed planimetrically. Based on ultrastructural observations, we characterized the secretory organelles in the ECL cells and classified them into granules (median profile diameter 120 nm), secretory vesicles (180 nm), micro-vesicles (70 nm), and vacuoles (more than 500 nm). The granules were unaffected by α-FMH and by acute gastrin stimulation. The secretory vesicles were reduced in number by α-FMH as well as by hypergastrinaemia. The microvesicles were increased in number in response to gastrin. Vacuoles were observed in response to long-term hypergastrinaemia; α-FMH prevented their formation. The findings support the view that histamine is stored in secretory vesicles and vacuoles and that granules develop into secretory vesicles by actively taking up preformed histamine from the cytoplasm. Gastrin accelerates several of the steps that control the birth and subsequent maturation of the storage/secretory organelles, namely the formation of granules, their transformation into secretory vesicles, the process of exocytosis and endocytosis (resulting in microvesicles), and the fusion of several secretory vesicles with each other (resulting in vacuoles).

Keywords: enterochromaffin-like cells, histamine, rat, secretory pathways

BACKGROUND

The histamine-containing enterochromaffin-like (ECL) cells in the gastric acid-producing mucosa can be demonstrated by light microscopy using argyrophil staining techniques [1]. Neither of these stainings demonstrates the ECL cells selectively. In fact, most of the endocrine cells of the digestive tract can be stained with the Grimelius technique. The ECL cells share the ability to be stained by argyrophil staining [1]. Due to their content of histamine and histamine-forming enzyme, histidine decarboxylase (HDC), the ECL cells can be demonstrated by immunocytochemistry using antibodies to histamine [2] or to HDC [3]. In rat, mouse and hamster, the ECL cells are quite numerous, while histamine-containing mast cells are comparatively few [2]. In these species, histamine immunostaining can be used to demonstrate the ECL cell popula-

This paper was presented at the Section of IUPHAR GI Pharmacology Symposium on 'Biochemical pharmacology as an approach to gastrointestinal disorders (basic science to clinical perspectives)', October 12–14, 1995, Pécs, Hungary.

tion. In addition, the ECL cells are known to produce and store other well-known constituents of neuroendocrine cells such as chromogranin/pancreastatin [4,5]. The ECL cells are restricted to the oxyntic mucosa and have been found in the stomach of all vertebrates from cartilaginous fish to man. In most mammals, the ECL cells occur in the basal half of the mucosa (Figure 1).

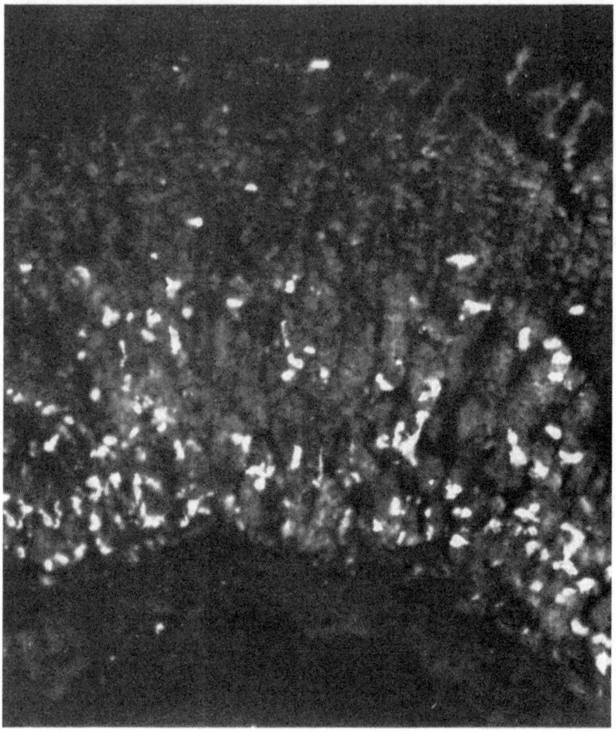

Figure 1. Histamine immunofluorescence of ECL cells in a transverse section of the oxyntic mucosa of rat stomach; mucosal surface upwards, ECL cells in the basal half of the mucosa. ×350

The ECL cells in the rat have an irregular shape and the cytoplasm contains numerous electron-lucent vesicles and a few electron-dense granules. Autoradiographic technique has been used to label ECL cells with [^{3}H]histidine [6]. However, [^{3}H]histamine could not be convincingly associated with either granules or vesicles. Furthermore, it has not been possible yet to demonstrate histamine in ECL-granules/vesicles by immunocytochemistry at the electron microscopic level [7]. Conceivably, the failure to demonstrate [^{3}H]histamine by autoradiography or histamine by immunocytochemistry in granules and vesicles at the electron microscopic level may reflect the loss of histamine from its storage site as a result of the processing of the tissue samples. Although direct evidence for the storage of histamine in the secretory organelles is still missing, available information (see below) seems to favour the view that histamine in the ECL cells is stored in secretory vesicles.

TABLE 1
Characteristic features of rat stomach ECL cells

Properties in common with known peptide hormone-producing cells	Special properties
Positive argyrophil staining	Production and release of histamine
APUD properties	Responsiveness to gastrin
Cytoplasmic (secretory) granules and/or vesicles	
Chromogranins in granules/vesicles	
Co-storage of amines and peptides in granules/vesicles	
Proteolytic 'processing' enzymes in granules/vesicles	

APUD = amine precursor uptake and decarboxylation

While histamine from the ECL cells is generally thought to play a role in the functional control of the parietal cells, activating acid secretion by binding to H_2-receptors [8–11], the anticipated peptide hormone, and consequently the endocrine function of the ECL cells, remains unidentified [12]. Probably the best clue to the unraveling of the biological and physiological significance of the ECL cells is the fact that they respond to gastrin with activation of secretion, hypertrophy and hyperplasia [12] (Table 1). The time course of the ECL cell response to gastrin has been studied from minutes up to two years [13]. The acute effect (within minutes) of gastrin is to stimulate histamine release from the gastric mucosa [4]. The more long-term effect of gastrin (manifested within hours) is the activation of HDC, which is present in rat ECL cells [4,14]. The long-term effect of gastrin (from days up to two years) includes trophic effects on the ECL cells, i.e. hypertrophy and hyperplasia [14–16]. The responses of ECL cells to gastrin are thought to be mediated through CCK-B/gastrin receptors [17–21] (Figure 2). However, the secretory pathways involved in the release of ECL-cell-histamine have not been elucidated. α-Fluoromethylhistidine (α-FMH, which depletes the ECL cell of histamine by inhibiting HDC [22]) and gastrin should provide excellent tools for such a study. α-FMH treatment reduced the oxyntic mucosal histamine content by more than 80% [22]. This reflected a loss of histamine from the ECL cells [22]. The remaining 20% seemed to reside in mast cells which appeared to be unaffected by α-FMH [9,22].

GRANULES AND VESICLES

Although the basic elements of secretion (i.e. Golgi sorting, packaging of secretory products, intracellular transport of granules/vesicles, and fusion of secretory organelles with the plasma membrane) are common to all secretory cells, it may be assumed that each class of secretory cells differs from all others as to the factors that regulate the

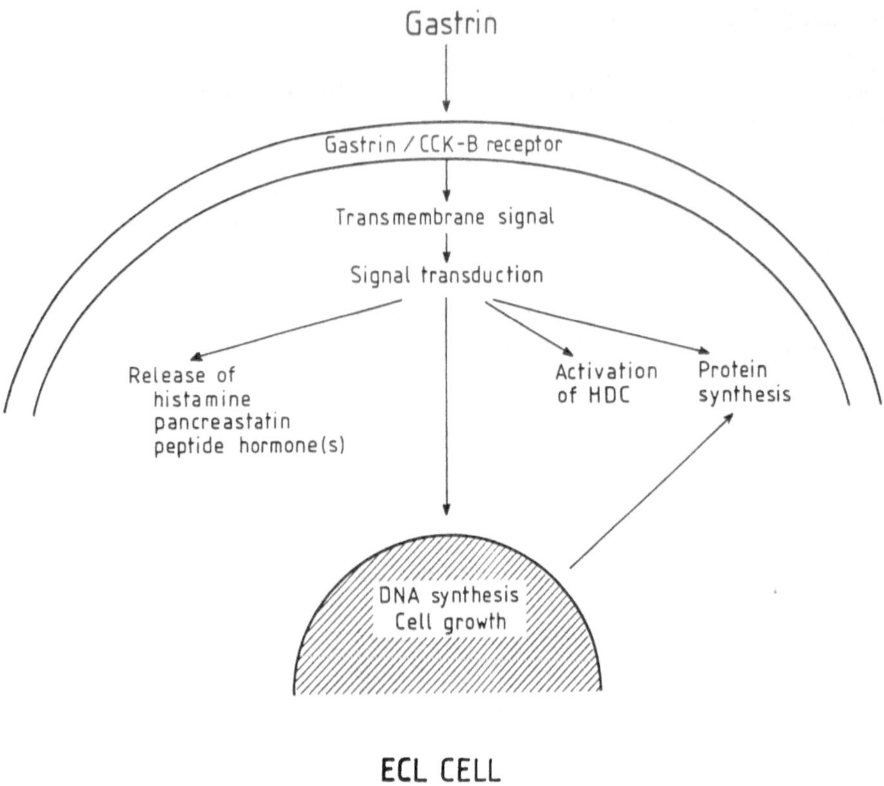

Figure 2. Diagram illustrating the effects of gastrin on the ECL cell. Gastrin stimulates the cell to release histamine, pancreastatin and the anticipated peptide hormone, and later it activates HDC, increases protein synthesis and accelerates DNA synthesis and cell growth. The responses are mediated via gastrin/CCK-B type receptors

discharge of the secretory products [23]. The ECL cells can be identified by their characteristic ultrastructure, i.e. the presence of typical electron-dense granules and electron-lucent vesicles in the cytoplasm [14,24–26] (Figure 3). By serial sectioning of ECL cells, we have found a small electron-dense core in empty-looking secretory vesicles; however, microvesicles lacked a dense core (Figure 4). Thus, we have classified and characterized the granules and vesicles in the ECL cells. The granules are defined as cytoplasmic membrane-enclosed organelles (with a diameter of 25–200 nm), displaying an electron-dense core and a thin electron-lucent halo between the membrane and the dense core, the diameter of the dense core representing more than 50% of the diameter of the entire organelle. The vesicles are membrane-enclosed electron-lucent organelles without a dense core or possessing a small, often eccentrically located, dense core, the diameter of the dense core being less than 50% of the diameter of the organelle. Based on profile size, vesicles belong to one of three populations: (1) secretory vesicles with a diameter of 125–500 nm (with a dense core),

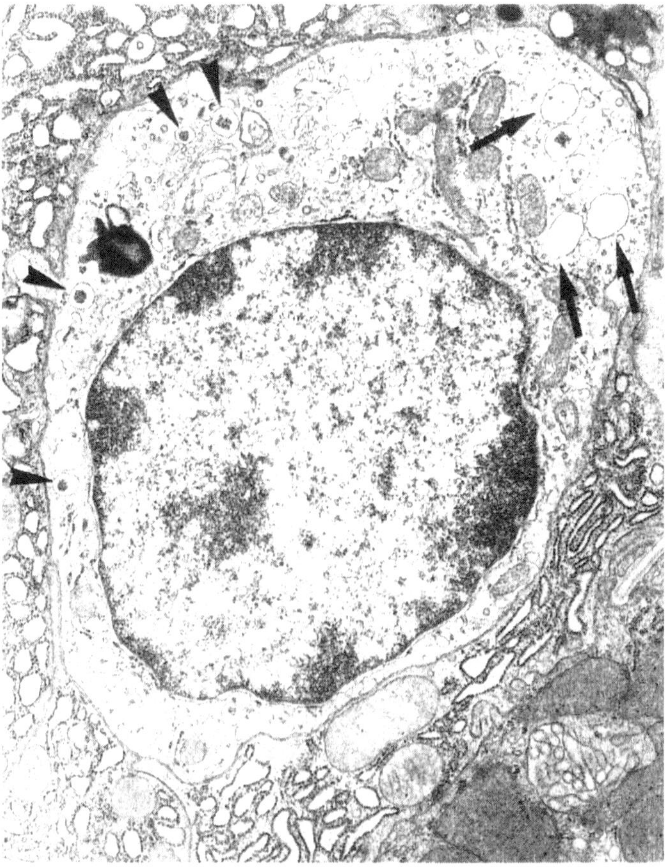

Figure 3. Electron micrograph showing an ECL cell profile in the stomach of a normal rat. Note the typical electron-lucent vesicles (indicated by arrows) and the electron-dense granules (indicated by arrowheads). ×9000

(2) vacuoles with a diameter of at least 500 nm (they were seen only in ECL cells of hypergastrinaemic rats; vacuoles invariably had one or more dense cores), and (3) clear electron-lucent microvesicles with a diameter of 25–200 nm (Figure 5).

Secretory vesicles represent a major storage site of histamine

α-FMH was given to adult rats by continuous subcutaneous infusion in a dose of 3 $mg\,kg^{-1}\,h^{-1}$ in 0.9% NaCl via osmotic minipumps (implanted in the neck) in order to eliminate histamine from the oxyntic mucosa [22,27]. The histamine-depletion (for 24 h or 6 weeks) was associated with a reduced number and volume density of secretory vesicles (Figures 6 and 7), indicating that ECL-cell histamine is stored predominantly in the secretory vesicles.

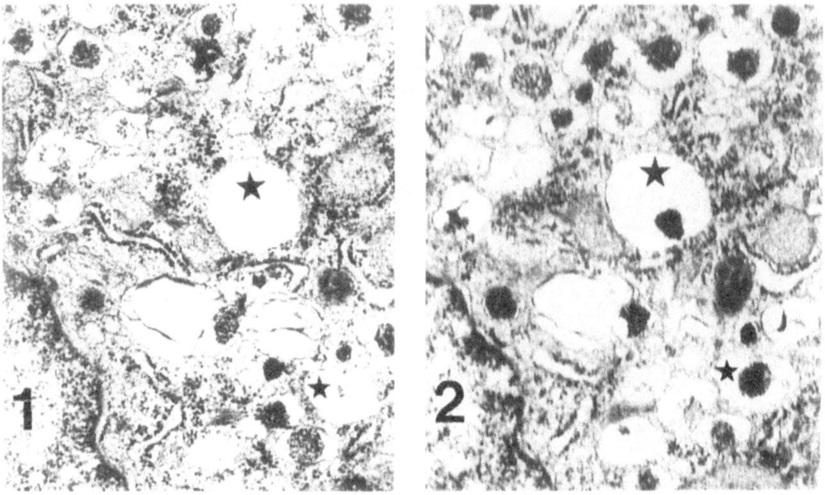

Figure 4. Serial sections (1 and 2) of an ECL cell. Note that apparently 'empty' vesicles (indicated by asterisks) turn out to have an electron-dense core. × 24 000

Secretory vesicles represent a readily releasable pool of histamine

Acute gastrin challenge with a maximal stimulated dose (human Leu^{15}-gastrin-17, 5 nmol/kg body weight per h i.v.) caused a prompt and marked loss of secretory vesicles (Figure 8). When we induced sustained gastrin stimulation with a half-maximally effective dose over days and weeks, the secretory vesicle number was reduced as well, suggesting that secretory vesicles are being released continuously in the presence of gastrin.

Granules may represent pro-secretory vesicles

The granules were unaffected by α-FMH-induced depletion of ECL-cell-histamine and by acute gastrin stimulation, suggesting that granules do not represent an important source of ECL-cell histamine. Thus, vesicles differ from granules by their content of histamine. However, both granules and secretory vesicles have a dense core (revealed by serial sectioning if not immediately apparent) and it cannot be excluded that they represent different manifestations of the same organelle; the granules, which are small in size, may be proforms of the secretory vesicles. Conceivably, vesicles are formed from granules as a result of histamine uptake. We propose that granules are new-born organelles, free of histamine, and that they mature into secretory vesicles, which are loaded with histamine.

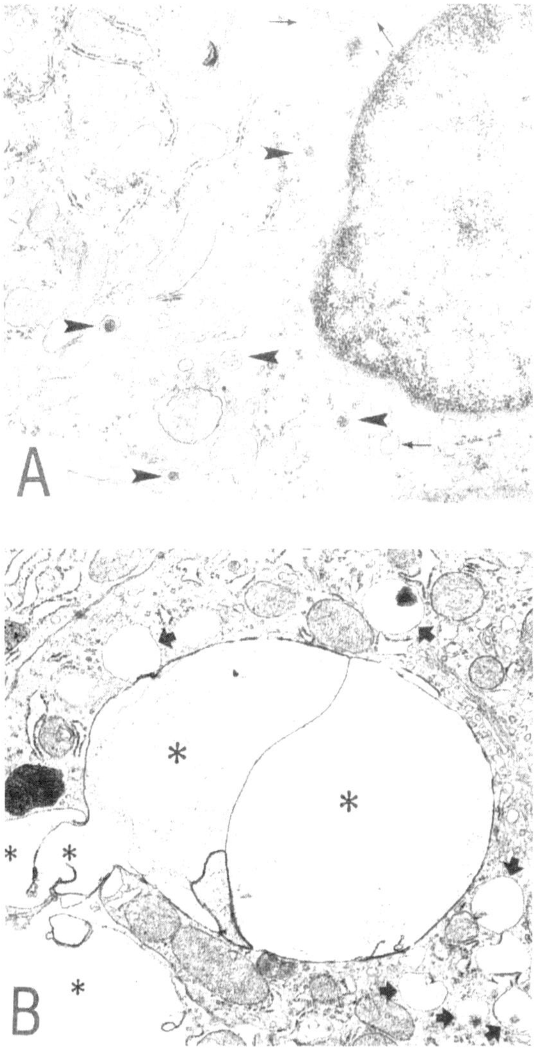

Figure 5. Electron micrographs of ECL cells in the stomach of an untreated rat (A) and of an omeprazole-treated (10 weeks) rat (B), showing granules (arrowheads) and microvesicles (small arrows) in A, and secretory vesicles (big arrows) and vacuoles (asterisks) in B. Note that the vacuoles in B are rich in membrane residues. × 18 000

Vacuoles are formed by fusion of several secretory vesicles

Vacuoles appeared in the ECL cells following long-term stimulation with gastrin (for days and weeks; e.g. evoked by omeprazole 400 μmol/kg per day p.o.). The appearance of vacuoles was associated with a decrease in the size of the secretory vesicle compartment, and the ratio of the number of secretory vesicles to the number of vacuoles was reduced

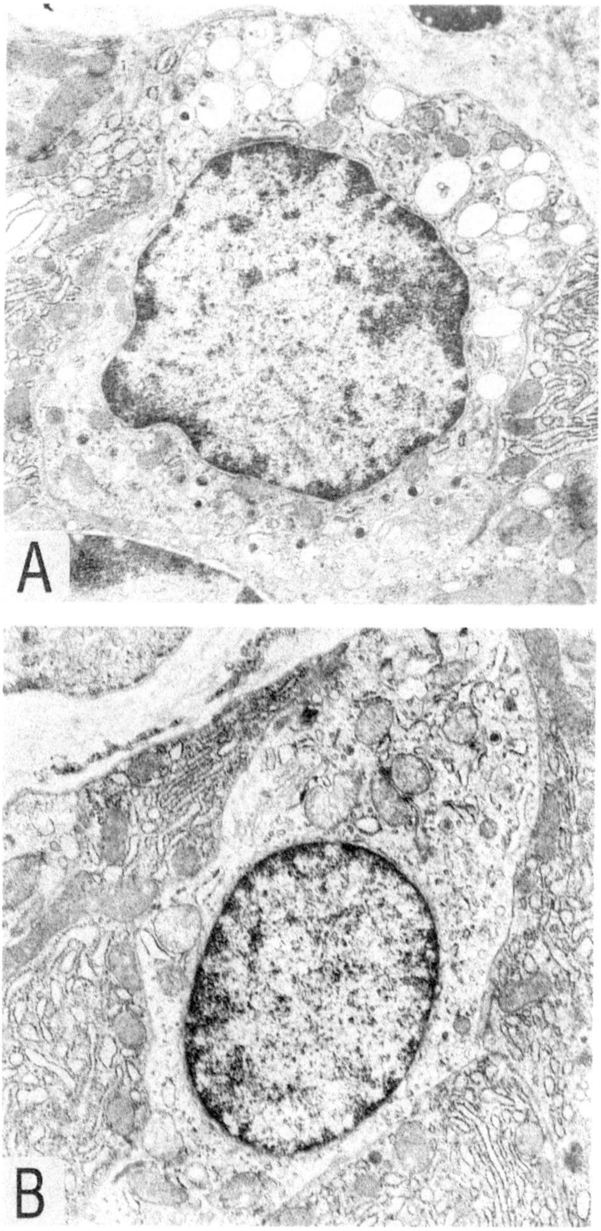

Figure 6. Electron micrographs showing ECL cells in the stomach of an untreated rat (A) and of an α-FMH-treated rat (B). α-FMH was given for 24 h. Note the loss of secretory vesicles in B. ×9000

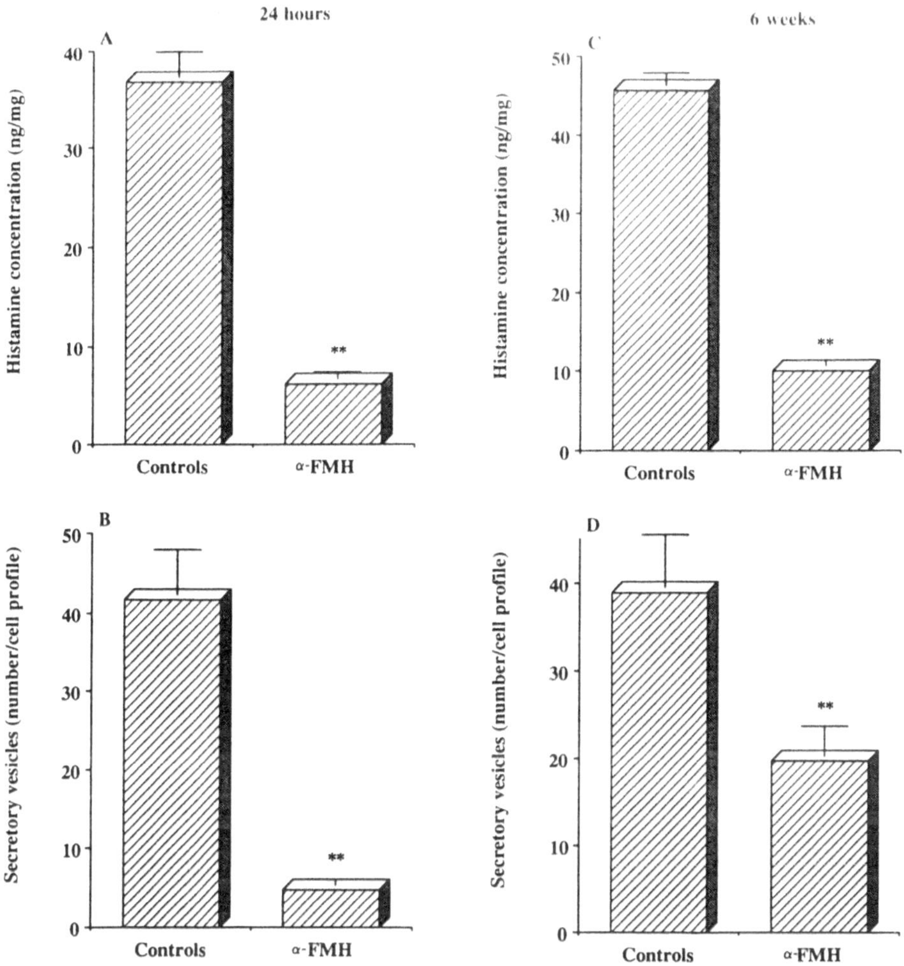

Figure 7. Histamine concentrations (A and C) in the oxyntic mucosa and number of secretory vesicles (B and D) in the ECL cells in the stomach of an untreated rat and of an α-FMH-treated rat. In A and B, the rats were given vehicle or α-FMH for 24 h, in C and D for 6 weeks. Mean ± SEM (vertical bars) of $n = 36$–41 cells and 7–8 rats in each group; **$p < 0.01$ (Student's t-test for two sides)

in response to long-term gastrin stimulation (Figure 9). No vacuoles were observed in normal rats or rats treated with α-FMH. In fact, α-FMH abolished the formation of the vacuoles induced by hypergastrinaemia (Figure 10), suggesting that vacuoles also contain histamine. Serial sectioning revealed that the vacuoles, which are irregular in shape and rich in membrane residues, sometimes have more than one dense core (Figure 11). These observations support the view that vacuoles are formed by fusion of several secretory vesicles [14,26]. The vacuoles may play a role (probably together with lysosomes) in the storage and/or degradation of superfluous secretory products (e.g. histamine, peptides) in the case of long-lasting stimulation.

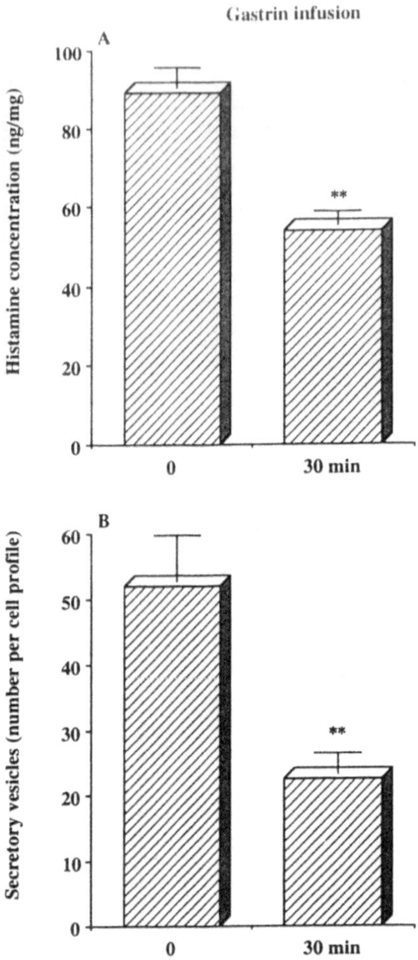

Figure 8. Histamine concentrations (A) in the oxyntic mucosa and number of secretory vesicles (B) in ECL cells of untreated and gastrin-infused rats. Human Leu[15]-gastrin-17 was infused for 30 min. Mean $\pm$ SEM (vertical bars) of $n = 35$–38 cells and 6–9 rats in each group; $^{**}p < 0.01$ (Student's t-test for two sides)

Microvesicles may represent retrieval vesicles

It is to be expected that the loss of secretory vesicles should be associated with an increased cell size since, upon exocytosis, the vesicle membrane is thought to be incorporated into the cell membrane. Such an increase in cell size could not be observed during the initial 1–2 days of gastrin stimulation. Conceivably, therefore, exocytosis is coupled with membrane retrieval (endocytosis), leaving the cell size unperturbed at this early stage. Microvesicles are relatively numerous in ECL cells and were found to increase greatly in number in response to gastrin stimulation (Figure

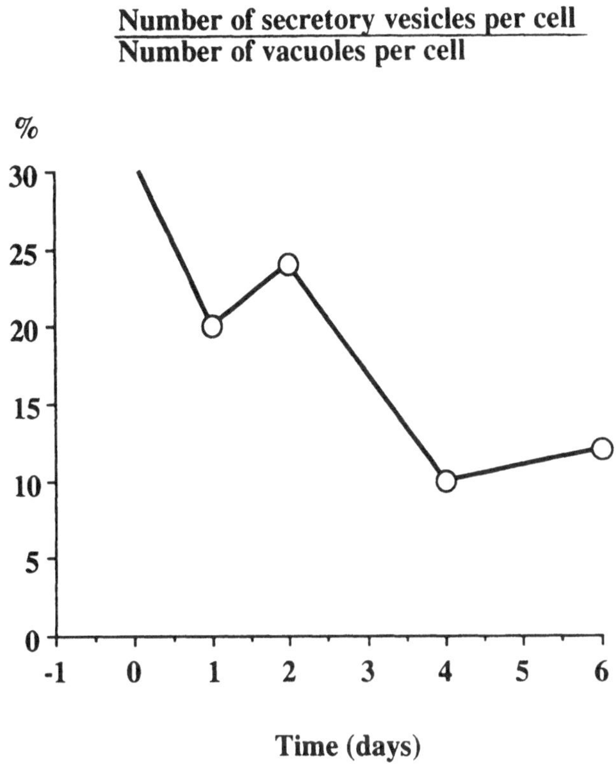

Figure 9. Time course of the decline in the ratio of the number of secretory vesicles to the number of vacuoles of the ECL cells in response to continuous subcutaneous infusion of human Leu^{15}-gastrin-17 (5 nmol kg^{-1} h^{-1}); 28–38 cells and 6–10 rats in each group

12). This is to be expected if the microvesicles are retrieval vesicles, engaged in the recycling of plasma membrane. Alternatively, some microvesicles may be also transport vesicles, pinched off from the endoplasmic reticulum to carry newly synthesized material to other intracellular sites or to shuttle material from the trans-Golgi network to the cell surface, where they may undergo exocytosis in a constitutive non-regulated fashion. Microvesicles have been identified in a number of endocrine cells and some of them may be analogous to the synaptic vesicles found in neurons [28].

In summary, granules and vesicles in the ECL cells can be classified and characterized into granules, secretory vesicles, vacuoles and microvesicles. Histamine is probably mainly stored in the secretory vesicles and vacuoles. Granules store proteins, e.g. chromogranin A, and peptide hormone precursors. Secretory vesicles contain secretory peptides, e.g. pancreastatin, peptide hormones (Table 2).

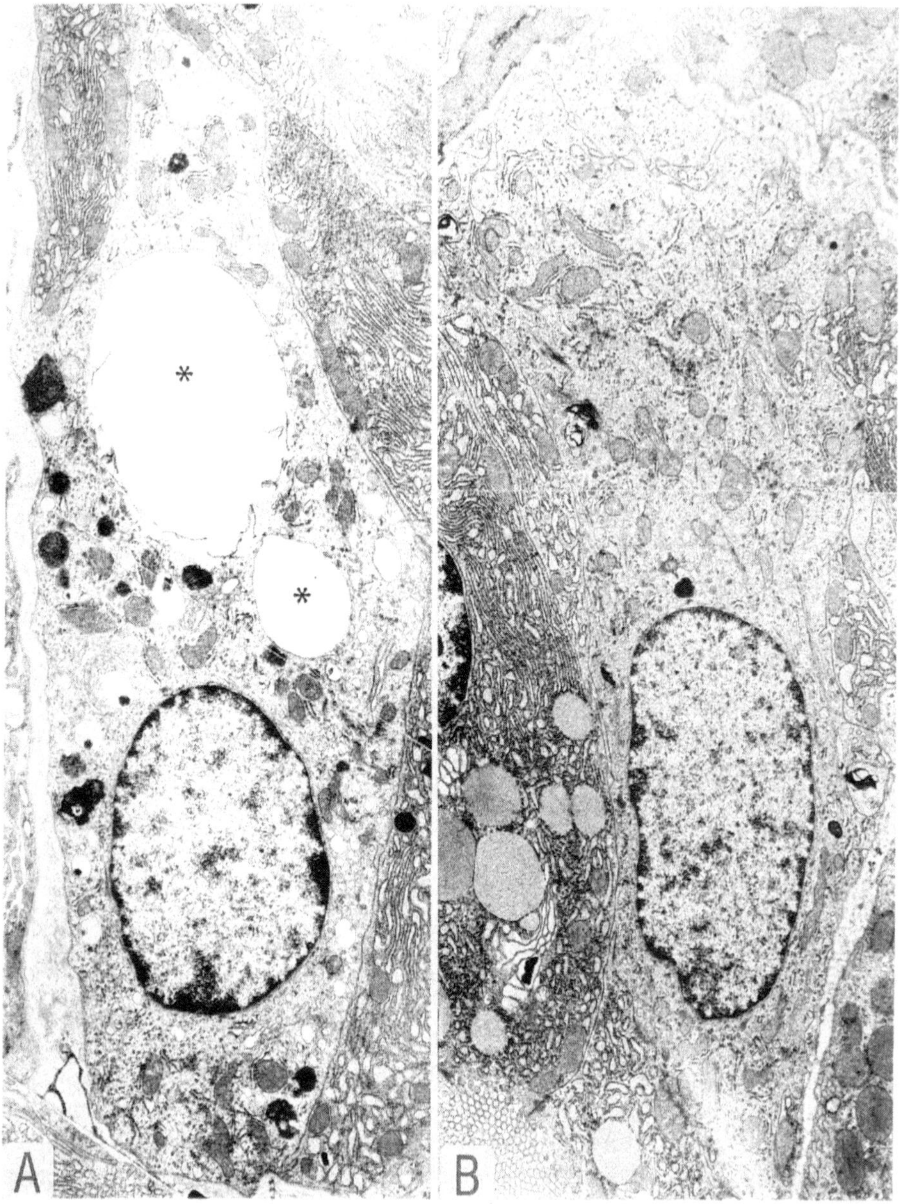

Figure 10. Electron micrographs showing ECL cells from an omeprazole-treated rat (A) and from an α-FMH + omeprazole-treated rat (B). Omeprazole or omeprazole + α-FMH were given for 6 weeks. Note that vacuoles (indicated by asterisks) appear following omeprazole treatment (A) and that α-FMH prevented the formation of such vacuoles (B). × 8400

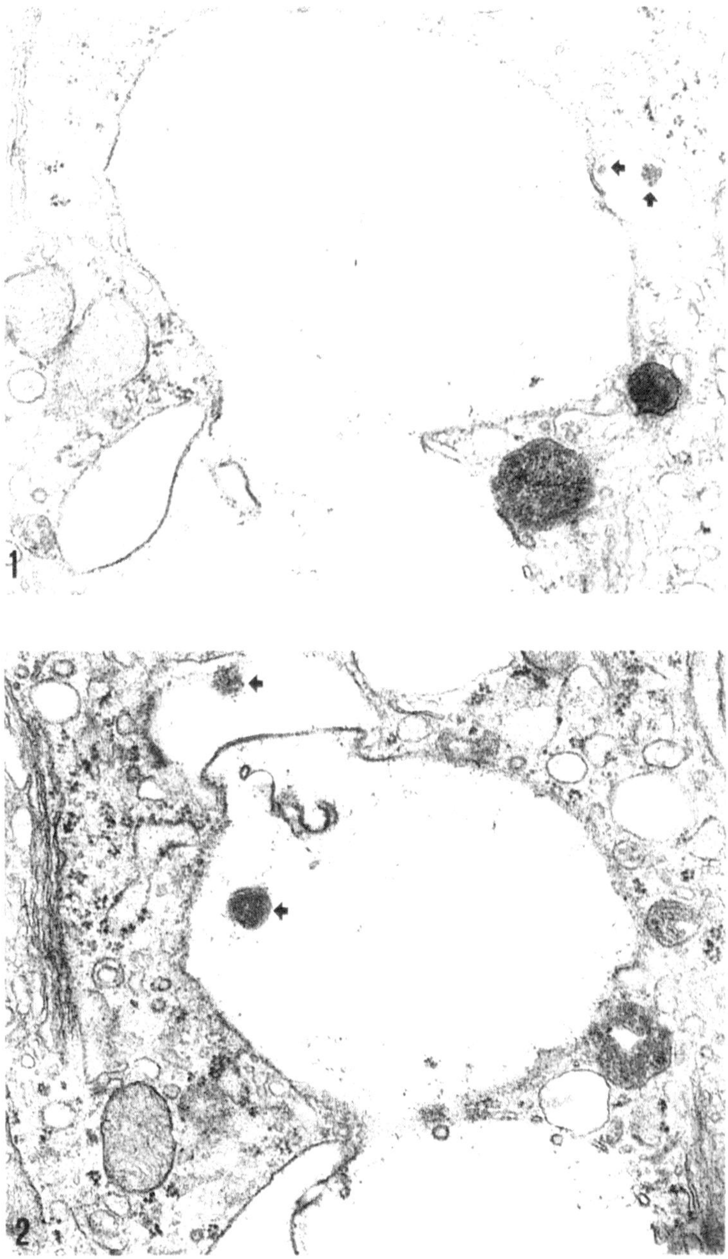

Figure 11. Serial sections (1 and 2) of an ECL cell from an omeprazole-treated (10 weeks) rat, revealing electron-dense cores in vacuoles (indicated by arrows). × 18 000

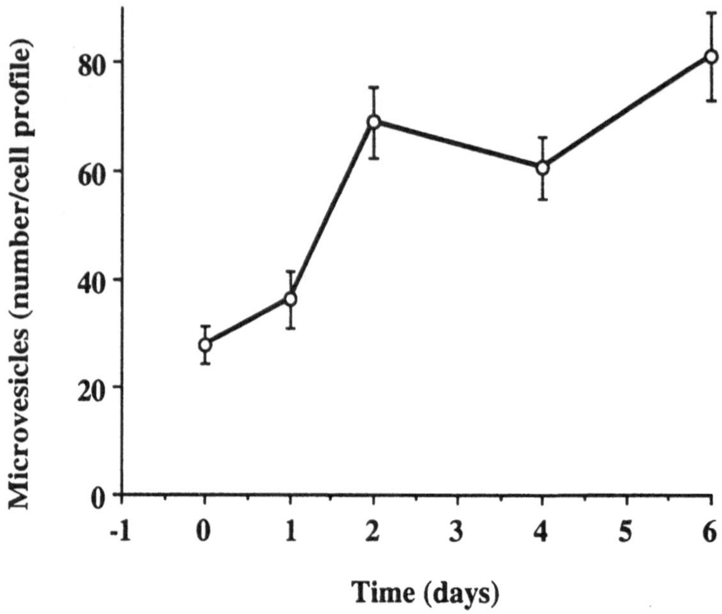

Figure 12. Time course of the increase in the number of ECL-cell microvesicles in response to continuous subcutaneous infusion of Leu[15]-gastrin-17 (5 nmol kg^{-1} h^{-1}); 28–38 cells and 6–10 rats in each group

TABLE 2
Classification and characterization of secretory organelles in the ECL cells

Microvesicles (Synaptic vesicles?)	Granules (Small dense core vesicles)	Secretory vesicles (Large dense core vesicles)	Vacuoles (Very large dense vesicles)
Histamine(?) No secretory protein	Histamine(?) Proteins (Chromogranin A, peptide hormone precursors)	Histamine Secretory peptides (Pancreastatin, peptide hormone)	Histamine Secretory peptides (degraded?)

A MODEL OF MEMBRANE FUSION IN THE ECL CELLS

The regulated secretory pathways in the ECL cells probably involve granules, secretory vesicles, vacuoles and microvesicles. Based on observations described above, we propose that the ECL-cell granules actively take up preformed histamine from the cytosol during transport from the Golgi zone to the more peripheral parts of the cells.

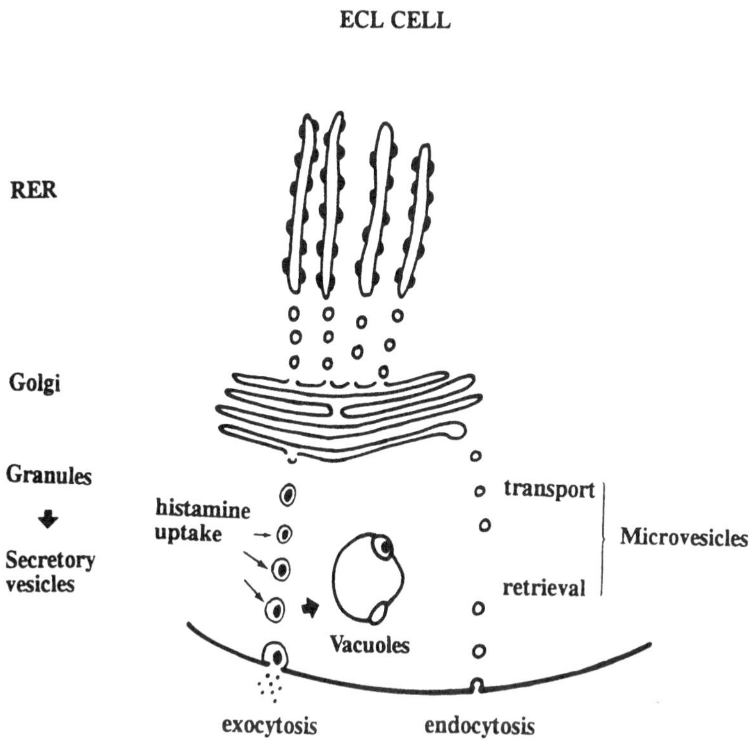

Figure 13. Proposed life cycle of granules and vesicles in the ECL cell. The prohormone is synthesized in a rough endoplasmic reticulum (RER) together with chromogranin A and other granular proteins. These products are packaged into prosecretory granules in the Golgi apparatus. The granules formed are small and electron-dense. As they are transported away from the Golgi area they actively take up preformed histamine from the cytoplasm. At the same time chromogranin A and the prohormone are being hydrolysed into small fragments, such as pancreastatin and peptide hormone. As a result of the accumulation of small molecules, osmotic forces are generated that will transform the granules into secretory vesicles. Microvesicles may represent retrieval or transport vesicles. Vacuoles are formed by fusion of several secretory vesicles in response to gastrin stimulation

In consequence, they turn into secretory vesicles, possibly through osmotic forces generated by the progressive accumulation of small molecules (histamine, peptides). This causes the granules to swell, turning them into secretory vesicles. Among the molecules that will accumulate in the secretory vesicles are histamine and cleavage products of chromogranin A (e.g. pancreastatin) and of the anticipated peptide hormone precursor, which are generated by proteolysis within the granules. According to this concept, we should expect the secretory vesicles to fuse with the cell membrane in response to stimulation and release their contents by exocytosis or to fuse with each other to form vacuoles. The microvesicles become numerous as a result of stimulated recycling, leading to increased number of retrieval vesicles. In fact, we have evidence that gastrin accelerates several of the steps that control the birth and subsequent maturation of storage/secretory organelles, namely the formation of granules, their transformation into secretory vesicles, exocytosis and endocytosis (resulting in microvesicles), and the fusion of several secretory vesicles with each other (resulting in vacuoles) (Figure 13).

CONCLUSIONS

1. Secretory vesicles in ECL cells develop from granules and represent a major storage site for histamine.

2. Granules develop into secretory vesicles, partly as a result of accumulation of histamine from the cytoplasm.

3. Vacuoles are formed by fusion of several secretory vesicles in response to gastrin stimulation.

4. Microvesicles may represent retrieval vesicles.

ACKNOWLEDGEMENTS

This study was supported by grants from the Swedish MRC (04X-1007), RmC (2542-B91-02XBB), the A. Påhlsson Foundation, the Royal Physiographic Society, the Novo Nordic Foundation, the Wenner-Gren Center Foundation and the Medical Faculty, University of Lund, Sweden.

REFERENCES

1. Sundler F, Håkanson R. Gastric endocrine cell typing at the light microscopic level. In: Håkanson R, Sundler F, eds. The Stomach as an Endocrine Organ. Fernström Symposium, No. 15. Amsterdam: Elsevier; 1991:9–26.
2. Håkanson R, Böttcher G, Ekblad E et al. Histamine in endocrine cells in the stomach: A survey of several species using a panel of histamine antibodies. Histochemistry. 1986;86:5–77.
3. Kubota H, Taguchi Y, Tohyama M et al. Electron microscopic identification of histidine decarboxylase-containing endocrine cells of the rat gastric mucosa: an immunohistochemical analysis. Gastroenterology. 1984;87:496–502.
4. Chen D, Monstein H-J, Nylander A-G, Zhao C-M, Sundler F, Håkanson R. Acute responses to rat stomach enterochromaffin like cells to gastrin: Secretory activation and adaptation. Gastroenterology. 1994;107:18–27.
5. Håkanson R, Ding X-Q, Norlén P, Chen D. Circulating pancreastatin is a marker for the enterochromaffin-like cells of the rat stomach. Gastroenterology. 1995;108:1455–52.
6. Rubin W, Schwartz B. Electron microscopic radioautographic identification of the ECL cell as the histamine-synthesis endocrine cell in the rat stomach. Gastroenterology. 1979;77:458–67.

7. Nissinen M, Panula P. Histamine-storing cells in the oxyntic mucosa of the rat stomach: A transmission electron microscopic study employing fixation with carbodiimide. J. Histochem Cytochem. 1993;41:1405–12.
8. Kahlson G, Rosengren E, Svensson SE. Histamine and gastric acid secretion with special reference to the rat. In: Holton P, ed. Pharmacology of Gastrointestinal Mobility and Secretion. Vol.I. Oxford: Pergamon; 1973:41–101.
9. Andersson K, Mattsson H, Larsson H. The role of gastric mucosal histamine in acid secretion and experimentally induced lesions in the rats. Digestion. 1990;46:1–9.
10. Andersson K, Cabero JL, Mattsson H, Håkanson R. Gastric acid secretion after depletion of enterochromaffin-like cell histamine. A study with α-fluoromethylhistidine in rats. Scand J Gastroenterol. 1996;31:24–30.
11. Waldum HL, Sandvik AK, Brenna E, Petersen H. Gastrin-histamine sequence in the regulation of gastric acid secretion. Gut. 1991;32:698–701.
12. Håkanson R, Chen D, Sundler F. The ECL cells. In: Johnson LR, ed. Physiology of the Gastrointestinal Tract, 3rd edn. New York: Raven Press; 1994:1171–84.
13. Chen D, Zhao C-M, Monstein H-J et al. A time table of rat stomach ECL cell responses to gastrin. In: Singer MV et al., eds. Gastrointestinal Tract and Endocrine System. Falk Symposium 77. Dordrecht, Boston, London: Kluwer Academic Publishers; 1994:178–85.
14. Håkanson R, Tielemans Y, Chen D, Andersson K, Mattsson H, Sundler F. Time-dependent changes in enterochromaffinlike cell kinetics in stomach of hypergastrinemic rats. Gastroenterology. 1993;105:15–21.
15. Böttcher G, Håkanson R, Nilsson G, Seensalu R, Sundler F. Effects of long-term hypergastrinemia on the ultrastructure of enterochromaffin-like cells in the stomach of the rat, hamster and guinea pig. Cell Tissue Res. 1989;256:247–57.
16. Håkanson R, Tielemans Y, Chen D et al. The biology and pathobiology of the ECL cells. Yale J Biol Med. 1992;65:761–74.
17. Sandvik AK, Waldum HL. CCK-B (gastrin) receptor regulates gastric histamine release and acid secretion. Am J Physiol. 1991;260:G925–8.
18. Nylander A-G, Chen D, Lilja I et al. Enterochromaffin-like cells in rat stomach respond to short-term infusion of high doses of cholecystokinin but not to long-term, sustained, moderate hyper CCKemia caused by continuous cholecystokinin infusion or pancreaticobiliary diversion. Scand J Gastroenterol. 1993;28:73–9.
19. Asahara M, Kinoshita Y, Nakata H et al. Gastrin receptor genes are expressed in gastrin parietal and enterochromaffin-like cells of *Mastomys natalensis*. Dig Dis Sci. 1994;39:2149–56.
20. Prinz C, Kajimura M, Scott DR, Mercier F, Helander HF, Sachs G. Histamine secretion from rat enterochromaffinlike cells. Gastroenterology. 1993;105:449–61.
21. Ding X-Q, Chen D, Håkanson R. Cholecystokinin-B receptor ligands of the dipeptoid series as agonists on rat stomach histidine decarboxylase. Gastroenterology. 1995;109:1181–7.
22. Andersson K, Chen D, Håkanson R, Mattsson H, Sundler F. Enterochromaffin-like cells in the rat stomach: effect of α-fluoromethylhistidine-evoked histamine depletion. A chemical, histochemical and electron-microscopic study. Cell Tissue Res. 1992;270:7–13.
23. Burgess TL, Kelly RB. Constitutive and regulated secretion of proteins. Ann Rev Cell Biol. 1987;3:243–93.
24. Capella C, Vassallo G, Solcia E. Light and electron microscopic identification of the histamine-storing argyrophil (ECL) cell in murine stomach and of its equivalent in other mammals. Z Zellforsch. 1971;118:68–84.
25. Solcia E, Capella C, Vassallo G, Buffa R. Endocrine cells of the gastric mucosa. Int Rev Cytol. 1975;42:223–86.
26. Chen D, Håkanson R, Sundler F. Effect of omeprazole-evoked hypergastrinemia on ultrastructure of enterochromaffin-like cells in the stomach of portacaval-shunted rats. Cell Tissue Res. 1993;272:71–7.
27. Andersson K, Håkanson R, Mattsson H, Ryberg B, Sundler F. Hyperplasia of histamine-depleted enterochromaffinlike cells in rat stomach using omeprazole and α-fluoromethylhistidine. Gastroenterology. 1992;103:897–904.
28. Thomas-Reetz AC, De Camilli P. A role for synaptic vesicles in non-neuronal cells: clues from pancreatic β cells and chromaffin cells. FASEB J. 1994;8:209–16.

Manuscript received 12 Oct. 95.
Accepted for publication 31 Oct. 95.

TS Gaginella et al. (eds.), Biochemical Pharmacology as an Approach to Gastrointestinal Disorders, 57–64

NITRIC OXIDE AS A MODULATOR OF FLUID ABSORPTION IN RAT JEJUNUM IN VIVO

E. BEUBLER AND A. SCHIRGI-DEGEN
Department of Experimental and Clinical Pharmacology, University of Graz, Universitätsplatz 4, A-8010 Graz, Austria

ABSTRACT

The role of nitric oxide (NO) as a regulator of intestinal fluid transport is still controversial. In part, the experimental work describes secretory properties of NO in vitro and in vivo; other investigators, however, demonstrate a proabsorptive role of NO.

In the present study, we present data to support the latter hypothesis, namely an absorptive effect of NO. We tested the effects of the NO-synthase inhibitor, L-NAME, and of the NO-donors, L-arginine and sodium nitroprusside, on basal fluid transport and on intestinal fluid secretion stimulated by 5-HT, PGE_2, *Escherichia coli* STa and cholera toxin. The experiments were performed in a tied-off loop of the anaesthetized rat in vivo. L-NAME was infused intravenously in the absence or presence of L-arginine or sodium nitroprusside. 5-HT (0.16 $\mu g\,min^{-1}$, 30 min) and PGE_2 (79 $ng\,min^{-1}$, 30 min) were infused close intra-arterially, and *E. coli* STa (10 $U\,ml^{-1}$, 30 min) and cholera toxin (0.5 $\mu g\,ml^{-1}$, 4 h) were administered intraluminally. Net fluid transport was determined gravimetrically.

The inhibitor of NO synthetase, L-NAME, dose-dependently (0.25–50 $mg\,kg^{-1}$, iv = 5.55 $\mu g\,kg^{-1}$–1.11 $mg\,kg^{-1}\,min^{-1}$) reversed net fluid absorption to net fluid secretion. L-NAME (0.55 $mg\,kg^{-1}\,min^{-1}$) furthermore significantly enhanced fluid secretion stimulated by 5-HT, PGE_2, *E. coli* STa and cholera toxin.

L-Arginine (8.88 $mg\,kg^{-1}\,min^{-1}$) and sodium nitroprusside (22.2 $\mu g\,kg^{-1}\,min^{-1}$) slightly, though not significantly, enhanced fluid absorption in controls but significantly inhibited 5-HT-, PGE_2-, *E. coli* STa- and cholera-toxin-induced fluid secretion.

These results indicate that exogenously administered or endogenously formed NO exerts a proabsorptive action in the intestine. This effect may also counteract the secretory response to secretagogues. NO thus may attenuate pathological secretory conditions in the intestine.

Keywords: nitric oxide, fluid absorption, jejunum

INTRODUCTION

Nitric oxide (NO) is established as an important mediator of neural, cardiovascular, immune and gastrointestinal function. Endogenous NO derives from enzymatic conversion of L-arginine through NO-synthase, a family of isoenzymes, at least one of which is present in the myenteric plexus of the intestine. The existence of the synthase enzyme within the enteric nervous system, in close proximity to the epithelium, suggests the possibility that NO could be a physiological regulator of intestinal ion transport.

This paper was presented at the Section of IUPHAR GI Pharmacology Symposium on 'Biochemical pharmacology as an approach to gastrointestinal disorders (basic science to clinical perspectives)', October 12–14, 1995, Pécs, Hungary.

The role of NO in intestinal fluid and electrolyte transport, however, remains controversial when the investigations performed in this relation are considered. Ussing-chamber experiments, using full-thickness preparations of intestine, support a proabsorptive role of NO [1]. In the isolated vascularly perfused rabbit ileum, inhibition of NO-synthase by L-NAME also caused secretion of water and ions which could be prevented by synchronous administration of L-arginine [2]. The observation that luminal administration of a NO-synthase inhibitor into the rat ileum also decreased net water absorption in vivo [3] gives further support to a proabsorptive role of NO. Other experiments, however, demonstrate exactly the opposite. In Ussing-chamber experiments, using stripped preparations, NO-donating compounds like sodium nitroprusside increased short circuit current, thus indicating a prosecretory role of NO [4–6]. Corresponding with the latter results, castor-oil-induced diarrhoea was prevented by intraperitoneal administration of NO-synthase inhibitors [7,8], and the secretory effect of sodium cholate was also inhibited by intraperitoneal administration of L-NAME [9]. Intraperitoneal administration of L-NAME furthermore inhibited *E. coli* STa-induced fluid secretion [10].

Our own experiments, summarized below, were performed to elucidate the significance of NO in the regulation of intestinal fluid transport in vivo under basal as well as under secretory conditions induced by the secretagogues prostaglandin E_2, 5-HT, *E. coli* STa and cholera toxin [11–12].

METHODS

The experiments were performed in a tied-off loop of anaesthetized rats in vivo. L-NAME was infused intravenously in the absence or presence of L-arginine or sodium nitroprusside. 5-HT (0.16 $\mu g\,min^{-1}$, 30 min) and PGE_2 (79 $ng\,min^{-1}$, 30 min) were infused close intra-arterially, and *E. coli* STa (10 $U\,ml^{-1}$, 30 min) and cholera toxin (0.5 $\mu g\,ml^{-1}$, 4 h) were administered intraluminally. Net fluid transport was determined gravimetrically. The cyclic nucleotides, cAMP and cGMP, were determined in mucosal scrapings by using commercial kits. PGE_2 was determined by radioimmunoassay.

Results are given as mean $\pm$ SEM and the data were analysed by the two-sample Student's *t*-test or by analysis of variance and Dunnett's test or the Student–Newman–Keuls test. Probability values <0.05 were considered significant.

RESULTS AND DISCUSSION

Effects of NO on basal fluid transport

Infusion of saline resulted in net absorption of luminal fluid in all rats. L-NAME dose-dependently (0.25–50 $mg\,kg^{-1} = 5.55\ \mu g\,kg^{-1}\,min^{-1}$–$1.11\ mg\,kg^{-1}\,min^{-1}$) reversed net absorption to net fluid secretion, whereas infusion of D-NAME in corresponding doses did not influence control net absorption significantly (Figure 1). Further experiments with L-NAME were performed at the dose of 0.55 $mg\,kg^{-1}\,min^{-1}$. L-NOARG (0.55

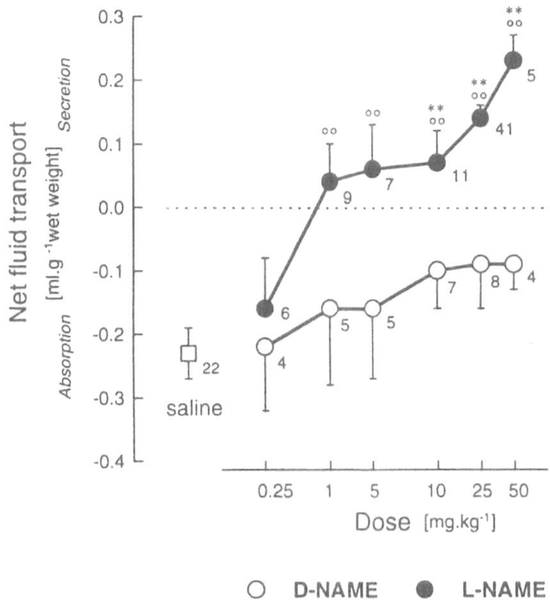

Figure 1. Effects of infusion of saline (□), L-NAME (●) and D-NAME (○) on net fluid transport in the rat jejunum in vivo. Each point represents the mean ± SEM. The figures indicate the number of experiments; $^{oo}p<0.01$ compared with saline, $^{**}p<0.01$ compared with D-NAME. (From Reference 11 with permission)

mg kg^{-1} min^{-1}), another NO-synthase inhibitor, also elicited net fluid secretion to an extent similar to the secretion evoked by an equivalent dose of L-NAME (data not shown).

Infusion of L-arginine (8.88 mg kg^{-1} min^{-1}) slightly but not significantly enhanced net fluid absorption compared with controls (Figure 2). L-Arginine reversed L-NAME-induced fluid secretion to net absorption. Infusion of sodium nitroprusside (22.2 μg kg^{-1} min^{-1}) showed no effect on control net absorption but also inhibited the secretory effect of L-NAME (Figure 2).

Effects of NO on PGE_2-induced fluid secretion

Close ia infusion of PGE_2 (79 ng min^{-1}, 30 min) reversed net fluid absorption to net secretion. Infusion of L-NAME markedly enhanced PGE_2-induced fluid secretion. Administration of L-arginine (8.88 mg kg^{-1} min^{-1} iv) as well as administration of sodium nitroprusside (22.2 μg kg^{-1} min^{-1} iv) significantly reduced PGE_2-induced fluid secretion (Figure 3).

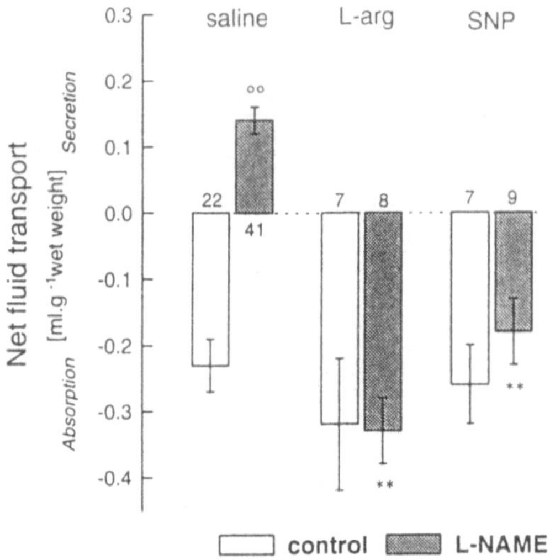

Figure 2. Effects of L-arginine (L-arg) and sodium nitroprusside (SNP) on basal (open columns) and on L-NAME-influenced (cross-hatched columns) net fluid transport in the rat jejunum in vivo. Each column represents the mean ± SEM. The figures indicate the number of experiments; $^{oo}p<0.01$ compared to saline, $^{**}p<0.01$ compared with L-NAME. (From Reference 11 with permission)

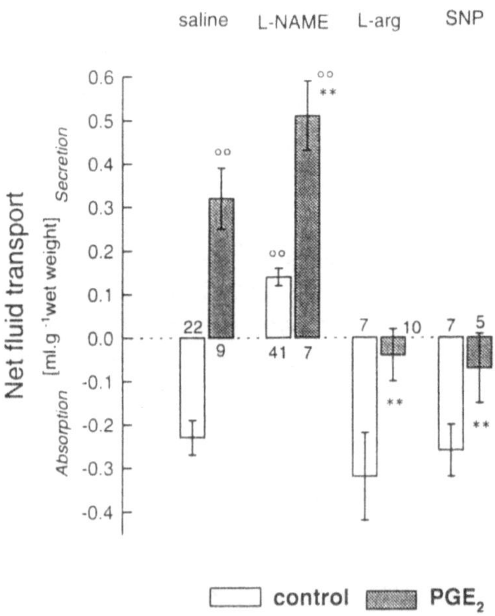

Figure 3. Effects of L-NAME, L-arginine (L-arg) and sodium nitroprusside (SNP) on basal (open columns) and PGE_2-influenced (cross-hatched columns) net fluid transport in the rat jejunum in vivo. Each column represents the mean ± SEM. The figures indicate the number of experiments; $^{oo}p<0.01$ compared with saline, $^{**}p<0.01$ compared with saline plus PGE_2. (From Reference 11 with permission)

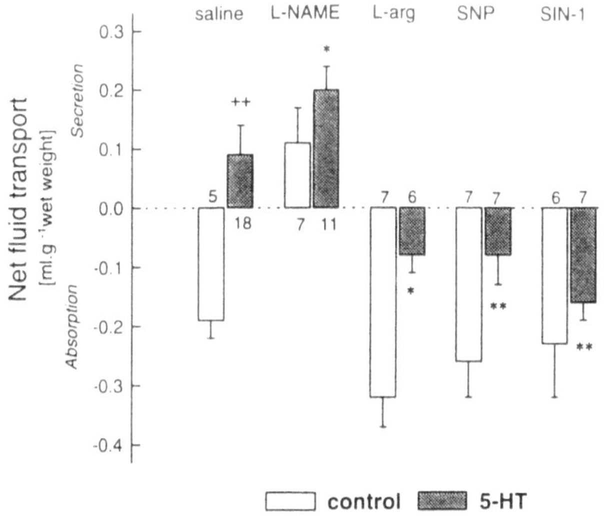

Figure 4. Effects of L-NAME, L-arginine (L-arg), sodium nitroprusside (SNP) and SIN-1 on net fluid transport in controls (open bars) and on 5-HT fluid secretion (cross-hatched bars). Each column represents the mean ± SEM. The figures indicate the number of experiments; $^{*}p<0.05$, $^{**}p<0.01$ compared with saline plus 5-HT, $^{++}p<0.01$ compared with the respective control.

Effects of NO on 5-HT-induced fluid secretion

Close ia infusion of 5-HT (0.16 μg min^{-1}) for 30 min reversed net fluid absorption to net fluid secretion. Infusion of L-NAME markedly, though not significantly, enhanced 5-HT-induced net fluid secretion. Infusion of L-arginine (8.88 mg kg^{-1} min^{-1}), sodium nitroprusside (22.2 μg kg^{-1} min^{-1}) and 3-morpholinosydnonimine (SIN-1) (22.2 μg kg^{-1} min^{-1}), another NO donor, all slightly, but not significantly, enhanced net fluid absorption compared with controls. All three NO donors, however, significantly reversed 5-HT-induced fluid secretion to fluid absorption (Figure 4).

Effect of NO on E. coli STa-induced fluid secretion

Intraluminal instillation of *E. coli* STa (10 U ml^{-1}) reversed net fluid absorption to net secretion. Infusion of L-NAME resulted in a pronounced enhancement of *E. coli* STa-induced secretion. Infusion of L-arginine (8.88 mg kg^{-1} min^{-1}) as well as infusion of sodium nitroprusside (22.2 μg kg^{-1} min^{-1}) significantly inhibited *E. coli* STa-induced net fluid secretion (Figure 5).

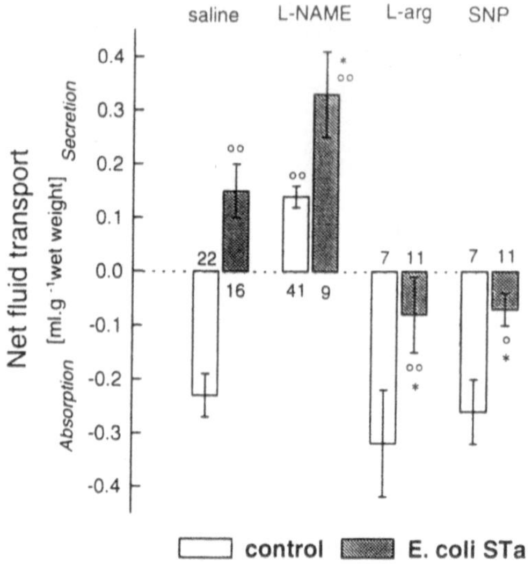

Figure 5. Effects of iv infusion of saline, L-NAME, L-arginine (L-arg) and sodium nitroprusside (SNP) on net fluid transport in controls (open bars) and on *E. coli* STa-induced fluid secretion (cross-hatched bars). Each column represents the mean ± SEM. The figures indicate the number of experiments; °$p<0.05$, °°$p<0.01$ compared with saline, *$p<0.05$ compared with saline plus *E. coli* STa. (From Reference 11 with permission)

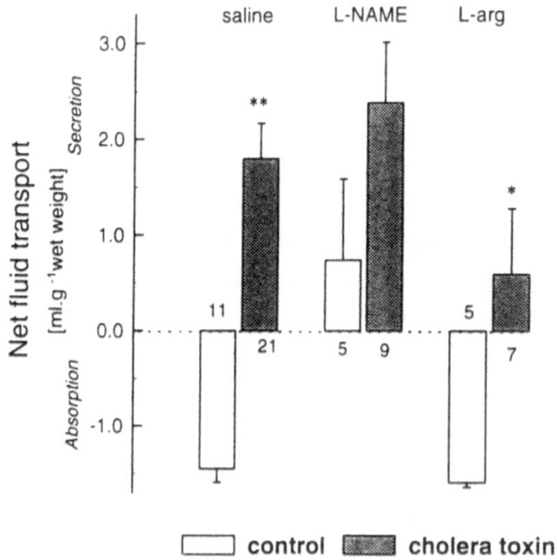

Figure 6. Effects of iv infusion of saline, L-NAME and L-arginine (L-arg) on net fluid transport in controls (open bars) and cholera-toxin-induced fluid secretion (cross-hatched bars). Each column represents the mean ± SEM. The figures indicate the number of experiments; *$p<0.05$, **$p<0.01$ compared with the respective control.

Effect of NO on cholera-toxin-induced fluid secretion

The 4-h exposure to cholera toxin (0.5 $\mu g\,ml^{-1}$) caused profuse net fluid secretion. Intravenous infusion of L-NAME reversed net absorption to net secretion and tended to enhance the secretory effect of cholera toxin. Infusion of L-arginine (8.88 mg $kg^{-1}\,min^{-1}$) as well as infusion of sodium nitroprusside (22.2 $\mu g\,kg^{-1}\,min^{-1}$) slightly enhanced net fluid absorption compared with controls and reduced cholera-toxin-induced fluid secretion (Figure 6).

Mechanism of action of NO

NO turned out to mediate the proabsorptive tone in the small intestine even in the conditions when the gut actively secretes fluid after challenge with PGE_2, 5-HT or enterotoxins. The mechanism of action of this proabsorptive effect of NO remains unexplained. L-NAME did not change cAMP levels or cGMP levels in mucosal scrapings nor did it enhance luminal PGE_2 output. The finding that the effect of L-NAME was inhibited by pretreatment of the rats with indomethacin, however, suggests the involvement of the cyclo-oxygenase pathway. The observation that, in Ussing-chamber experiments, stripped preparations reveal a prosecretory role of NO and full-thickness preparations demonstrate a proabsorptive role of NO implicates the involvement of myenteric nerves in the NO effect, finally determining the direction of transport changes. Further experiments will be necessary to evaluate the role of NO in transport processes under physiological and pathophysiological conditions.

ACKNOWLEDGEMENTS

This work was supported by the Austrian Scientific Research Funds Nos. 3630, 4920, 6087, 7877 and 10007.

REFERENCES

1. Rao RK, Riviere PJM, Pascaud X, Junien JL, Porreca F. Tonic regulation of mouse ileal ion transport by nitric oxide. J Pharmacol Exp Ther. 1994;269:626–31.
2. Barry MK, Aloisi JD, Pickering SP, Yeo CJ. Nitric oxide modulates water and electrolyte transport in the ileum. Ann Surg. 1994;219:382–8.
3. Mailman D. Differential effects of luminal L-arginine and N-ω-nitro L-arginine on blood flow and water fluxes in rat ileum. Br J Pharmacol. 1994;112:304–10.
4. Wilson KT, Xie Y, Musch MW, Chang EB. Sodium nitroprusside stimulates anion secretion and inhibits sodium chloride absorption in rat colon. J Pharmacol Exp Ther. 1993;266:224–30.
5. MacNaughton WK. Nitric oxide-donating compounds stimulate electrolyte transport in the guinea-pig intestine in vitro. Life Sci. 1993;53:585–93.
6. Tamai H, Gaginella TS. Direct evidence for nitric oxide stimulation of electrolyte secretion in the rat colon. Free Rad Res Commun. 1993;19:229–39.
7. Mascolo N, Izzo AA, Barbato F, Capasso F. Inhibitors of nitric oxide synthetase prevent castor-oil-induced diarrhoea in the rat. Br J Pharmacol. 1993;108:861–4.

8. Mascolo N, Izzo AA, Autore G, Barbato F, Capasso F. Nitric oxide and castor-oil-induced diarrhea. J Pharmacol Exp Ther. 1994;268:291–5.
9. Mascolo N, Gaginella TS, Izzo AA, Dicarlo G, Capasso F. Nitric oxide involvement in sodium choleate-induced fluid secretion and diarrhoea in rats. Eur J Pharmacol. 1994;264:21–6.
10. Rolfe V, Levin RJ. Enterotoxin Escherichia coli STa activates a nitric oxide-dependent myenteric plexus secretory reflex in the rat ileum. J Physiol. 1994;475:531–7.
11. Schirgi-Degen A, Beubler E. Significance of nitric oxide in the stimulation of intestinal fluid absorption in the rat jejunum in vivo. Br J Pharmacol. 1995;114:13–18.
12. Beubler E, Schirgi-Degen A. Proabsorptive effect of nitric oxide in cholera toxin and 5-HT-induced fluid secretion in the rat jejunum in vivo. Gastroenterology. 1995;108:A274.

Manuscript received 12 Oct. 95.
Accepted for publication 31 Oct. 95.

TS Gaginella et al. (eds.), Biochemical Pharmacology as an Approach to Gastrointestinal Disorders, 65–72

MECHANISM OF CHOLERA

E. BEUBLER AND A. SCHIRGI-DEGEN
Department of Experimental and Clinical Pharmacology, University of Graz, Universitätsplatz 4, A-8010 Graz, Austria

ABSTRACT

The effect of cholera toxin on intestinal fluid secretion is commonly considered to be mediated by cyclic adenosine monophosphate. Also, 5-hydroxytryptamine (5-HT), prostaglandin E_2 (PGE_2) and the action of neuronal structures have been implicated in the pathogenesis of cholera.

To elucidate the role of 5-HT and PGE_2 in mediating cholera secretion, experiments were performed in the rat jejunum in vivo. Cholera toxin was administered intraluminally (0.1–0.5 $\mu g/ml^{-1}$, 1–5 h). 5-HT receptor antagonists and indomethacin were administered subcutaneously and calcium antagonists intra-arterially. 5-HT was measured by HPLC and PGE_2 by radioimmunoassay.

Cholera toxin caused a dose-dependent and time-dependent increase in mean net fluid secretion with a peak at 4 h. It also caused a dose-dependent release of 5-HT and PGE_2 into the luminal fluid. The 5-HT_2 receptor antagonist, ketanserin, and the cyclo-oxygenase inhibitor, indomethacin, both partially reduced cholera-toxin-induced fluid secretion but not 5-HT release. The 5-HT_3 receptor antagonists, tropisetron, ondansetron and granisetron, reduced in a dose-dependent manner and at higher doses totally blocked cholera-toxin-induced secretion. The most potent blocker was granisetron. Both nifedipine and verapamil also dose-dependently inhibited cholera-toxin-induced secretion.

In conclusion, our results provide evidence for a predominant role of 5-HT in cholera-toxin-induced secretion. Our data suggest a model in which cholera toxin may activate the adenylate cyclase–cAMP system in enterochromaffin cells, resulting in 5-HT release. 5-HT then activates 5-HT_2 receptors, which cause PGE_2 formation, as well as 5-HT_3 receptors on neuronal structures. The stimulation of 5-HT_2 and 5-HT_3 receptors leads to profuse secretion, probably via Ca^{2+} as final mediator.

Keywords: cholera toxin; intestinal fluid secretion ; cAMP system, enterochromaffin cells; 5-HT_2 and 5-HT_3 receptors

INTRODUCTION

The diarrhoea of cholera is commonly considered to depend on a cyclic adenosine monophosphate (cAMP)-mediated active secretory mechanism. Several other mediators have, however, been implicated in the mediation of cholera-toxin-induced intestinal fluid secretion. In 1970, Bhide and co-workers [1] demonstrated an increase in 5-HT blood levels in choleraic rabbits. Cholera toxin introduced into the duodenum of rabbits caused severe degranulation of enterochromaffin cells as revealed by electron microscopy [2]. From these experiments, a hypothesis was proposed that cholera toxin stimulates an apical receptor on the enterochromaffin cells and that serotonin and a polypeptide released by the stimulus may mediate the diarrhoeagenic action of cholera toxin. After these observations, a lot of evidence accumulated to prove the involvement

This paper was presented at the Section of IUPHAR GI Pharmacology Symposium on 'Biochemical pharmacology as an approach to gastrointestinal disorders (basic science to clinical perspectives)', October 12–14, 1995, Pécs, Hungary.

of 5-HT in the genesis of cholera-toxin-induced fluid and electrolyte secretion. The involvement of 5-HT in choleraic secretion was proved by inducing tachyphylaxis against 5-HT in the experimental animals, cats and rats, by intravenous infusion of increasing doses of 5-HT. In these animals, cholera-toxin-induced secretion was inhibited [3]. In a histochemical study, cholera toxin was shown to cause a significant depletion of 5-HT from enterochromaffin cells in the feline small intestine [4].

It has been further suggested that cholera toxin may cause diarrhoea by stimulating prostaglandin (PG) synthesis [5]. This concept is supported by the observations that cholera toxin is apparently associated with increased local PG synthesis [6–9] and that PG-synthetase inhibitors impair the secretory effect of cholera toxin [10–13]. The finding that indomethacin in some studies has been reported to inhibit cholera-toxin-induced secretion but not mucosal cAMP accumulation [13,14] favours the notion that PGs may play a primary role in the secretory mechanism. This view is supported by the observation that low concentrations of PGs exert a secretory effect by facilitating the entry of calcium into the cell, rather than by stimulating the adenylate cyclase–cAMP system [15]. On the other hand, PGE_2 has been shown to be an important intermediate in the transduction mechanism which leads to 5-HT-induced intestinal secretion [15].

This review summarizes the results of several papers which aimed to elucidate the role of 5-HT and prostaglandin PGE_2 in mediating cholera secretion.

METHODS

The experiments were performed in a tied-off loop model in the rat jejunum in vivo. Net fluid transfer rates were determined gravimetrically after the instillation of Tyrode's solution into the gut lumen. Cholera toxin was administered intraluminally (0.1–0.5 $\mu g\,ml^{-1}$, 1–5 h). 5-HT receptor antagonists and indomethacin were administered subcutaneously and calcium antagonists intra-arterially. 5-HT was measured by HPLC, and PGE_2 by radioimmunoassay. cAMP was measured in mucosal scrapings with a cAMP assay kit. Sodium and potassium were determined by flame photometry and chloride was measured in a chloride meter. The experiments in each series were performed in balanced blocks. The results were given as mean$\pm$SEM and the data were analysed by the two-sample Student's *t*-test or by using analysis of variance and Duncan's multiple range test. Probability values <0.05 were considered significant.

RESULTS AND DISCUSSION

In the rat jejunum in vivo, cholera toxin dose-dependently increased intestinal fluid (Figure 1) and electrolyte secretion as well as luminal 5-HT (Figure 2) and prostaglandin E_2 output (Figure 3) [16,17]. The dose–response curve for cholera-toxin-induced fluid secretion was shifted to the right by ketanserin and by indomethacin, neither of which caused a change in cholera-toxin-induced release of 5-HT; however, both reduced the release of PGE_2 [16]. The 5-HT_3 blocker, tropisetron, also partially inhibited cholera-toxin-induced fluid secretion in these experiments. A

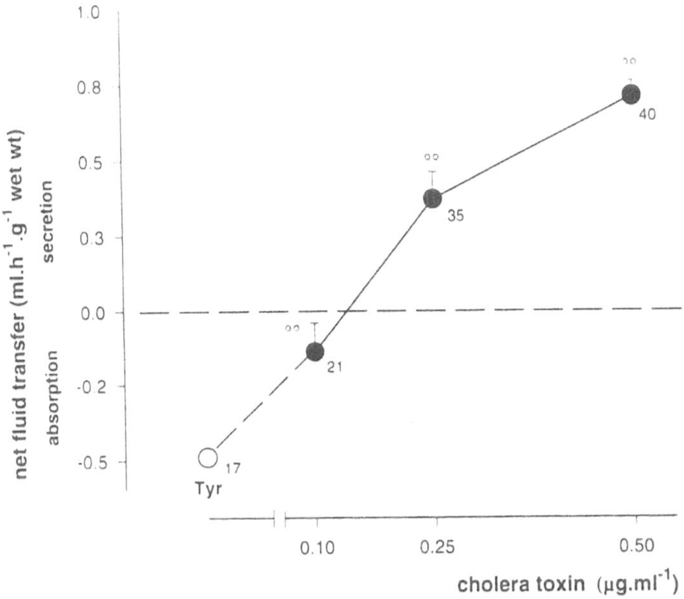

Figure 1. Dose–response relationship for the effect of cholera toxin (4 h) on net fluid transport in the rat jejunum in vivo. Each point represents the mean ± SEM. The figures indicate the number of experiments; $^{oo}p<0.01$ compared with control. (From Reference 16 with permission)

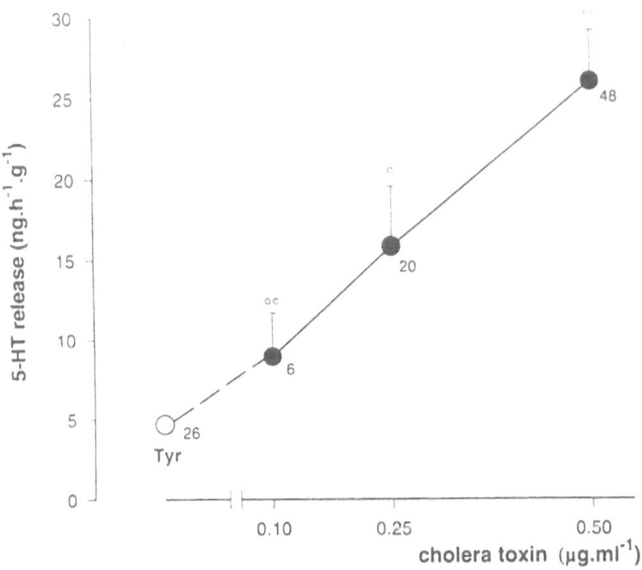

Figure 2. Dose–response relationship for the effect of cholera toxin (4 h) on luminal 5-HT output in the rat jejunum in vivo. Each point represents the mean ± SEM. The figures indicate the number of experiments; $^{o}p<0.05$, $^{oo}p<0.01$ compared with control. (From Reference 17 with permission)

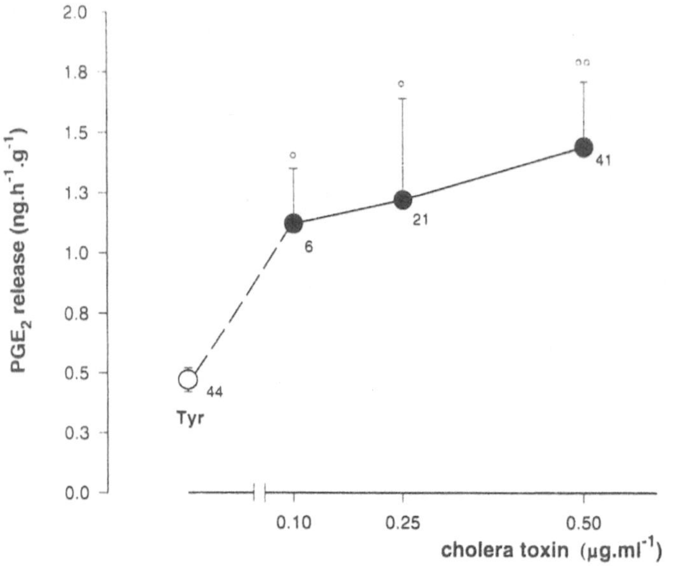

Figure 3. Dose–response relationship for the effect of cholera toxin (4 h) on luminal PGE_2 output in the rat jejunum in vivo. Each point represents the mean ± SEM. The figures indicate the number of experiments; $^{\circ}p<0.05$, $^{\circ\circ}p<0.01$ compared with control. (From Reference 16 with permission)

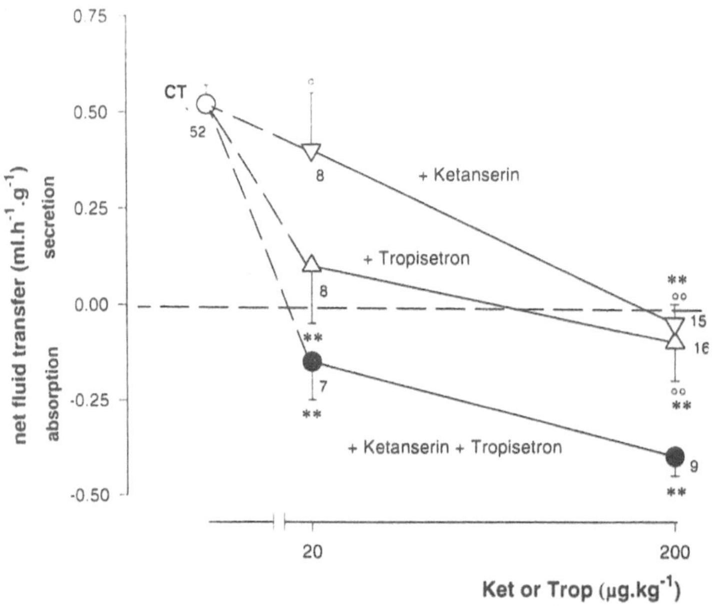

Figure 4. Effects of ketanserin, tropisetron and the combination of ketanserin plus tropisetron on cholera-toxin-induced net fluid secretion in the rat jejunum in vivo. Each point represents the mean ± SEM. The figures indicate the number of experiments; $^{**}p<0.01$ compared with cholera toxin (CT); $^{\circ}p<0.05$, $^{\circ\circ}p<0.01$ compared with cholera toxin in the presence of ketanserin plus tropisetron (From Reference 17 with permission)

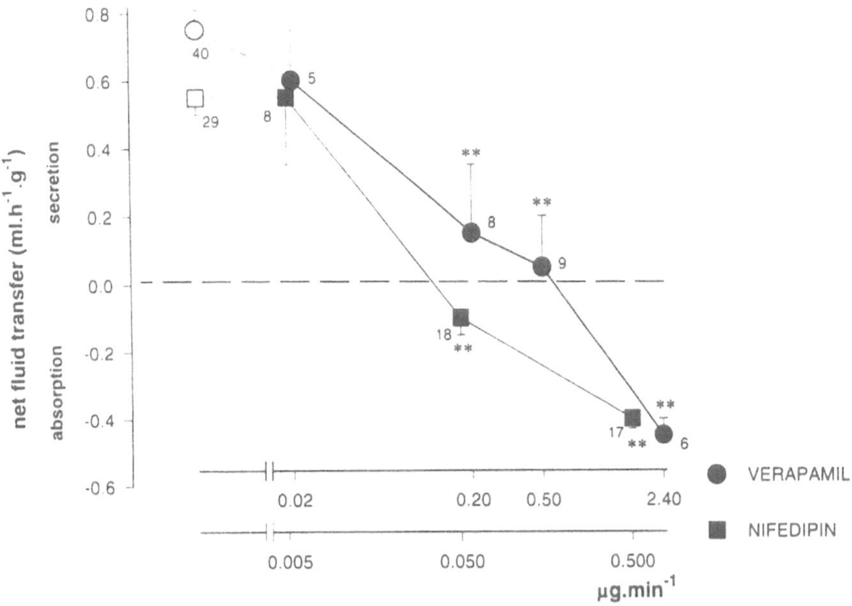

Figure 5. Effects of verapamil and nifedipine on cholera-toxin-induced fluid secretion in the rat jejunum in vivo. Each point represents the mean ± SEM. The figures indicate the number of experiments; $^{**}p<0.01$ compared with cholera toxin plus saline (○, □). (From Reference 16 with permission)

combination of ketanserin and tropisetron completely abolished choleraic secretion, indicating the involvement of $5\text{-}HT_2$ and $5\text{-}HT_3$ receptors in the mediation of the secretory response to cholera toxin [17] (Figure 4). Furthermore, the calcium-channel blockers verapamil and nifedipine also dose-dependently inhibited the secretory effect of cholera toxin (Figure 5) [16]. Cholera toxin enhanced mucosal cAMP levels by about 70% in this study. The combination of ketanserin plus tropisetron, which totally abolished the secretory effect of cholera toxin (Figure 4) [17], failed to influence elevated cAMP levels (Figure 4) [18]. Similarly, the calcium-channel blocker, verapamil, which also abolished cholera-toxin-induced secretion, did not influence elevated cAMP levels. Because the stimulation of the adenylate cyclase in enterochromaffin cells results in 5-HT release from these cells [18,20], the elevated cAMP levels may indicate that cholera toxin causes serotonin release from enterochromaffin cells via this mechanism.

Observations concerning the involvement of 5-HT in cholera-toxin-induced secretion were also obtained in other species: in dogs with chronic Thiry-Vella loops, intraluminally administered cholera toxin significantly increased jejunal output and effluent concentration of 5-HT [21]. Circulating serotonin levels did not change and the $5\text{-}HT_2$ receptor antagonist, ketanserin, failed to inhibit cholera-toxin-induced secretion in these experiments. In mice, ketanserin and tropisetron reduced cholera-toxin-

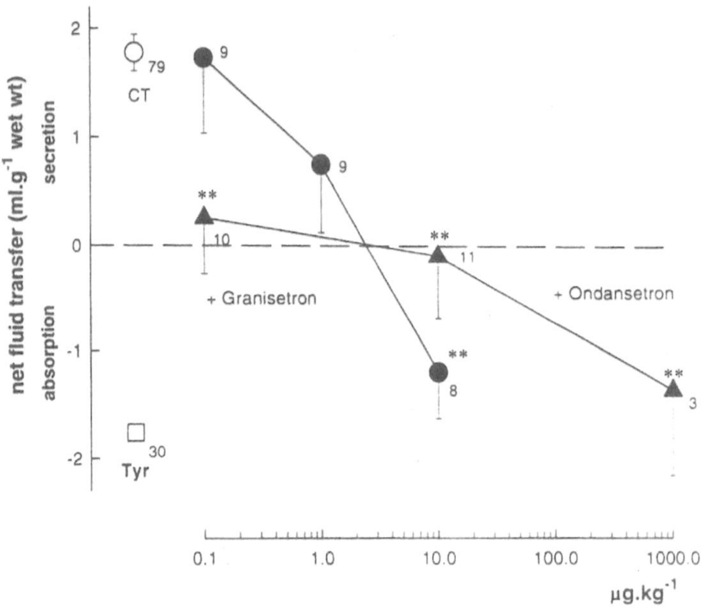

Figure 6. Effects of ondansetron and granisetron on cholera-toxin-induced fluid secretion in the rat jejunum in vivo. Each point represents the mean ± SEM. The figures indicate the number of experiments; $^{**}p<0.01$ compared with cholera toxin alone. (From Reference 24 with permission)

induced intestinal fluid accumulation [22]. The inhibitory effect of tropisetron was also partly confirmed in a conscious rat model [23].

In a further investigation, dose–response curves of the different 5-HT antagonists, ketanserin, tropisetron, ondansetron and granisetron, were compared concerning their inhibitory potency on 5-HT- and cholera-toxin-induced secretion [24]. The named 5-HT antagonists all dose-dependently inhibited 5-HT-induced fluid secretion in the rat jejunum in vivo. Ketanserin dose-dependently, but even at the highest dose of 2 mg kg^{-1} only partially, inhibited the secretory effect of cholera toxin. Tropisetron, ondansetron and granisetron all dose-dependently inhibited cholera-toxin-induced secretion, granisetron revealing total inhibition at only 10 µg kg^{-1} (Figure 6) [24]. The observation that 5-HT_2 receptor antagonists are more potent in inhibiting enterotoxin-induced fluid secretion than 5-HT_2 receptor antagonists implicates the involvement of 5-HT_3 receptors on enterochromaffin cells, the blockade of which lowers 5-HT release [25]. It is therefore suggested that 5-HT_3 receptors located on enterochromaffin cells and on certain nervous structures are more important in mediating fluid secretion than 5-HT_2 receptors, which are located on the epithelial cell.

In another study in the anaesthetized rat, granisetron and ondansetron markedly diminished cholera-toxin-evoked secretion, whereas ketanserin was without any effect [26]. The selective 5-HT_3 receptor antagonist, Y-25130, which dose-dependently inhibited net fluid secretion induced by 5-HT, also inhibited net fluid secretion induced by cholera toxin in rats [27]. So did granisetron and, to a lesser extent, ondansetron in the same study. Similar results supporting the involvement of 5-HT in cholera-toxin-induced secretion were obtained by using 5-HT antagonists to reduce cholera-toxin-induced hypersecretion in pig jejunum [28].

In human volunteers, cholera toxin caused an increase in serum 5-HT levels [29] and secretion of 5-HT into the gut lumen [30]. 5-HT antagonists, however, were without inhibitory effect on cholera-toxin-induced secretion in human volunteers [31].

In conclusion, our results provide evidence for a predominant role of serotonin in cholera-toxin-induced secretion. Our data suggest a model in which cholera toxin may activate the adenylate cyclase–cAMP system in enterochromaffin cells, resulting in 5-HT release. 5-HT then activates 5-HT_2 receptors which cause PGE_2 formation, and 5-HT_3 receptors on neuronal structures. Stimulation of both 5-HT_2 and 5-HT_3 receptors finally leads to the profuse fluid secretion that can be totally blocked by the combination of 5-HT_2 and 5-HT_3 blockers.

ACKNOWLEDGEMENTS

This work was supported by the Austrian Scientific Research Funds Nos. 3630, 4920, 6087, 7877 and 10007.

REFERENCES

1. Bhide MB, Aroskar VA, Dutta NK. Release of active substances by cholera toxin. Indian J Med Res. 1970;58:548–50.
2. Osaka M, Fujita T, Yanatori Y. On the possible role of intestinal hormones as the diarrhoeagenic messenger in cholera. Virchows Arch B Cell Pathol. 1975;18:287–96.
3. Cassuto J, Jodal M, Tuttle R, Lundgren O. 5-Hydroxytryptamine and cholera secretion. Physiological and pharmacological studies in cats and rats. Scand J Gastroenterol. 1982;17:695–703.
4. Nilsson O, Cassuto J, Larsson PA et al. 5-Hydroxytryptamine and cholera secretion: a histochemical and physiological study in cats. Gut. 1983;24:542-8.
5. Bennett A. Cholera and prostaglandins. Nature. 1971;231:536.
6. Okpako D. Prostaglandins and cholera: the occurrence of prostaglandin-like smooth muscle contracting substances in cholera diarrhoea. Prostaglandins. 1975;10:769–77.
7. Speelmann P, Rabbani GH, Bukhave K, Rask-Madsen J. Increased jejunal prostaglandin E_2 concentrations in patients with acute cholera. Gut. 1985;26:188–93.
8. Bedwani JR, Okpako D. Effects of crude and pure cholera toxin on prostaglandin release from the rabbit ileum. Prostaglandins. 1975;10:117–27.
9. Tothill A. Prostaglandin E_2: a factor in the pathogenesis of cholera. Prostaglandins. 1975;10:117–27.
10. Jacoby HI, Marshall CH. Antagonism of cholera enterotoxin by anti-inflammatory agents in the rat. Nature. 1972;235:163–4.
11. Finck AD, Katz RL. Prevention of cholera-induced intestinal secretion in the cat by aspirin. Nature. 1972;238:273–4.
12. Gots RE, Dormal SB, Giannella RA. Indomethacin inhibition of Salmonella typhimurium, Shigella flexneri and cholera-mediated rabbit ileal secretion. J Infect Dis. 1974;130:280–4.
13. Wald A, Gotterer GS, Rajendra GR, Turjman NA, Hendrix TR. Effect of indomethacin on cholera-induced fluid movements, unidirectional sodium fluxes and intestinal cAMP. Gastroenterology. 19777;72:106–10.

14. Wilson DE, El Hindi S, Tao P, Poppe L. Effects of indomethacin on intestinal secretion, prostaglandin E and cyclic cAMP. Evidence against a role for prostaglandins in cholera toxin-induced secretion. Prostaglandins. 1975;10:581–7.
15. Beubler E, Bukhave K, Rask-Madsen J. Significance of calcium for the prostaglandin E_2-mediated secretory response to 5-hydroxytryptamine in the small intestine of the rat in vivo. Gastroenterology. 1986;90:1972–7.
16. Beubler E, Kollar G, Saria A, Bukhave K, Risk-Madsen J. Involvement of 5-hydroxytryptamine, prostaglandin E_2, and cyclic adenosine monophosphate in cholera toxin-induced fluid secretion in the small intestine of the rat in vivo. Gastroenterology. 1989;96:368–76.
17. Beubler E, Horina G. 5-HT_2 and 5-HT_3 receptor subtypes mediate cholera toxin-induced intestinal fluid secretion in the rat. Gastroenterology. 1990;99:83–9.
18. Forsberg EJ, Miller RJ. Regulation of serotonin release from rabbit intestinal enterochromaffin cells. J Pharmacol Exp Ther. 1983;227:755–66.
19. Schwörer H, Racke K, Kilbinger H. Spontaneous release of endogenous 5-hydroxytryptamine and 5-hydroxyindoleacetic acid from the isolated vascularly perfused ileum of the guinea-pig. Neuroscience. 1987;21:297–303.
20. Racke K, Schwörer H, Kilbinger H. Adrenergic modulation of the release of 5-hydroxytryptamine from the vascularly perfused ileum of the guinea-pig. Br J Pharmacol. 1988;95:923–31.
21. Larosa CA, Sherlock D, Kimura K, Pimpl W, Money SR, Jaffe BM. The role of serotonin in the canine secretory response to cholera toxin in vivo. J Pharmacol Exp Ther. 1989;251:71–6.
22. Buchheit KH. Inhibition of cholera toxin-induced intestinal secretion by the 5-HT_3 receptor antagonist ICS 205-930. NS Arch Pharmacol. 1989;339:704–5.
23. Ku P, Lee CH, Smith WL, Jett MF. Effect of 5-hydroxytryptamine agonists and antagonists on cholera toxin-induced intestinal fluid accumulation in conscious rats. Proc West Pharmacol. 1992;35:221–6.
24. Beubler E, Schirgi-Degen A, Gamse R. Inhibition of 5-hydroxytryptamine- and enterotoxin-induced fluid secretion by 5-HT receptor antagonists in the rat jejunum. Eur J Pharmacol. 1993;248:157–62.
25. Gebauer A, Merger M, Kilbinger H. Modulation by 5-HT_3 and 5-HT_4 receptor of the release of 5-hydroxytryptamine from the guinea-pig small intestine. NS Arch Pharmacol. 1993;347:137–40.
26. Sjoqvist A, Cassuto J, Jodal M, Lundgren O. Actions of serotonin antagonists on cholera-toxin-induced intestinal fluid secretion. Acta Physiol Scand. 1992;145:229–37.
27. Ooe M, Asano K, Haga K, Setoguchi M. Effect of Y25130, a selective 5-HT_3 receptor antagonist, on the intestinal fluid secretion in rats. Nippon Yakurigaku Zasshi. 1993;101:299.
28. Hansen MB, Skadhauge E. Combination of ketanserin and granisetron reduce cholera toxin-induced hypersecretion in pig jejunum. Scand J Gastroenterol. 1994;29:908–15.
29. Thillainayagam AV, Dias JA, Schirgi-Degen A, Beubler E, Clark ML, Farthing MJG. Supportive evidence that 5-hydroxytryptamine (5-HT) is a mediator of cholera toxin (CT) induced secretion in man. Gastroenterology. 1991;100:A706.
30. Bearcroft CP, Taylor TM, Perrett D, Farthing MJG. 5-Hydroxytryptamine release into human jejunum by cholera toxin. Gastroenterology. 1992;102:A199.
31. Eherer AJ, Hinterleitner TA, Petritsch W, Holzer-Petsche U, Beubler E, Krejs GJ. Effect of 5-hydroxytryptamine antagonists on cholera toxin induced secretion in the human jejunum. Eur J Clin Gastroenterol. 1994;24:664.

Manuscript received 12 Oct. 95.
Accepted for publication 31 Oct. 95.

TS Gaginella et al. (eds.), Biochemical Pharmacology as an Approach to Gastrointestinal Disorders, 73–82

CRITICAL EVALUATION OF ACINAR, DUCTAL, VASCULAR AND INTESTINAL INTRALUMINAL FACTORS INFLUENCING PANCREATIC CYTOPROTECTION

M. PAPP, B. BURGHARDT, K. KISFALVI AND G. VARGA*
Institute of Experimental Medicine, Hungarian Academy of Sciences, 1450 Budapest, PO Box 67, Hungary
*Correspondence

ABSTRACT

This paper gives a brief survey on adaptive pancreatic cytoprotection and vasoprotection in the framework of which noxious agents and factors of defensive mechanism are made known and critically evaluated. In development of acute pancreatitis, intra-acinar redistribution of lysosomal hydrolases, colocalization of digestive and lysosomal enzymes, escape of digestive and lysosomal enzymes from pancreatic ductal system into the interstitium, inflammatory modulators released from macrophages and evoking local inflammation, ischaemia, and furthermore feedback regulation of pancreatic secretion can be regarded as motives. Factors of defensive mechanism include prostaglandins, nitric oxide and unobstructed juice flow which promote the repair of injured membranes in acinar and vascular endothelial cells, respectively. Their whole sum may be called adaptive pancreatic cyto- and vasoprotection or pancreatic 'self-defence mechanism'.

Keywords: pancreatic, adaptation, cytoprotection, vasoprotection, inflammatory mediators, nitric oxide, intestinal luminal factors

INTRODUCTION

The aim of this overview is to direct attention to some pathogenic agents which may cause acute pancreatitis (AP) and discuss some aspects of the rapid adaptive or cytoprotective mechanisms of action against these agents. The original concept of cytoprotection implies prostaglandins (PG) in short-term adaptation of gastric epithelium, or in other words rapid gastric mucosal repair [1]. Later, this concept was widened and extended to other organs: exogenous prostaglandins evoke direct cytoprotection, and release of endogenous prostaglandins results in adaptive cytoprotection [2–4]. Preservation of vascular integrity is called vasoprotection in which release of nitric oxide can be assigned [5] (Figure 1).

Nitric oxide (NO) is a mediator by which macrophages exert their cytotoxic activity against, among others, micro-organisms. Activation of macrophages results in expression of NO-synthase (Figure 2). This enzyme converts L-arginine to L-citrulline and NO [5]. Vasoactive agents (like acetylcholine, kinins, histamine, etc.) acting on

This paper was presented at the Section of IUPHAR GI Pharmacology Symposium on 'Biochemical pharmacology as an approach to gastrointestinal disorders (basic science to clinical perspectives)', October 12–14, 1995, Pécs, Hungary.

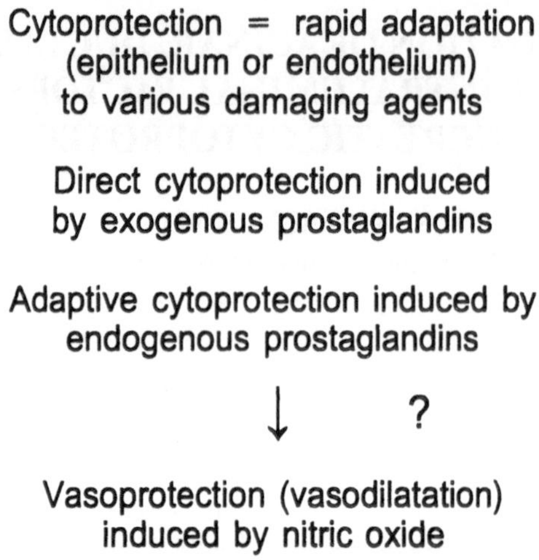

Cytoprotection = rapid adaptation
(epithelium or endothelium)
to various damaging agents
Direct cytoprotection induced
by exogenous prostaglandins
Adaptive cytoprotection induced by
endogenous prostaglandins
?
Vasoprotection (vasodilatation)
induced by nitric oxide

Figure 1. Terms of cytoprotection and vasoprotection

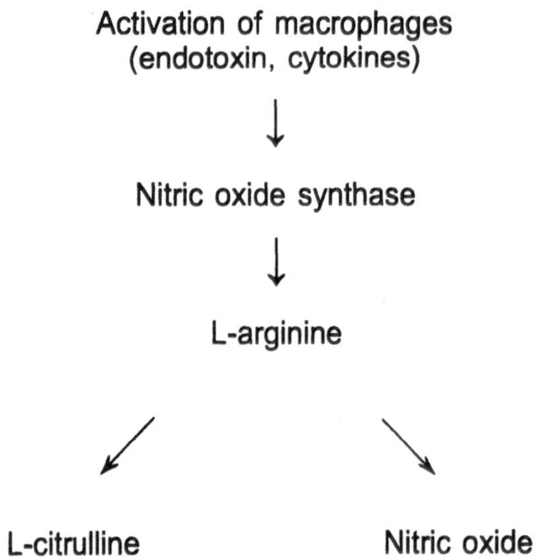

Figure 2. Genesis of nitric oxide

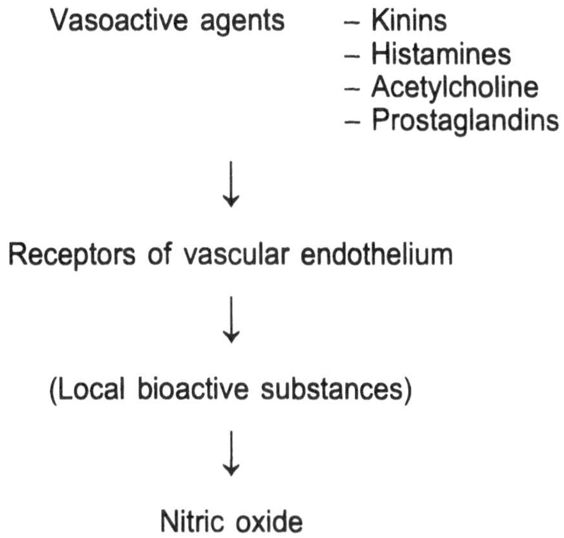

Figure 3. Relationship between vasoactive agents and nitric oxide

superficial receptors of vascular endothelial cells, release NO which evokes relaxation of vascular smooth muscle cells. NO is thought to be an endogenous vasodilator (Figure 3). It inhibits platelet aggregation, adherence of neutrophils to endothelium and, by these means, release of inflammatory modulators [2,5].

Within the framework of pancreatic cytoprotection and vasoprotection, pathogenic and protective factors in AP are discussed in relation to acinar–enzymatic, ductal–interstitial, vascular and intestinal luminal components [6,7].

ACINAR–ENZYMATIC COMPONENTS

In most recent investigations, hyperstimulation of the exocrine pancreatic function by the CCK-analogue, octapeptide caerulein, is used to induce AP.

The most characteristic feature of this AP is glandular oedema. Ultrastructure of early cellular and subcellular events reveals development of intra-acinar enlarged secretory and large autophagic vacuoles which contain both digestive and lysosomal enzymes as a result of fusion of condensing vacuoles and zymogen granules. Due to the co-localization and interaction of digestive enzyme zymogens and lysosomal hydrolases, e.g. cathepsin B, inactive trypsinogen is activated to active trypsin which leads to acinar cell necrosis [8–10]. However, the pancreas regenerates in hormone-induced AP within 6 days [9] and the acinar cell destruction never leads to haemorrhagic necrotic AP [11]. In ex-vivo isolated and perfused canine pancreas, intra-arterial caerulein infusion produced depletion of zymogen granules, formation of condensing vacuoles and basolateral exocytosis. The ex-vivo perfused canine pancreatitis model seems to be morphologically and biochemically identical to findings seen in an in-vivo model [12]. In vitro, a supramaximal concentration of caerulein evoked cathepsin B redistribution in a subcellular fraction of rat pancreas only when it was combined with blood plasma from a rat exposed in vivo to supramaximal caerulein stimulation. This phenomenon was attributed to a 10–30 kDa plasma protein and its effect was abolished by a protease inhibitor [13]. Extraluminal trypsinogen activation was demonstrated with a direct test of trypsin activation measuring the trypsinogen activation peptide. This peptide is released when trypsinogen is activated to trypsin. Tissue and plasma concentration of this peptide rises significantly in different AP models in rodents [14].

By contrast with the aforementioned, colocalization of digestive and lysosomal enzymes is absent in AP of opossums induced by pancreatic duct ligation [15]. Induction of AP results in the rapid and massive rearrangement of the pattern of gene expression [16].

Ethanol is the best known inducer of human AP. It increases the fragility of zymogen granules without morphological evidence of glandular injury by permitting contact between digestive and lysosomal hydrolases [17]. So far, it is suspected that elastase destroys the vessel walls in AP. It has been published, however, that active elastase cannot be a principal factor in AP of pigs while its inhibition capacity is higher in biological fluids than that of trypsin [18]. Reduction of pancreatic digestive enzyme stores seems to be protective in AP of rats [11,19].

In different models of experimental AP in the rat, an acute-phase protein can be detected in large amounts in the pancreas. It is synthesized in the rough endoplasmic reticulum and stored in zymogen granules. Its molecular weight is 12 kDa [20], and the pathogenic role of such protein has been mentioned before [13].

Inhibition of trypsin activity is believed to block the enzymatic chain reaction related to activation of zymogen of digestive enzymes. Urinary trypsin inhibitor, as well as other new synthetic protease inhibitors, such as E3123 [21] and ONO3307 [22], applied before and during caerulein-induced AP in rats, each exert cytoprotective effects by stabilizing lysosomal membranes and preventing redistribution of lysosomal enzymes. Although the low molecular weight protease inhibitor ONO3307 and PG are each effective in secretagogue-evoked AP, as stabilizers of lysosomal membranes, their combination is greater and more effective against pancreatic injury [22].

PGE_2 inhibits CCK-8-, bombesin-, carbachol-, VIP- and secretin-stimulated amylase secretion from isolated rat pancreatic acini. This function is mediated via specific receptors for PGE [23,24]. On the other hand, intragastric administration of a synthetic analogue of PGE_2 increases pancreatic enzyme secretion while its intravenous administration counteracts it in the conscious rat. This effect is not influenced by CCK-antagonist, secretin antibody or bilateral vagotomy, but is completely inhibited by atropine showing the role of gastropancreatic reflex in this phenomenon [25]. In the very early phase of sodium taurocholate-induced pancreatitis, glandular tissue levels of some PGs (E_2, D_2) increase significantly, while PGE_1 remains unchanged [26]. PGE_2, but not PGE_1, prevents dose-dependently the redistribution of cathepsin B and the intra-acinar increase in amylase and trypsin in secretagogue-induced AP in rats [27]. Other authors find that PGE_1 is protective in taurocholate-evoked pancreatitis in the rat [28]. PGE_2 decreases pancreatic oedema induced by a supramaximal dose of caerulein and inhibits secretion-stimulated pancreatic secretion in the rat [29]. In the early phase of sodium taurocholate treatment of rats, PGE_2 counteracts, while superoxide dismutase partially influences the conversion of xanthine dehydrogenase to xanthine oxidase and, by this means, the subsequent production of free radicals which may extend damage of acinar parenchyma [30].

INFLAMMATORY MEDIATORS

Inflammatory mediators are regarded as markers of severity of AP or common effectors of acinar cell damage [31]. Markers of severity of AP are: C-reactive protein, interleukin-6, polymorphonuclears, elastase, trypsin activation peptide and urinary immunoglobulin G (Figure 4). Suspected mediators of AP are tumour necrosis factor-α, phospholipase A_2, a rate-limiting enzyme in prostaglandins, and platelet-activating factor formation (Figure 5). Adhesion molecules facilitate leucocyte migration, oxygen free radicals and mediate tissue damage. Finally, some authors suppose that AP is a result of an ischaemia–reperfusion injury [31,32].

Blockade of tumour necrosis factor (TNFα) by anti-TNFα antibody, in contrast with the expected findings, increases oedema formation in caerulein-induced AP [33]. Inflammatory mediators seem to be important in sepsis or in septic complications of AP. They participate in induction of local or systemic acute-phase response, rather than in onset of AP.

- C-reactive protein
- Interleukin-6
- Polymorphonuclear elastase
- Trypsinogen activation peptide
- Urinary immunoglobulin G

Figure 4. Inflammatory markers of severity of acute pancreatitis

- Tumour necrosis factor alpha
- Phospholipase A2
  (formation of prostaglandin and
  platelet activating factor)
- Platelet activating factor
  (activated endothelial cells)
- Adhesion molecules
  (leukocyte migration)
- Cytokines
  (released by endothelial cells)
- Oxygen free radicals
- Hypoperfusion
  (ischaemia-reperfusion injury)

Figure 5. Inflammatory mediators of acute pancreatitis

DUCTAL AND INTERSTITIAL FACTORS

In different models of AP, both basal and CCK-stimulated pancreatic secretion are reduced. Recovery of secretory capacity takes longer in necrotizing than in oedematous AP [34]. Caerulein stimulates the secretion of both amylase and cathepsin B in pancreatic juice of rats and rabbits. Significantly more cathepsin B is secreted in pancreatic juice evoked by stimulation when the temporary ductal obstruction is released. The lysosomal enzymes seem to be present in zymogen granules under normal conditions [35,36]. The epithelium lining pancreatic ducts is the main barrier [37] preventing the secreted enzymes from entering pancreatic interstitium and coming into contact with acinar cells. The increase in ductal permeability induced by different agents helps the initiation of experimental AP [38]. Transient ductal ligation decreases protein synthesis and output in the rat [39]; when pancreatic ducts are ligated pancreatic oedema develops. Digestive enzyme activity in oedema interstitial fluid reaches 20–30% of the stimulated pancreatic juice collected before duct ligation [40]. Digestive enzymes may reach the pancreatic interstices at the basolateral membranes too [41]. These findings are important because pancreatic oedema is thought to be the first stage of acute pancreatic necrosis [42].

VASCULAR FACTORS

It is suspected that vasoactive agents, like acetylcholine, kinins and histamines, release nitric oxide (NO) from the vascular endothelial cells; NO relaxes vascular smooth muscle cells, evoking vasodilatation [2,5]. Caerulein increases pancreatic blood flow (PBF) [43]. The specific NO synthase inhibitor (LNNA; *N*-omega-nitro-L-arginine) inhibits completely the caerulein-induced increase in PBF but this inhibition is reversed by L-arginine in rats [44]. LNNA causes a significant reduction in canine PBF [45] and decreases the secretin plus cholecystokinin-stimulated pancreatic secretion [45,46].

In experimental AP, pancreatic blood flow decreases and pancreatic ischaemia develops [47,48]. In AP, changes of intrapancreatic vascular pattern are: early dilatation of pancreatic capillaries followed by increased permeability, with extravasation of plasma resulting in capillary stasis. Obstruction of the pancreatic duct system results in pancreatic oedema, which slows capillary blood flow and leads to ischaemia, haemorrhages and venous congestion [47]. Both vasoactive substances and inflammatory mediators which are released in the inflamed pancreas take part in the production of local and systemic vascular changes and inflammatory reactions. Such inflammatory mediators can be demonstrated in pancreatic exudate, pancreatic venous and peripheral blood [31,47,48]. Ischaemia aggravates, but does not initiate pancreatitis [47,48]. Arterial hypotension aggravates histological damage in experimental haemorrhagic pancreatitis in rats [49] and accelerates lysosomal and mitochondrial fragility [50]. Hypovolaemia exerts a deleterious effect on the pancreas [51]. Concentration of vasoactive substances, like kallikrein, bradykinin and PGE_2, increases gradually after induction of AP in portal venous blood; bradykinin reduces PBF [52,53].

In acute endotoxaemia, inhibition of NO synthesis by LNNA decreases perfusion of the pancreas in rats [54]. NO may damage pancreatic islet cells and the cells can be protected by LNNA which inhibits the generation of NO by activated macrophages [55].

INTESTINAL LUMINAL FACTORS

Reduction in the secretion of pancreatic enzymes is mediated by the presence of digestive enzymes in the duodenum. The process is termed negative feedback regulation [56]. As the concentration of enzymes in the duodenum increases, proteases in the upper small intestine suppress pancreatic exocrine secretion. Suppression of the exocrine secretion by proteases is attributed to restrained release of CCK and secretin [56]. Release of CCK and secretin are mediated by peptides secreted from mucosal cells into the intestinal lumen. These peptides are inactivated by pancreatic proteases, mainly by trypsin [57,58]. As a consequence, when proteases are inactivated or are absent from the duodenal lumen – for example by diversion of pancreatic juice – both CCK and secretin plasma levels increase and they enhance pancreatic secretion [59].

In relapsing chronic pancreatitis, failure of enzyme secretion and its elimination from the duodenum, due to obstructed outflow of the juice, does occur. In therapy of relapsing chronic pancreatitis, the goals of treatment are pain relief and control of maldigestion by administration of enzyme replacement therapy. Enzyme preparations in the form of enteric-coated microspheres in hard gelatine capsules and combined with prostaglandins have a significant advantage over commercial enzyme preparations: they improve maldigestion and pain relief by diminishing the secretion of juice and, in this way, decrease the pain induced by distension of the pancreatic ductal system [60]. Enzyme preparations alone with proteolytic activity seem to control pancreatic secretion [61]. However, application of pure proteases or enzymes in high concentrations of proteases as a treatment seems to be ineffective [62] in the treatment of chronic pancreatitis.

CONCLUSIONS

The total sum of agents promoting rapid repair of injured pancreatic acinar, ductal and vascular membranes constitutes the basis of pancreatic cyto- and vasoprotection which may be called the pancreatic 'self-defence mechanism' [40].

ACKNOWLEDGEMENTS

This work was supported in part by grants OTKA T5429 and OTKA T017104.

REFERENCES

1. Robert A. Cytoprotection by prostaglandins. Gastroenterology. 1979;77:761–7.
2. Konturek SJ, Konturek JW. Gastric adaptation: basic and clinical aspects. Digestion. 1994;55:131–8.
3. Papp M. Pancreatic cytoprotection: a survey. Acta Physiol Hung. 1989;73:305–10.
4. Papp M. Pancreatic cytoprotection: new approaches. Acta Physiol Hung. 1992;80:399–406.
5. Gibaldi M. What is nitric oxide and why are so many people studying it. J Clin Pharmacol. 1993;33:488–96.
6. Papp M. Les facteurs acineux et enzymatiques, vasculaires et inflammatoires, lymphatil et interstitiels du déclenchement de la nécrose aiguë du pancreas. Lyon Chir. 1972;68:260–4.
7. Papp M. Pathogenesis of acute pancreatitis: pancreatic ductal–interstitial–vascular and lymphatic pathways. Acta Med Acad Sci Hung. 1976;33:191–200.
8. Willemer I, Adler G. Mechanism of acute pancreatitis (cellular and subcellular events). Int J Pancreatol. 1991;9:21–30.
9. Willemer I, Elsässer HP, Adler G. Hormone-induced pancreatitis. Eur Surg Res. 1992;24(Suppl.1):29–39.
10. Steer ML. How and where does acute pancreatitis begin. Arch Surg. 1992;127:1350–3.
11. Kisfalvi K, Papp M, Friess HM, Gorácz G. Beneficial effects of preventive oral administration of camostate on caerulein-induced pancreatitis in rats. Dig Dis Sci. 1995;40:546–7.
12. Clemens JA, Olson J, Cameron JL. Caerulein-induced pancreatitis in the ex vivo isolated perfused canine pancreas. Surgery. 1991;104:515–22.
13. Saluja M, Saluja A, Lerch MM, Steer ML. A plasma protease which is expressed during supramaximal stimulation causes in vitro subcellular redistribution of lysosomal enzymes in rat exocrine pancreas. J Clin Invest. 1991;87:1280–5.
14. Foitzik T, Lewandrowski KB, Fernandez-del Castillo C, Rattner DW, Warshaw AL. Evidence for extraluminal trypsinogen activation in three different models of acute pancreatitis. Surgery. 1994;115:698–702.

15. Samuel I, Wilcockson DP, Regan JP, Joehe RI. Ligation-induced acute pancreatitis in opossums: acinar cell necrosis in the absence of colocalization. J Surg Res. 1995;58:64–74.
16. Iovanna JL, Keim V, Michel R, Dagorn JC. Pancreatic gene expression is altered during acute experimental pancreatitis in the rat. Am J Physiol. 1991;261:G485–9.
17. Haber PS, Wilson JS, Apte MV, Korsten MA, Pirola RC. Chronic ethanol consumption increases the fragility of rat pancreatic zymogen granules. Gut. 1994;35:1474–8.
18. Hakansson H, Borgstrom A, Ohlsson K. Pancreatic cationic elastase in porcine experimental pancreatitis. Eur Surg Res. 1991;23:73–84.
19. Coelho AM, Kubrusky MS, Bonizzia A, Goncalez Y, Abdo EE, Machado MC. Protective effect of pancreatic enzyme depletion in the course of acute pancreatitis – experimental study in rats. Rev Hosp Clin Fac Med Sao Paolo. 1993;48:106–11.
20. Keim V, Iovanna JL, Rorh G, Usadel KH, Dagorn JC. Characterization of a rat pancreatic secretory protein associated with pancreatitis. Gastroenterology. 1991;100:775–82.
21. Sata N, Atomi Y, Kimura W, Kuroda A, Muto T, Mines C. Intracellular activation of an exogenous low-molecular-weight synthetic protease inhibitor, E 3123, in caerulein-induced acute pancreatitis in rats. Int J Pancreatol. 1994;15:119–27.
22. Hirano T, Manabe T, Tobe T. Cytoprotective effect of prostaglandins and a new potent protease inhibitor in acute pancreatitis. Am J Med Sci. 1992;304:154–63.
23. Ogami Y, Kimura T, Nawata H. Role of prostaglandin E2 in stimulus-secretion coupling in rat exocrine pancreas. Pancreas. 1990;5:598–605.
24. Mössner J, Secknus R, Spiekermann GM et al. Prostaglandin E2 inhibits secretagogue-induced enzyme secretion from rat pancreatic acini. Am J Physiol. 1991;260:G711–19.
25. Masuda M, Miyasaka K, Funakoshi A. Cholinergic stimulatory effect of intragastric administration of a prostaglandin E2 analogue in pancreatic exocrine secretion in conscious rats. Pancreas. 1995:10:395–400.
26. Closa D, Rosell-Catafu J, Fernandez-Cruz L, Gelpi E. Prostaglandin D2, F2 alpha, E2, and E1 in early phase of experimental acute necrohaemorrhagic pancreatitis in rats. Pancreas. 1994;9:73–7.
27. Hirano T, Manabe T, Yotsumoto F, Ando K, Imanishi K, Tobe T. Effect of prostaglandin E on redistribution of lysosomal enzymes in caerulein-induced pancreatitis. Hepatogastroenterology. 1993;40:155–8.
28. Sakai Y, Hayakawa T, Kondo T et al. Protective effects of prostaglandin E1 oligomer on taurocholate-induced rat pancreatitis. J Gastroenterol Hepatol. 1992;7:591–5.
29. Ando K, Manabe T, Tobe T. Protective effect of prostaglandin E2 on caerulein-induced rat pancreatitis. Nippon Geka Hokan. 1992;61:259–67.
30. Closa D, Bulbena D, Rosello-Catafau J, Fernandez-Cruz L, Gelpi E. Effect of prostaglandins and superoxide dismutase administration on oxygen free radical production in experimental acute pancreatitis. Inflammation. 1993;17:563–75.
31. Formela LJ, Galloway JN, Kingsnorth AN. Inflammatory mediators in acute pancreatitis. Br J P Surg. 1995;82:6–13.
32. Müller MK, Keim V, Chari S. Pathophysiologishe Konzepte und protektive Möglichkeiten bei experimentellen Pankreasläsionen. Z Gastroenterol. 1993;31:621–8.
33. Giuce KS, Oldham Kt, Remich DG, Kunkel SL, Ward PA. Anti-tumor necrosis factor antibody augments oedema formation in caerulein-induced acute pancreatitis. J Surg Res. 1991;51:495–9.
34. Niederau C, Niederau M, Luthen R, Strohmeyer G, Ferrel LD, Grendell JH. Pancreatic exocrine secretion in acute experimental pancreatitis. Gastroenterology. 1990:99:1120–7.
35. Hirano T, Manabe T, Printz H, Saluja A, Steer ML. Secretion of lysosomal and digestive enzymes into pancreatic juice under physiological and pathological conditions in rabbits. Nippon Geka Hokan. 1992;61:103–24.
36. Hirano T. Lysosomal enzyme secretion into pancreatic juice in rats injected with pancreatic secretagogues and augmented secretion after short-term pancreatic duct obstruction. Nippon Geka Hokan. 1994;63:21–35.
37. Papp M, Somogyi J, Virágh Sz, Szabó D. Fine structural relation between pancreatic excretory ductules and intracellular spaces. Experientia. 1976;32:1580–1.
38. Reber HA. Acute pancreatitis; the role of duct permeabilities. In: Gyr KE, Singer MV, Sarles H, eds. Pancreatic Concepts and Classification. Excerpta Med Internat Congress Series 642:Elsevier Sci Publ; 1984:149–52.
39. Papp M, Varga G, Folly G. Pancreatic secretion. II. Pancreatic duct ligation and protein secretion in caerulein-stimulated pancreatic juice of rats. Mt Sinai J Med. 1983;50:441.
40. Papp M, Fodor I, Varga G, Folly G. Pancreatic oedema: its effect on the function and morphology of the pancreas in dogs and rats. Mt Sinai J Med. 1982;49:456–64.

41. Adler G, Rohr G, Kern HF. Alteration of membrane fusion as a cause of acute pancreatitis in the rat. Dig Dis Sci. 1982;27:993–1002.
42. Zoepffel H. Das akute Pankreasödem, eine Vorstafe der akuten Pankreasnekrose. Dtsch Z Chir. 1992;175:301–2.
43. Papp M, Fehér J, Varga G, Folly G. Humoral influences on local blood flow and external secretion of the resting dog pancreas. Acta Med Acad Sci Hung. 1977;34:185–98.
44. Satoh A, Shimosegawa T, Abe T et al. Role of nitric oxide in the pancreatic blood flow response to caerulein. Pancreas. 1994;9:574–9.
45. Konturek SJ, Bilski J, Konturel PK, Cieszkowski M, Pawlik W. Role of endogenous nitric oxide in the control of canine pancreatic secretion and blood flow. Gastroenterology. 1993;104:896–902.
46. Patel AG, Toyama MT, Nguyen TN et al. Role of nitric oxide in the relationship of pancreatic blood flow and exocrine secretion in cats. Gastroenterology. 1995;108:1215–20.
47. Papp M. Role of the circulation in acute pancreatitis. In: Kvietys PR, Barrowman JA, Granger DN, eds. Pathophysiology of the Splanchnic Circulation. Vol II, Chapter 10. Boca Raton, Florida: CRC Press Inc; 1987:119–35.
48. Prinz RA. Mechanism of acute pancreatitis. Int J Pancreatol. 1991;9:31–8.
49. Németh Éva P, Fodor I, Folly G, Papp M. Arterial hypotension as a factor aggravating the histological damage in experimental acute haemorrhagic pancreatitis. Acta Morphol Acad Sci Hung. 1973;21:319–32.
50. Robert JH, Toledano AE, Huang G et al. The pancreas and oxygen consumption. 1. Pancreatic oxygen consumption in normo- and hypovolemic dogs. Int J Pancreatol. 1989;4:51–63.
51. Hirano T, Manabe T. A new experimental model for gallstone pancreatitis: short-termed pancreatico-biliary duct obstruction and exocrine stimulation with systemic hypotension in rats. Nippon Geka Hokan. 1993;62:3–15.
52. Waldner H, Vollmar B, Conzen P et al. Enzymfreizetzung und Aktivierung der Kallikrein-Kinin Systeme in experimenteller Pancreatitis. Untersuchung in Pfotaderblut, Pancreaslymphe und Peritonealexudat. Langebecks Arch Klin. 1993;378:154–9.
53. Yotsumoto F, Manabe T, Ohshio G et al. Role of pancreatic blood flow and vasoactive substances in the development of canine acute pancreatitis. J Surg Res. 1993;55:331–6.
54. Mulder NF, van Lambalgen AA, Huisman E, Visser JJ, van den Bos BC, Thijs LG. Protective role of NO in the regional hemodynamic changes during acute endotoxaemia in rats. Am J Physiol. 1994;266:H1558–64.
55. Kroncke KD, Kolb-Bachofen V, Bersicht B, Burkart V, Kolb H. Activated macrophages kill pancreatic syngeneic islet cells via arginine-dependent nitric oxide generation. Biochem Biophys Res. 1991;175:752–8.
56. Chey WY. Regulation of pancreatic secretion. Int J Pancreatol. 1991;9:7–20.
57. Lu L, Louie D, Owyang C. A cholecystokinin releasing peptide mediates feedback regulation of pancreatic secretion. Am J Physiol. 1989;256:G430–5.
58. Miyasaka K, Guan D, Liddle RA, Green GM. Feedback regulation by trypsin: evidence for intraluminal CCK-releasing peptide. Am J Physiol. 1989;257(Gastrointest Liver Physiol 20):G175–81.
59. Li P, Lee KY, Ren XS, Chang TM, Chey WY. Effect of pancreatic protease on plasma cholecystokinin, secretin, and pancreatic exocrine secretion in response to sodium oleate. Gastroenterology. 1990;98:1642–8.
60. Dobrilla G. Management of chronic pancreatitis. Focus on enzyme replacement therapy. Int J Pancreatol. 1989;5(Suppl):17–29.
61. Malfertheiner P, Dominguez-Maunoz JE. Effect of exogenous pancreatic enzymes on gastrointestinal and pancreatic hormone release and gastrointestinal motility. Digestion. 1993;54(Suppl 2):15–20.
62. Mössner J. Is there a place for pancreatic enzymes in the treatment of pain in chronic pancreatitis? Digestion. 1993;54(Suppl.2):35–9.

Manuscript received 30 Oct. 95.
Accepted for publication 9 Nov. 95.

TS Gaginella et al. (eds.), Biochemical Pharmacology as an Approach to Gastrointestinal Disorders, 83–94

PEPTIDE RECEPTOR ANTAGONISTS AND MONOCLONAL ANTIBODIES RAISED AGAINST PEPTIDES: TOOLS TO STUDY PHYSIOLOGICAL REGULATION OF PANCREATIC FUNCTION

G. VARGA
Institute of Experimental Medicine, Hungarian Academy of Sciences, H-1450 Budapest, Hungary

ABSTRACT

This work is an attempt to demonstrate the applicability of peptide antagonists and monoclonal antibodies for blocking certain regulatory elements of pancreatic function in vivo. Data from the experiments using these tools suggest that circulating CCK, indeed, is a primary factor in regulating pancreatic enzyme secretion acting on CCK-A receptors in rats. Bombesin-like peptides play a minor role in mediating pancreatic function under physiological conditions, although gastrin-releasing peptide-preferring receptors are located on pancreatic acini. Immunoneutralization of circulating somatostatin led to an increased pancreatic secretory response to CCK stimulation, suggesting an inhibitory role of endogenous somatostatin. Receptor antagonists that antagonize the actions of galanin in the central nervous system, behaved as partial agonists of the peptide on the exocrine pancreas. Therefore, these antagonists are not suitable for evaluation of the physiological role of galanin in this organ. In conclusion, regulation of exocrine pancreatic function is complex, involving several bioactive peptides, and this control is not completely understood, as yet. Selective receptor antagonists and monoclonal antibodies are useful tools to identify the role of bioactive peptides in this function.

Keywords: pancreas, regulation, antagonist, immunoneutralization, CCK, bombesin, somatostatin, galanin

INTRODUCTION

It is now well established that cholecystokinin (CCK) exerts a major role in the physiological regulation of pancreatic enzyme secretion, but the role of other putative peptide regulators, such as gastrin, bombesin-like peptides, somatostatin and galanin, is less clear [1]. A specific approach to evaluate the importance of bioactive peptides in the physiological regulation of pancreatic exocrine function is that specific blockade of the binding of the peptide to its receptor should lessen or abolish the biological function to endogenous stimulants thought to act through the release of the given peptide. Immunoneutralization (i.e. administration of specific, high-affinity antibodies) is one approach to this [2], but the use of a specific and competitive receptor blocker is generally better. Unfortunately, clear definition of the role of bioactive peptides in the physiology of pancreatic enzyme secretion has long been hampered by the lack of

This paper was presented at the Section of IUPHAR GI Pharmacology Symposium on 'Biochemical pharmacology as an approach to gastrointestinal disorders (basic science to clinical perspectives)', October 12–14, 1995, Pécs, Hungary.

specific and potent receptor antagonists. The availability of such compounds [3–5] has stimulated a broad array of investigations into the physiological actions of bioactive substances and examination of their putative role in certain diseases. In a series of our experiments, selective receptor blockade by CCK/gastrin, bombesin, and galanin receptor antagonists, as well as immunoneutralization of circulating CCK and somatostatin were achieved while pancreatic enzyme secretion was evaluated in different in-vivo and in-vitro test systems.

CHARACTERIZATION OF PEPTIDE RECEPTOR ANTAGONISTS

Application of selective peptide antagonists in physiological experiments can be performed only after careful characterization of the antagonists both in vivo and in vitro. As an example, the following investigation with two CCK antagonists is described. The effect of two recently developed pentanoic acid derivatives, namely dexloxiglumide (Dex) [6,7] and spiroglumide (Spiro) [7,8] (both gifts of Dr L. Rovati, Rotta Research Laboratorium, Monza, Italy), on pancreatic enzyme secretion, gastric emptying and secretion, as well as their selectivity towards CCK-A and CCK-B receptors in vivo, was studied in the rat.

Pancreatic enzyme secretion was studied in urethane-anaesthetized rats supplied with a jugular vein catheter and pancreatic cannula. Gastric emptying and acid secretion were measured in conscious rats surgically prepared with jugular vein and gastric cannulas. Emptying of 1% methylcellulose was evaluated using phenol red as a non-absorbable colour marker. Gastric acid was collected in 30-min periods, and acidity of samples was determined by titration.

The putative CCK-A receptor antagonist, Dex, administered by the intravenous route, was able to inhibit CCK-8-induced pancreatic enzyme secretion and delay of gastric emptying in a dose-dependent fashion, with ID_{50}s of 0.64 and 1.14 mg/kg iv bolus, respectively. Similarly, the putative CCK-B/gastrin antagonist, Spiro, proved to be capable of inhibiting dose-dependently pentagastrin-induced (16 $\mu g\,kg^{-1}\,h^{-1}$) acid hypersecretion, its ID_{50} being 20.1 mg/kg. On the other hand, Dex, at doses able to almost completely block CCK-A-mediated effects (i.e. delay of gastric emptying), was ineffective against pentagastrin-induced acid hypersecretion. Similarly, Spiro, at doses which inhibit by 55% CCK-B/gastrin-mediated effects (i.e. acid secretion), was inactive when tested against CCK-8-induced delay of gastric empyting. Table 1 summarizes the effect of the antagonists during agonist administration.

These results demonstrate that dexloxiglumide is a selective antagonist for CCK-A receptors whereas spiroglumide is selective for CCK-B/gastrin receptors. The observations are in line with findings of other authors [6,8]. These compounds are therefore useful tools for discriminating between different subclasses of CCK receptors in vivo.

In the following investigation, the effect of Dex on gastric and pancreatic adaptation in response to both exogenous and endogenous CCK was studied in rats. Caerulein (1 µg/kg sc, three times daily) was used as a CCK agonist whereas camostate (200 mg/kg ig, once daily), a potent trypsin inhibitor, was employed as an endogenous CCK releaser. These compounds were administered to rats alone or in combination with Dex

TABLE 1
Effect of dexloxiglumide (Dex, 7.5 mg/kg iv) and spiroglumide (Spiro, 25 mg/kg iv) on CCK-stimulated pancreatic amylase secretion, CCK-evoked delay of gastric emptying and pentagastrin-stimulated gastric acid secretion

Treatment	Amylase output (U/30 min)	Gastric emptying (% delay)	Acid output (μEq/30 min)
Saline	1241 ± 251	46.9 ± 4.0	222 ± 31
Dex	219 ± 33*	5.2 ± 1.5*	198 ± 25
Spiro	1589 ± 354	41.2 ± 5.3	111 ± 10*

*$p < 0.01$ vs saline

TABLE 2
Effect of dexloxiglumide (Dex, 25 mg/kg sc) on caerulein- (1 μg/kg sc) and camostate- (200 mg/kg ig) induced pancreatic growth in rats

Treatment	Pancreas weight	Pancreas DNA	Pancreas protein
Caerulein	125 ± 5†*	124 ± 6*	151 ± 9*
Caerulein + Dex	101 ± 6	108 ± 7	108 ± 5
Camostate	159 ± 6*	126 ± 8*	173 ± 7*
Camostate + Dex	112 ± 6	100 ± 9	128 ± 6*

†% of control; *$p < 0.01$ vs control

(25 mg/kg sc, 20 min before each stimulation) for one week. Rats were then sacrificed, and the gastric corpus and antrum, as well as the pancreas, were excised, weighed and analysed for tissue DNA and protein contents. Neither exogenous nor endogenous CCK affected growth of the corpus and the antrum of the stomach but both caerulein and camostate treatment resulted in pancreatic hypertrophy and hyperplasia (Table 2). Dex suppressed both caerulein- and camostate-induced increases in pancreatic weight, DNA and protein contents (Table 2).

Our results demonstrate the ability of Dex to antagonize the growth-promoting effects of both exogenous and endogenous CCK on the pancreas, and confirm early observations [9] that CCK induces pancreatic growth through activation of CCK-A receptors. In conclusion, results from our laboratories demonstrate that dexloxiglumide is a selective and competitive CCK receptor antagonist. With this compound, direct evidence was provided for the presence of specific CCK receptors (of the A subtype) in rat exocrine pancreas and of their involvement in both secretory and trophic actions of the hormonal peptide. Dexloxiglumide, therefore, can be considered a useful tool for characterizing CCK-receptor interactions in peripheral organs.

USE OF CCK IMMUNONEUTRALIZATION AND SELECTIVE CCK-A RECEPTOR ANTAGONIST TO DIFFERENTIATE BETWEEN ENDOCRINE AND NON-ENDOCRINE ACTIONS

In the next set of experiments we used well-characterized antagonists and antibodies in physiological studies. Previous work had revealed that CCK-A blockade inhibits the pancreatic secretory response to food intake [10] and induces an increased intake of food [11].

A CCK monoclonal antibody (CCK MAb) was used to immunoneutralize CCK to test the hypothesis that endogenous CCK stimulates pancreatic enzyme secretion and produces satiety by an endocrine mechanism [12]. We first characterized the effect of CCK MAb on pancreatic secretion. Conscious rats with jugular vein and bile-pancreatic duct cannulas received CCK MAb or control antibody intravenously 30 min before a 2-h maximal dose of CCK-8 (200 pmol kg^{-1} h^{-1}) or access to food. CCK MAb caused a dose-dependent inhibition of amylase secretion. CCK MAb (2 mg/kg) completely blocked the response to CCK-8 and inhibited the response to food by 89% (Table 3). In feeding experiments, rats with free access to food received CCK MAb or control antibodies (2 mg/kg iv) 2 h after lights off. CCK MAb had no effect on 1.5-h or 3.5-h food intake. Another group of rats received CCK MAb (4 mg/kg iv) or a combined injection of type A and B CCK receptor antagonists devazepide and L-365,260 (1 mg/kg each iv). CCK MAb had no effect on feeding whereas the receptor antagonists stimulated 1-, 2-, 3- and 4-h intake by 62, 45, 43 and 29%.

These results suggest that endogenous CCK stimulates pancreatic enzyme secretion at least partially by an endocrine mechanism. These data confirm that elimination of the actions of CCK inhibits pancreatic secretory response to food intake [10]. In addition, we confirmed that blockade of CCK receptors induces an increased intake of food [11] and provided evidence that CCK produces satiety by a non-endocrine mechanism.

TABLE 3
Effect of CCK monoclonal antibody (MAb) and control antibody (2 mg.kg iv each) on cumulative amylase secretory (kU/120 min, basal secretion sustracted) response to CCK-8 (200 pmol kg^{-1} h^{-1}) and liquid diet (Sustacal HC)

Stimulation	Control antibody (2 mg/kg)	CCK MAb (2 mg/kg)
CCK-8	15.6 ± 2.1	0.5 ± 2.1*
Liquid food	6.4 ± 1.5	0.9 ± 1.0*

*$p < 0.01$ vs control

ROLE OF BOMBESIN RECEPTORS IN REGULATING PANCREATIC FUNCTION

Recent synthesis of specific potent bombesin receptor antagonists allows examination of the role of bombesin-like peptides in physiological processes in vivo [4]. We characterized the effects of D-Phe^6-bombesin(6-13)-methyl-ester (BME) on pancreatic enzyme secretion stimulated by the C-terminal decapeptide of gastrin-releasing peptide (GRP-10), food intake and diversion of bile-pancreatic juice in rats [13].

In isolated pancreatic acini, BME had no agonistic effects on amylase secretion but competitively inhibited responses to GRP-10, yielding a pA_2 value of 8.89 ± 0.19 (Figure 1a). In conscious rats with gastric, jugular vein, bile-pancreatic and duodenal

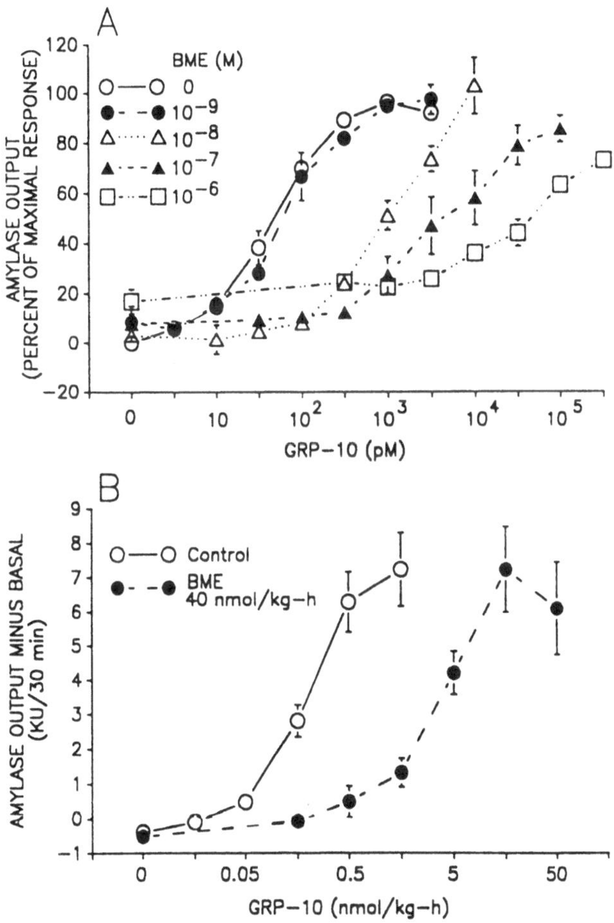

Figure 1. Effect of bombesin antagonist BME on gastrin-releasing peptide-10 (GRP-10)-stimulated amylase secretion from isolated rat pancreatic acini (A) and in conscious rats (B). Values are mean ± SEM

cannulas, basal enzyme secretion (bile-pancreatic juice recirculated) was not affected by the antagonist. Maximal amylase response to GRP-10 (0.5 nmol $kg^{-1} h^{-1}$) was inhibited dose-dependently by BME, reaching 97% inhibition at a dose of 400 nmol $kg^{-1} h^{-1}$. The dose–response curve of amylase secretion stimulated by GRP-10 was shifted to the right by 40 nmol $kg^{-1} h^{-1}$ BME but maximal amylase response was unaltered, suggesting competitive inhibition in vivo (Figure 1b). Liquid food intake and bile-pancreatic juice diversion caused substantial increases in amylase secretion; neither response was altered during administration of 400 pmol $kg^{-1} h^{-1}$ BME. Cumulative amylase responses to food intake (minus basal secretion) during vehicle and BME infusion were 9.98 ± 1.88 and 10.21 ± 2.22 kU/120 min, respectively.

Our results demonstrated that BME is a potent competitive antagonist of pancreatic responses to bombesin-like peptides in vitro and in vivo. This observation was confirmed subsequently by others [14]. Lack of effect of BME on basal pancreatic secretion or responses to liquid food intake or diversion of bile-pancreatic juice in rats suggested that endogenous bombesin-like peptides do not act either directly or indirectly to mediate these responses. Characterization of BME was still very useful since we were able to use this compound to investigate the role of bombesin-like peptides in other functions of the gut [15–17].

IMMUNONEUTRALIZATION OF CIRCULATING SOMATOSTATIN

It has been reported that exogenous somatostatin inhibits CCK-stimulated pancreatic enzyme secretion in rats [18–20]. The involvement of somatostatin in urethane-anaesthesia-evoked suppression of gastric acid secretion has also been previously described [2]. In our study [21], we have examined the role of endogenous somatostatin in diminished pancreatic enzyme secretion during anaesthesia, while monitoring acid secretion concurrently.

Rats were anaesthetized with urethane or sodium pentobarbital. An indwelling catheter (PE50) was placed into the right jugular vein. After laparotomy, the oesophagus and the pylorus were ligated, and two polyethylene cannulas (PE240) were inserted through an incision in the forestomach. The stomach was continuously perfused with saline (1 ml/min), the effluent was collected in 10-min fractions, and acid output was determined. The common bile duct was ligated at the hepatic hilum, and a cannula (PE50) was introduced into the duodenal end of the duct for collecting pure pancreatic juice. Pancreatic juice was collected in 30-min fractions and amylase activity was determined. After monitoring basal pancreatic and gastric secretions for 60 min, purified somatostatin monoclonal antibody (CURE.S6) was injected iv in increasing doses (0.05, 0.15, 0.5 and 1.5 mg) every 30 min ($n = 6$). Gastric acid and pancreatic amylase secretions were measured. A control group received control antibody (keyhole limpet haemacyanin, KLH) instead of CURE.S6 ($n = 5$).

Somatostatin antibody induced a dose-dependent increase in acid output during urethane anaesthesia. Basal acid secretion averaged 12.3 ± 1.8 μEq/30 min, while acid secretion reached 30.5 ± 6.4 μEq/30 min after 1.5 mg CURE.S6 ($p < 0.01$; Figure 2a). Control antibody did not change acid output. Basal pancreatic amylase secretion

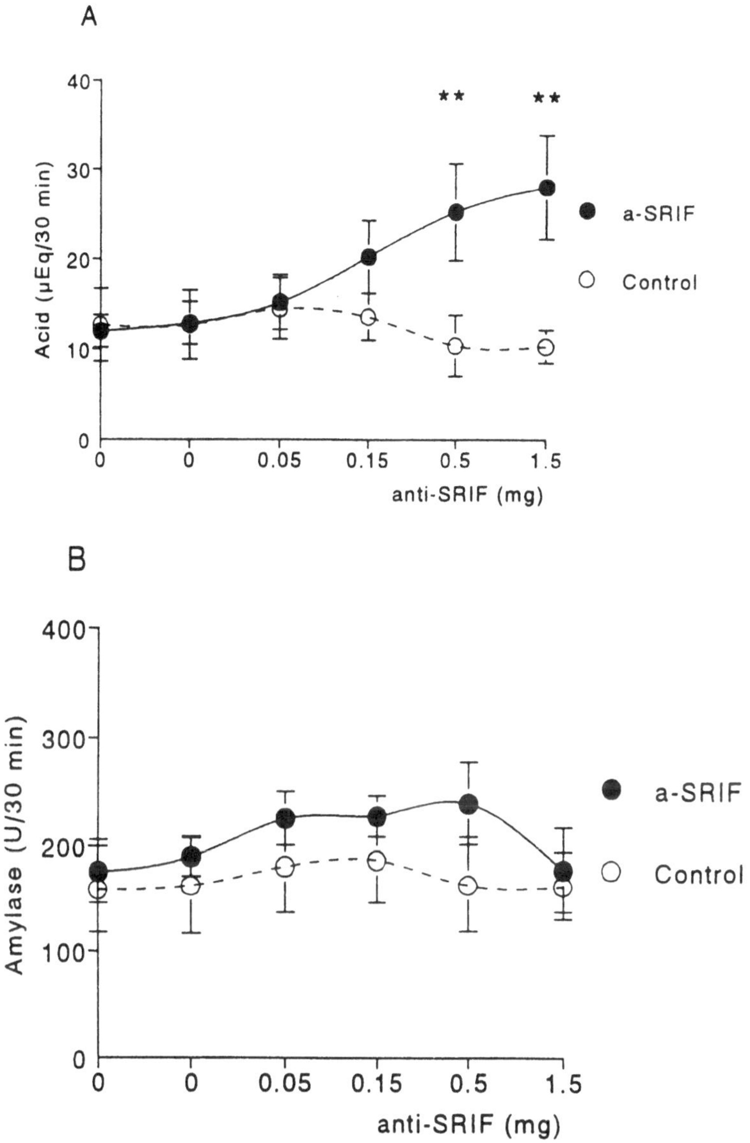

Figure 2. Dose-dependent effect of somatostatin antibody (a-SRIF) on basal gastric acid secretion (A) and basal pancreatic amylase secretion (B) in urethane-anaesthetized rats. Values are mean ± SEM; $^{**}p<0.01$ vs control

(190 ± 18 U/30 min) was not affected by either CURE.S6 (179 ± 18 U/30 min after injection of the highest dose, $p>0.05$) or by KLH (Figure 2b). When sodium pentobarbital anaesthesia was used instead of urethane, similar modulations were observed during neutralization of circulating somatostatin: basal acid secretion

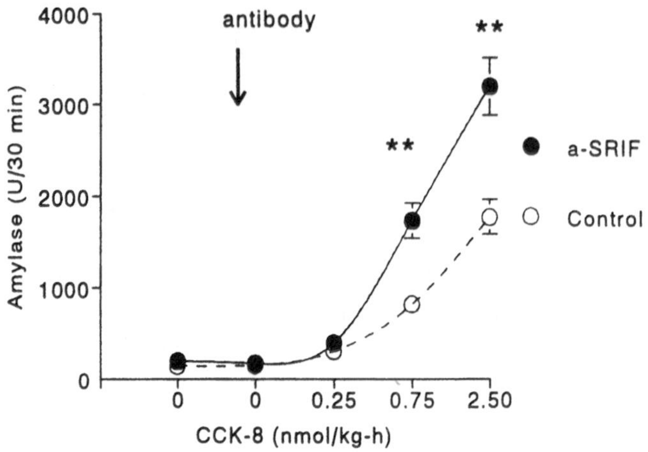

Figure 3. Effect of somatostatin antibody (a-SRIF) on CCK-stimulated pancreatic amylase secretion in urethane-anaesthetized rats. Values are mean ± SEM; $^{**}p < 0.01$ vs control

increased; pancreatic amylase secretion did not change. Pancreatic secretory response to CCK, however, was found to be elevated following elimination of somatostatin from the circulation by immunoneutralization (Figure 3).

The results indicate that endogenous somatostatin mediates, at least in part, suppression of basal gastric acid secretion, as described previously [2], but not that of pancreatic amylase secretion in anaesthetized rats. Our findings also suggest that this phenomenon does not depend on the type of anaesthesia. Finally, the data provide evidence that during stimulation by CCK in vivo, not only exogenous [18–20] but also endogenous somatostatin plays an inhibitory role in controlling enzyme secretion.

PUTATIVE GALANIN RECEPTOR ANTAGONISTS DO NOT ANTAGONIZE THE EFFECTS OF GALANIN ON THE PANCREAS

Galanin, a recently described neuropeptide, has a wide range of biological actions [5]. Extensive work led to the discovery of selective galanin receptor antagonists, such as M15 (galanin$_{1-12}$-Pro-substance-P$_{5-11}$), M35 (galanin$_{1-12}$-Pro-bradykinin$_{2-9}$-amide) and C7 (galanin$_{1-12}$-Pro-spantide-amide). These antagonists have blocked the actions of galanin on flexor-reflex, glucose-induced insulin secretion and acetylcholine release from the hippocampus [5]. Galanin is also known for its actions in the gut, such as inhibition of pancreatic enzyme secretion [22] and modulation of intestinal smooth muscle activity [23]. Our experiment [24,25] was designed to investigate whether M15, M35 and C7 can affect galanin-induced inhibition of pancreatic enzyme secretion and stimulation of jejunal smooth-muscle contractions in rats.

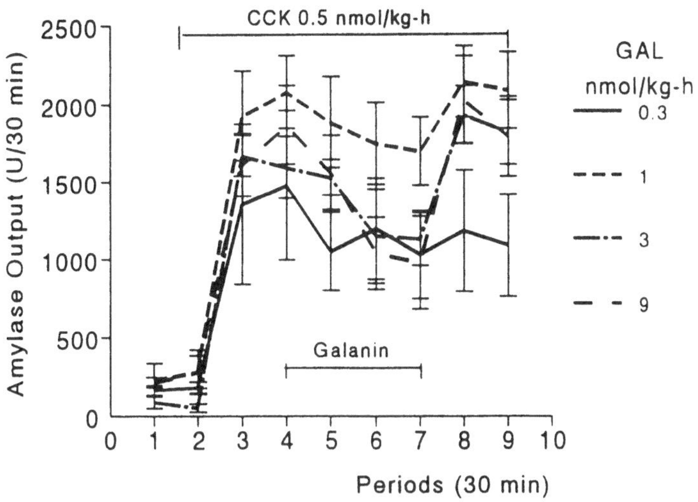

Figure 4. Effect of galanin (GAL) on 0.5 nmol $kg^{-1} h^{-1}$ CCK-stimulated pancreatic amylase secretion in urethane anaesthetized rats. Values are mean $\pm$ SEM

Pancreatic enzyme secretion was studied in urethane-anaesthetized rats supplied with a jugular-vein catheter and pancreatic cannula. Jejunal muscle strips were isolated from rats and set up in organ baths filled with modified Krebs solution. Isometric contractions were recorded. Amylase secretion evoked by submaximal CCK-8 stimulation (0.5 nmol $kg^{-1} h^{-1}$) was inhibited dose-dependently by galanin ($ID_{50} = 1.5 \pm 0.4$ nmol $kg^{-1} h^{-1}$) in anaesthetized rats (Figure 4). Galanin stimulated the contractions of isolated rat jejunal strips ($EC_{50} = 45 \pm 7$ nmol/L) (Figure 5a). Surprisingly, neither M15, M35 nor C7 (up to 9 nmol $kg^{-1} h^{-1}$ in vivo, and up to 100 nmol/L in vitro) were able to modify responses of the exocrine pancreas and the isolated jejunal smooth muscle to galanin (Figure 5a). However, both putative galanin receptor antagonists have shown some degree of agonistic effects in our experimental models (Figure 5b).

The data presented here confirm earlier studies that galanin inhibits pancreatic enzyme secretion [22] and stimulates jejunal smooth muscle activity [23] in the rat. Our results with the putative antagonists suggest that the effects of galanin on pancreatic enzyme secretion and jejunal contractions are not mediated by M15-, M35- or C7-sensitive galanin receptors. This observation is original regarding the pancreas and confirms the findings of Gu and co-workers [23] on the jejunum. Therefore, the galanin receptors located on the pancreas seem to belong to the same subclass as jejunal receptors for the peptide. Since heterogeneity of galanin receptors has already been suggested in the central nervous system [26], it is probable that there are at least three distinct galanin receptor subclasses. The antagonists that we used in our experiments are not suitable for blockade of pancreatic galanin receptors.

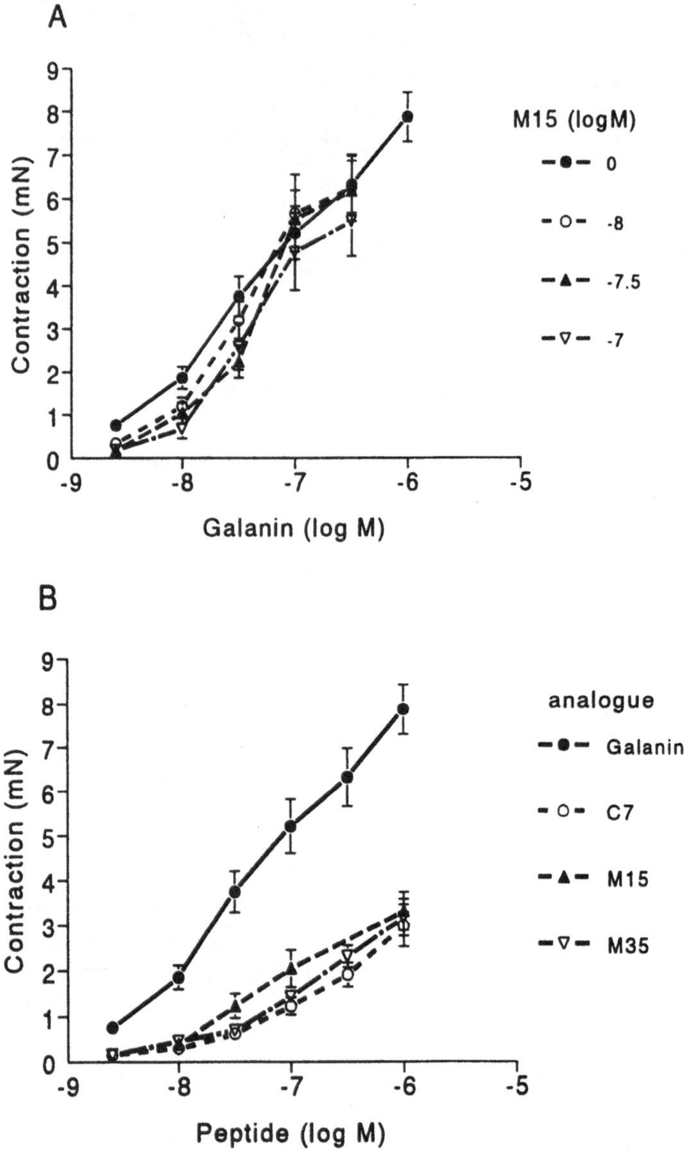

Figure 5. Dose-dependent effects of galanin analogue M15 on galanin-induced contractions (A), and of analogues M15, M35 and C7 on basal tone (B) of isolated rat longitudinal jejunal muscle. Values are mean ± SEM

CONCLUSIONS

In conclusion, regulation of the exocrine function of the pancreas is complex, involving several bioactive peptides, and this control is not completely understood, as yet. Selective peptide receptor antagonists and monoclonal antibodies raised against peptides are useful tools to identify the role of bioactive peptides in this function. The studies described in this paper could help to improve understanding of the mechanisms that control the exocrine pancreas.

ACKNOWLEDGEMENTS

This work was supported by grants ETT T-02 149/93, OTKA T-5429 and OTKA T-017104.

REFERENCES

1. Walsh JH, Dockray GJ. Gut Peptides. New York: Raven Press; 1994.
2. Yang H, Wong H, Wu V, Walsh JH, Tache Y. Somatostatin monoclonal antibody immunoneutralization increases gastrin and gastric acid secretion in urethane-anesthetized rats. Gastroenterology. 1990;99:659–65.
3. Scarpignato C, Varga C, Corradi C. Effect of CCK and its antagonists on gastric emptying. J Physiol. 1993;87:335–44.
4. Jensen RT, Coy DH. Progress in the development of potent bombesin receptor antagonists. Trends Pharmacol Sci. 1991;12:13–18.
5. Bartfai T, Fisone G, Langel U. Galanin and galanin antagonists: molecular and biochemical perspectives. Trend Pharmacol Sci. 1992;13:312–17.
6. D'Amato M, Makovec F, Mennuni L, Rovati LC. In vitro and in vivo evaluation of the anti-cholecystokinin activities of the D- and L-enantiomers of the potent and selective CCK-A antagonist loxiglumide. Br J Pharmacol. 1996.
7. Varga G, Kisfalvi K, Scarpignato C. CR-2194 and CR-2017: new tools to differentiate between CCK-A and CCK-B/gastrin receptors in vivo. Gut. 1993;34(S3):S21.
8. Revel L, Ferrari F, Makovec F, Rovati LC, Impicciatore M. Characterization of antigastrin activity in vivo of CR2194, a new R-4-benzamido-5-oxo-pentanoic acid derivative. Eur J Pharmacol. 1992;216:217–24.
9. Scarpignato C, Varga G, Dobronyi I, Papp M. Effect of a new potent CCK antagonist, lorglumide, on caerulein- and bombesin-induced pancreatic secretion and growth in the rat. Br J Pharmacol. 1989;96:661–9.
10. O'Rourke MF, Reidelberger RD, Solomon TE. Effect of CCK antagonist L364718 on meal-induced pancreatic secretion in rats. Am J Physiol. 1990;258:G179–84.
11. Reidelberger RD, O'Rourke MF. Potent cholecystokinin antagonist L 364718 stimulates food intake in rats. Am J Physiol. 1989;257:R1512–6.
12. Reidelberger RD, Varga G, Liehr R-M et al. Cholecystokinin suppresses food intake by a non-endocrine mechanism in rats. Am J Physiol. 1994;267:R901–8.
13. Varga G, Reidelberger RD, Liehr R-M, Bussjaeger LJ, Coy DH, Solomon TE. Effect of potent bombesin antagonist on exocrine pancreatic secretion in rats. Peptides. 1991;12:493–7.
14. Coy DH, Mungan Z, Rossowski WJ et al. Development of a potent bombesin receptor antagonist with prolonged in vivo inhibitory activity on bombesin-stimulated amylase and protein release in rat. Peptides. 1992;13:775–81.
15. Kortezova N, Mizhorkova Z, Milusheva E, Coy DH, Vizi ES, Varga G. GRP-preferring bombesin receptor subtype mediates contractile activity in cat terminal ileum. Peptides. 1994;15:1331–3.

16. Varga G, Adrian TE, Coy DH, Reidelberger RD. Bombesin receptor subtype mediation of gastro-enteropancreatic hormone secretion in rats. Peptides. 1994;15:713–18.
17. Varga G, Liehr R-M, Scarpignato C, Coy DH. Distinct receptors mediate gastrin-releasing peptide and neuromedin B induced delay of gastric empyting of liquids in rats. Eur J Pharmacol. 1995;286:109–12.
18. Chariot J, Roze C, Vaille C, Debray C. Effects of somatostatin on basal and stimulated pancreatic secretion of the pancreas of the rat. Gastroenterology. 1978;75:832–7.
19. Singh M. Effect of somatostatin on amylase secretion from in vivo and in vitro rat pancreas. Dig Dis Sci. 1983;28:456–68.
20. Shiratori K, Watanabe S, Takeuchi T. Somatostatin analog, SMS 201-995, inhibits pancreatic exocrine secretion and release of secretin and cholecystokinin in rats. Pancreas. 1991;6:23–30.
21. Varga G, Wong H, Walsh JH, Campbell DR, Solomon TE. Gastric acid but not pancreatic enzyme secretion is stimulated by immunoneutralization of somatostatin in anesthetized rats. Dig Dis Sci. 1994;39:1805.
22. Yagci RV, Alpetkin N, Zacharia S, Coy DH, Ertan A, Rossowski WJ. Galanin inhibits pancreatic amylase secretion in the pentobarbital-anesthetized rat. Regul Peptides. 1991;34:275–82.
23. Gu Z-F, Rossowski WJ, Coy DH, Pradhan TK, Jensen RT. Chimeric galanin analogs that function as antagonists in the CNS are full agonists in gastrointestinal smooth muscle. J Pharmacol Exp Ther. 1993;266:912–18.
24. Kisfalvi I Jr, Bartfai T, Langel Ü, Vizi ES, Varga G. Actions of galanin and its antagonists M15, M35 and C7 on exocrine pancreatic and jejunal muscle contractions. Gut. 1995;37(Suppl.2):A220.
25. Burghardt B, Bartfai T, Langel U, Varga G. Secretory and motor effects of galanin and its putative antagonists M15, M35 and C7 on the stomach in rats. Gut. 1995;37(Suppl.2):A220.
26. Örgen SO, Pramanik A, Land T, Langel Ü. Differential effects of the putative galanin receptor antagonists M15 and M35 on stiatal acetylcholine release. Eur J Pharmacol. 1993;242:59–64.

Manuscript received 4 Nov. 95.
Accepted for publication 9 Nov. 95.

TS Gaginella et al. (eds.), Biochemical Pharmacology as an Approach to Gastrointestinal Disorders, 95–102

MECHANISMS AND REGULATION OF Cl^- SECRETION IN THE LARGE INTESTINE: STUDIES WITH THE RAT DISTAL COLON

M. DIENER
Institut für Veterinär-Physiologie, Universität Giessen, Frankfurter Strasse 100, D-35392 Giessen, Germany

ABSTRACT

Chloride secretion is under the intracellular control of at least three intracellular second messenger pathways, the cAMP-, the Ca^{2+}- and the cGMP-system. An increase in the intracellular cAMP concentration causes the opening of apical Cl^- channels and a stimulation of the basolateral Na^+-K^+-Cl^--cotransporter responsible for intracellular Cl^- accumulation. In contrast, the effect of intracellular Ca^{2+} is, at least in isolated crypts from the rat distal colon, restricted to the opening of a basolateral Ca^{2+}-dependent K^+ conductance, which leads to a hyperpolarization of the membrane and thereby increases the driving force for Cl^- exit across spontaneously open apical Cl^- channels. In the rat distal colon, there is evidence for a modulation of cAMP-mediated secretion by intracellular cGMP, which affects Cl^- secretion indirectly via a cGMP-sensitive phosphodiesterase, an enzyme which is responsible for cAMP degradation. These studies suggest a complex interaction of all three signalling pathways in the intracellular regulation of Cl^- secretion.

Keywords: chloride secretion, colon, calcium, cAMP, cGMP, Cl^- channels, K^+ channels

The epithelium of the colon is able to absorb and secrete water and electrolytes. One of the quantitatively most important anions actively secreted is Cl^-. Chloride secretion is activated under physiological conditions, e.g. after distension of the gut wall, and plays a prominent role under pathophysiological conditions, i.e. during secretory diarrhoea. Chloride secretion is performed by the colonic epithelial cells, i.e. by polarized cells with a more or less smooth basolateral membrane and an apical membrane enlarged by microvilli facing the colonic lumen. Both membranes are equipped with different transporters, ion channels and pumps in order to secrete Cl^- (Figure 1). The main active, energy-consuming enzyme among these transporters is the basolateral Na^+-K^+-ATPase, which pumps Na^+ out of the cell in exchange for K^+, thereby keeping the intracellular Na^+ concentration low. Potassium ions pumped into the cell recycle by basolateral quinine- and barium-sensitive K^+ channels. These channels are mainly responsible for the height of the membrane potential, which is predominated by a K^+ diffusion potential. The Cl^- ions to be secreted enter the epithelium via a basolateral bumetanide-sensitive Na^+-K^+-Cl^--cotransporter. This cotransporter, which is energized by the Na^+ gradient established by the Na^+K^+-ATPase, accumulates Cl^- in the cell above electrochemical equilibrium. The Cl^- ions leave the cell by Cl^- channels in

---

This paper was presented at the Section of IUPHAR GI Pharmacology Symposium on 'Biochemical pharmacology as an approach to gastrointestinal disorders (basic science to clinical perspectives)', October 12–14, 1995, Pécs, Hungary.

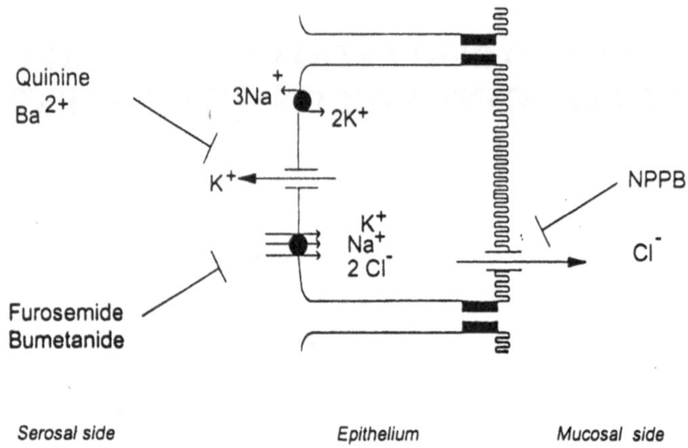

Figure 1. Ion transporters involved in colonic Cl^- secretion

the apical membrane. These channels can be inhibited by NPPB (5-nitro-2-[3-phenylpropylamino]benzoate) [1], a typical Cl^- channel blocker [2]. The final driving force for the exit of Cl^- is the membrane potential because the intracellular Cl^- concentration is lower than the extracellular concentration.

The colon is the final station of the gastrointestinal tract, where the organism has the last chance to alter the electrolyte contents of the faeces and thereby to regulate water and salt balance. Therefore, electrolyte transport across the colonic mucosa is under close control of the enteric nervous system, hormones and paracrine substances. The topic of this review is the extra- and intracellular regulation of ion secretion in the colon. The experimental data presented were obtained at the rat distal colon using electrophysiological and pharmacological approaches.

Secretagogues can be classified mainly into four categories (Table 1). The first group is those stimulating enteric secretomotor neurons and thereby inducing secretion indirectly. Typical examples are ion secretion induced by electric field stimulation or that induced by prostaglandin I_2, which can be suppressed by the neurotoxin, tetrodotoxin [3,4]. The secretion induced by prostaglandin I_2 or electric field stimulation can be partially inhibited by atropine, suggesting the mediation by acetylcholine. The main non-cholinergic secretory transmitter may be vasoactive intestinal polypeptide as revealed by studies with an antibody against this peptide (Diener and Rummel, unpublished observation). The second group of secretagogues are those acting via an increase in the intracellular cAMP concentration, like forskolin, vasoactive intestinal polypeptide or prostaglandin E_2. The third group of secretagogues, e.g. acetylcholine, its stable analogue, carbachol, serotonin and substance P, acts via intracellular Ca^{2+}. The effect of the last group is mediated by cGMP. Typical examples are guanylin or the heat-stable enterotoxin (STa) of *Escherichia coli.*

TABLE 1
Classification of secretagogues in the colon

Secretion induced by neuronal stimulation	
	Electric field stimulation
	Prostaglandin I_2
Secretion mediated by cAMP	
	Forskolin, vasoactive intestinal polypeptide
	Prostaglandin E_2
Secretion mediated by Ca^{2+}	
	Acetylcholine, carbachol
	Serotonin
	Substance P
Secretion mediated by cGMP	
	Heat-stable toxin (STa) of *Escherichia coli*
	Guanylin

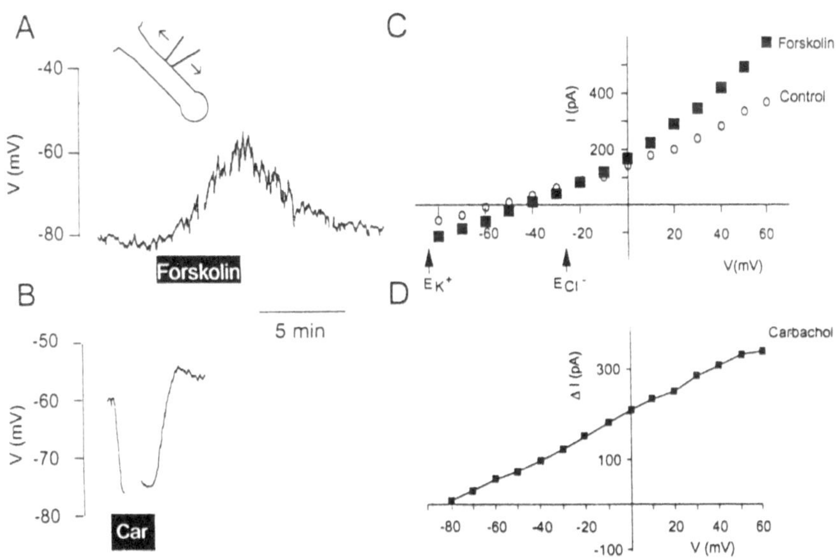

Figure 2. Effect of forskolin (5×10^{-6} mol/L; **A**) or carbachol (Car; 5×10^{-5} mol/L; **B**) on the membrane potential of cells in isolated crypts studied with the whole-cell patch-clamp technique as indicated by the symbol. **C**) Current–voltage relationship of a crypt cell in the absence (control) and presence of forskolin. For comparison, the equilibrium potentials for K^+ (E_{K^+}) and Cl^- (E_{Cl^-}) are given. **D**) Current–voltage relationship of the current induced by carbachol (Δ I)

An adequate method to study the effect of secretagogues at the native colonic epithelium is to measure membrane currents and membrane voltage at isolated colonic crypts with the patch-clamp technique [5,6]. Basal potentials in the crypt cells can vary between –40 and –70 mV. Basal membrane potential is more negative towards the fundus of the crypts, i.e. the position where the undifferentiated cells are located [5]. Administration of forskolin, the agonist of the cAMP-pathway, induces a membrane depolarization (Figure 2A). This effect is completely reversible after wash-out and can be demonstrated repeatedly on the same cells without loss of sensitivity. The effect of forskolin is mimicked by vasoactive intestinal polypeptide [7], one of the most important natural secretagogues acting on the cAMP pathway. Measurements of current–voltage relationships revealed an increase in membrane current in the presence of forskolin (Figure 2B), suggesting that forskolin opens a Cl^- conductance which would shift the membrane potential closer to the Cl^- equilibrium potential of about –25 mV under these experimental conditions. Indeed, the current stimulated by forskolin has a reversal potential identical to the Cl^- reversal potential and forskolin has no more effect if the experiment is performed in the absence of Cl^-. Interestingly, the effect of forskolin shows some dependence on the localization of the patched cell along the longitudinal axis of the crypt. A Cl^- current cannot be stimulated at the very bottom of the crypt, that is near the localization of the stem cells [5]. The response is most pronounced in the middle of the crypt but it can still be induced at cells very close to the opening of the crypt. In other words, the differentiated cells at the surface of the epithelium also conserve the ability to secrete Cl^- ions. Indeed, we have found single Cl^- channels at the apical membrane of the surface epithelium of the intact mucosa [6] and also recent experiments by Fromm and co-workers [8] with a vibrating microelectrode confirm that the surface epithelium is able to secrete. The stimulation of Cl^- current by forskolin can be suppressed by injecting an inhibitor peptide of the protein kinase A into the cell, demonstrating that the effect of cAMP is mediated by protein phosphorylation, presumably of the apical Cl^- channels [5].

The nature of the single channels carrying this cAMP-stimulated whole-cell current is still a matter of debate. Most recent evidence suggests that the final target of cAMP-stimulated Cl^- secretion is the CFTR channel, the cystic fibrosis transmembrane regulator, which acts as a 8–10 pS Cl^- channel [9]. Also, in the rat distal colon, the current stimulated by forskolin can be blocked by a typical blocker of CFTR Cl^- currents, glibenclamide [10]. However, a Cl^- channel with a somewhat higher conductance, the so-called outward rectifier, which seems to be under control of CFTR [11], may contribute to Cl^- secretion. Other evidence from the group of Greger and Kunzelmann [12] points to a subpicosiemens channel, which seems to carry most of the cAMP-stimulated Cl^- current in a colonic tumour cell line, the HT29 cells. Therefore, it is not yet clear whether a single set of Cl^- channels is regulated by cAMP-dependent phosphorylation.

Activation of apical Cl^- channels is not the only action of cAMP. In addition, an increase in the intracellular cAMP concentration leads to a stimulation of the basolateral Na^+-K^+-Cl^- cotransporter. This can be demonstrated when measuring the serosal uptake of $^{86}Rb^+$ as a marker for K^+ transport. Forskolin causes a significant increase in basolateral Rb^+ uptake in the rat distal colon (Figure 3). This effect can be completely prevented by prior administration of an inhibitor of the Na^+-K^+-Cl^-

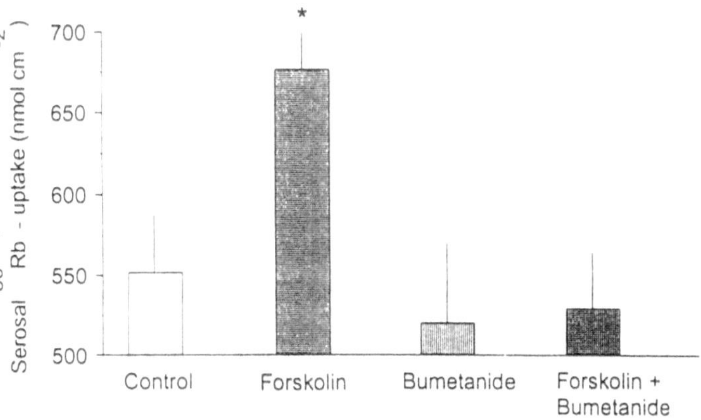

Figure 3. Serosal uptake of $^{86}Rb^+$ under control conditions (open bar), in the presence of forskolin (5×10^{-6} mol/L; horizontally dashed bar), bumetanide (10^{-4} mol/L; vertically dashed bar), and in the combined presence of bumetanide and forskolin (crossed bar). Values are means ± SEM, $n = 6$–7, $*p < 0.05$ vs. control

cotransporter, bumetanide. Thus, in addition to stimulation of apical efflux of Cl^-, cAMP also controls the rate of basolateral entry of Cl^- [13].

In contrast to forskolin, carbachol, a typical agonist of Ca^{2+}-dependent secretion, induces a strong hyperpolarization of the crypt cells (Figure 2B). This effect is not dependent on the localization of the patched cells along the crypt axis; it can be evoked in the very young cells at the bottom of the crypt. The current stimulated by carbachol has a reversal potential near –80 mV, i.e. very close to the theoretical K^+ equilibrium potential (Figure 2D). The effect of carbachol is completely blocked by a typical K^+ channel blocker like Ba^{2+} [5]. There is no direct indication for stimulation of Cl^- conductance by carbachol in the isolated colonic crypts.

Measurements at crypts loaded with the Ca^{2+}-sensitive dye, fura-2, confirmed that the effect of carbachol is mediated by intracellular Ca^{2+} [14]. Carbachol induces a biphasic increase in the intracellular Ca^{2+} concentration: an initial peak in intracellular Ca^{2+} is followed by a long-lasting plateau phase, which lasts as long as the agonist is present in the perfusion. The Ca^{2+} ions responsible for the induction of the hyperpolarization, i.e. the opening of Ca^{2+}-sensitive basolateral K^+ channels, seem to originate predominantly from the release of intracellular Ca^{2+} from cellular stores [5].

Consequently, in the native colonic epithelium, the effect of intracellular Ca^{2+} is restricted to the opening of a Ca^{2+}-dependent K^+ conductance. This will, however, increase the driving force for Cl^- secretion across apical Cl^- channels and thereby stimulate Cl^- secretion indirectly. This model was originally proposed from radioisotope efflux studies by Dharmsathaphorn and Pandol [15]. We have no indication for a direct activation of apical Cl^- channels by intracellular Ca^{2+}. This contrasts with results obtained at airway epithelium [16] and at colonic tumour cell lines like T_{84} [17] or HT29 cells [12,18], where there is no doubt about the functional significance of Ca^{2+}-dependent Cl^- channels.

When comparing these patch-clamp data obtained at the isolated crypts, which point to an indirect effect of carbachol, and the response in the intact mucosa mounted in the Ussing chamber, there is an apparent contradiction, i.e. in the intact mucosa carbachol is one of the most efficient secretagogues [19], whereas the data from the isolated crypts suggests only an indirect action. The question arises, therefore, of what the reason may be for this discrepancy. Two fundamental differences between the intact mucosa and the isolated crypt exist: (1) the presence of subepithelial connective tissue, producing eicosanoids like prostaglandins, and (2) the presence of the enteric nervous system, spontaneously releasing neurotransmitters. Prostaglandins or neurotransmitters might either mediate the activation of Cl^- secretion by carbachol or, alternatively, they might create a facilitative influence on the epithelium, which makes the epithelium sensitive for stimulation of Cl^- secretion by carbachol. Consequently, in a recent study [10], we re-evaluated the effect of carbachol in the Ussing chamber with a special look at the prostaglandin and neuronal system.

Carbachol induces a biphasic increase in short-circuit current due to Cl^- secretion as confirmed by blocker experiments and anion substitution [10]. This response is completely blocked when the tissue is pretreated with a combination of both indomethacin, a cyclo-oxygenase inhibitor, and tetrodotoxin. None of the blockers alone is able to completely suppress the carbachol response. Elevation of intracellular cAMP by a low concentration of forskolin, a membrane-permeable cAMP-derivative, or prostaglandin E_2 completely overcomes the inhibition induced by the combination of indomethacin and tetrodotoxin. Consequently, carbachol does not act by releasing prostaglandins or neurotransmitters because both processes were blocked by indomethacin or tetrodotoxin, respectively; i.e. the effect of carbachol in the intact mucosa is not *mediated* by nerves or prostaglandins. Instead, the continuous release of both stimulates basal cAMP production in the enterocytes, which brings the epithelium to a state in which it can respond to carbachol with Cl^- secretion. This interaction of the Ca^{2+} and the cAMP pathways takes place presumably at the Cl^- channel in the apical membrane, which is kept open by a sufficient cAMP concentration in the cell as suggested in the original model by Dharmsathaphorn and Pandol [15]. Only if the epithelial cells possess spontaneously open apical Cl^- channels can the hyperpolarization induced by carbachol induce Cl^- secretion due to an increase in the driving force for Cl^- exit across these channels. This conclusion is further supported by recent genetic experiments with a CFTR –/– mouse [20], which demonstrate that, in contrast to airway epithelium, the intestine does not possess Ca^{2+}-regulated Cl^- channels. It is also further supported by electrophysiological experiments on isolated crypts from the guinea-pig small intestine [21] and rabbit colon [22]. Thus, the native intestinal epithelium, in contrast to airway epithelium or colonic tumour cell lines, does not express Ca^{2+}-activated Cl^- channels, a fact, which is quite important for cystic fibrosis, a disease with a defect in cAMP-stimulated Cl^- channels.

The third intracellular pathway responsible for the regulation of ion transport is the cGMP-pathway. A typical agonist of this pathway is the heat-stable enterotoxin of *Escherichia coli* (STa). This toxin has a segment-specific anion in the rat colon; its response increases from the distal to the proximal colon [23]. In the distal colon, the effect of STa can be inhibited by indomethacin. However, as in the case of carbachol,

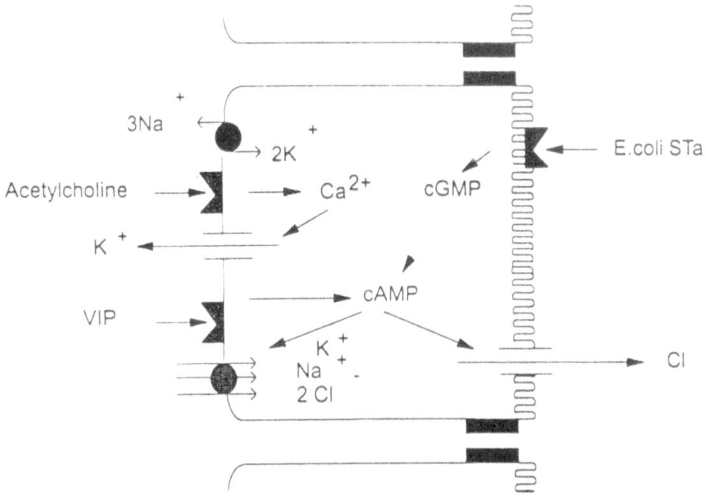

Figure 4. Model for the presumed action sites of cAMP, cGMP and Ca^{2+} during the induction of Cl^- secretion in the rat distal colon

this is an indirect effect. Inhibition by indomethacin can be overcome by prostaglandin E_2. It can also be overcome by forskolin but not by CPT-cAMP (8-[4-chlorophenylthio]-cAMP), a hydrolysis-resistant cAMP analogue. This observation led to the hypothesis that the effect of cGMP may be related to the inhibition of cAMP metabolism, mediated, for example, by a cGMP-sensitive phosphodiesterase as it has been shown for other tissues like the heart (for references see [23]). Indeed, amrinone and trequinsin, two inhibitors of cGMP-sensitive phosphodiesterases, mimic the effect of STa in the distal colon and prevent the effect of a subsequent administration of STa [23]. They have, however, no effect in the proximal colon, a segment where the response to STa is not inhibited by indomethacin and may consist of a direct activation of CFTR Cl^- channels as suggested by Goldstein et al. [24]. There is controversy in the literature about whether the effect of cGMP on the apical Cl^- channels is mediated by protein kinase G-dependent phosphorylation of the Cl^- channel [25] or whether it is mediated by protein kinase A, which discriminates only poorly between cAMP and cGMP [26].

To come to the conclusions (Figure 4), these results suggest that, in the rat colonic epithelium, the cAMP pathway plays the central role in the control of Cl^- secretion by regulating the apical Cl^- conductance and the activity of the basolateral Na^+-K^+-Cl^--cotransporter. The only effect of intracellular Ca^{2+} is the regulation of a basolateral K^+ conductance, which determines the driving force for Cl^- exit via cAMP-controlled Cl^- channels by membrane hyperpolarization. There is, in addition, a control by cGMP, regulating, at least in the rat distal colon, the hydrolysis of cAMP, and, in other intestinal segments, regulating apical Cl^- channels either by protein kinase G or by the ability of cGMP to stimulate the protein kinase A.

REFERENCES

1. Diener M, Rummel W. Actions of the Cl^- channel blocker NPPB on absorptive and secretory transport processes of Na^+ and Cl^- in rat descending colon. Acta Physiol Scand. 1989;137:215–22.
2. Wangemann P, Wittner M, DiStefano A et al. Cl^--channel blockers in the thick ascending limb of the loop of Henle. Structure activity relationship. Pflügers Arch. 1986;407(Suppl.2):S128–41.
3. Diener M, Bridges RJ, Knobloch SF, Rummel W. Neuronally mediated and direct effects of prostaglandins on ion transport in rat colon descendens. Naunyn-Schmiedeberg's Arch Pharmacol. 1988;337:74–8.
4. Diener M, Mestres P, Bridges RJ, Rummel W. Functional and morphological changes during electric field stimulation of rat colon descendens. In: Singer MV, Goebell H, eds. Nerves and the Gastro-intestinal Tract. Lancaster: MTP Press; 1989:705–12.
5. Böhme M, Diener M, Rummel W. Calcium- and cyclic-AMP-mediated secretory responses in isolated colonic crypts. Pflügers Arch. 1991;419:144–51.
6. Diener M, Rummel W, Mestres P, Lindemann B. Single chloride channels in colon mucosa and isolated colonic enterocytes of the rat. J Membrane Biol. 1989;108:21–30.
7. Diener M, Gartmann V. Effect of somatostatin on cell volume, Cl^- currents, and transepithelial Cl^- transport in rat distal colon. Am J Physiol. 1994;266:G1043–53.
8. Köckerling A, Fromm M. Origin of cAMP-dependent Cl^- secretion from both crypts and surface epithelium of rat intestine. Am J Physiol. 1993;264:C1285–301.
9. Bear CE, Li C, Kartner N et al. Purification and functional reconstitution of the cystic fibrosis transmembrane conductance regulator (CFTR). Cell. 1992;68:808–18.
10. Strabel D, Diener M. Evidence against direct activation of chloride secretion by carbachol in the rat distal colon. Eur J Pharmacol. 1995;274:181–91.
11. Egan M, Flotte T, Afione S et al. Defective regulation of outwardly rectifying Cl^- channels by protein kinase A corrected by insertion of CFTR. Nature. 1992;358:581–4.
12. Kunzelmann K, Grolik K, Kubitz R, Greger R. cAMP-dependent activation of small-conductance Cl^- channels in HT29 colon carcinoma cells. Pflügers Arch. 1992;421:230–7.
13. Diener M, Hug F, Strabel D, Scharrer E. Cyclic AMP-dependent regulation of K^+ transport in the rat distal colon. Br J Pharmacol. 1996 [in press].
14. Diener M, Eglème C, Rummel W. Phospholipase C-induced anion secretion and its interaction with carbachol in the rat colonic mucosa. Eur J Pharmacol. 1991;200:267–76.
15. Dharmsathaphorn K, Pandol S. Mechanism of chloride secretion induced by carbachol in a colonic epithelial cell line. J Clin Invest. 1986;77:348–54.
16. Frizzell RA, Halm DR, Rechkemmer G, Shoemaker RL. Choride channel regulation in secretory epithelia. Fed Proc. 1986;45:2727–31.
17. Cliff WH, Frizzell RA. Separate Cl^- conductances activated by cAMP and Ca^{2+} in Cl^--secreting cells. Proc Natl Acad Sci USA. 1990;87:4956–60.
18. Morris AP, Frizzell RA. Ca^{2+}-dependent Cl^- channels in undifferentiated human colonic cells (HT-29). I. Single-channel properties. Am J Physiol. 1993;264:C968–76.
19. Nobles M, Diener M, Mestres P, Rummel W. Segmental heterogeneity of the rat colon in the response to activators of secretion on the cAMP-, the cGMP- and the Ca^{2+}-pathway. Acta Physiol Scand. 1991;142:375–86.
20. Cuthbert AW, MacVinish LJ, Hickman ME, Ratcliff R, Colledge WH, Evans MJ. Ion-transporting activity in the murine colonic epithelium of normal animals and animals with cystic fibrosis. Pflügers Arch. 1994;428:508–13.
21. Walters RJ, Sepúlveda FV. A basolateral K^+ conductance modulated by carbachol dominates the membrane potential of small intestinal crypts. Pflügers Arch. 1991;419:537–9.
22. Lohrmann E, Greger R. The effect of secretagogues on ion conductances of in vitro perfused, isolated rabbit colonic crypts. Pflügers Arch. 1995;429:494–502.
23. Nobles M, Diener M, Rummel W. Segment-specific effects of the heat-stable enterotoxin of E. coli on electrolyte transport in the rat colon. Eur J Pharmacol. 1991;202:201–11.
24. Goldstein JL, Sahi J, Bhuva M, Layden TJ, Rao MC. Escherichia coli heat-stable enterotoxin-mediated colonic Cl^- secretion is absent in cystic fibrosis. Gastroenterology. 1994;107:950–6.
25. Lin M, Nairn AC, Guggino SE. cGMP-dependent protein kinase regulation of a chloride channel in T84 cells. Am J Physiol. 1992;262:C1304–12.
26. Forte LR, Thorne PK, Eber SL et al. Stimulation of intestinal Cl^- transport by heat-stable enterotoxin: activation of cAMP-dependent protein kinase by cGMP. Am J Physiol. 1992;263:C607–15.

Manuscript received 12 Oct. 95.
Accepted for publication 8 Jan. 96.

Section II

GASTROINTESTINAL MOTILITY

TS Gaginella et al. (eds.), Biochemical Pharmacology as an Approach to Gastrointestinal Disorders, 105–114

PROSTAGLANDIN E_2: ACTIONS ON THE CIRCULAR AND LONGITUDINAL CONTRACTIONS OF THE CANINE COLON

T. WITTMANN[1*], O. SANCHES[2], A. LAMBERT[2], G. BULIARD[2] AND J.F. GRENIER[2]
[1]First Department of Medicine, Albert Szent-Györgyi Medical University, Szeged, Hungary; [2]INSERM U.61 and Department of General and Digestive Surgery, Civil Hospital, Strasbourg, France
*Correspondence

This paper was first published in: Inflammopharmacology. 1997;5:67–76.

ABSTRACT

The effect of prostaglandin E_2 (PGE_2) on the circular and longitudinal contractions of the canine colon was studied in chronic conditions. A mechanical transducer capable of recording simultaneously the variations of length in two perpendicular directions at 90° to each other was developed and implanted on the canine colon 10 cm distal to the ileocaecal junction. The recording sessions started on the 6th postoperative day. The colonic motility was recorded two hours before (control period) and two hours after the intravenous injection of PGE_2 in three different doses (0.1, 1.0 and 10 μg/kg). Two sorts of mechanical activity were identified: contractile phases (mean duration: 8.8 min for longitudinal and 6.7 min for circular contractions) and sporadic contractions (mean duration: 0.37 min for longitudinal and 0.28 min for circular contractions).

PGE_2 in the three different doses used induces an important reduction in the duration and in the amplitude of the circular contractions. These reductions become important only in the 2nd hour after the injection of PGE_2. The duration of the longitudinal contractions was modified by 10 μg/kg of PGE_2, provoking an important and immediate increase of this value. Although the amplitude of longitudinal contractions remains constant, each dose of PGE_2 induces strong premature bursts of longitudinal colonic contractions.

It is concluded that PGE_2 has a regulating effect on colonic motility, even at small doses, with a different action on the two muscular layers. According to the dose used, it leads to hypokinesia (relaxation) in the circular and to strong contractions in the longitudinal colonic muscles.

Keywords: motility, prostaglandins, colon

INTRODUCTION

In the last decade, research on prostaglandins (PGs) has provided a large series of information concerning the physiological role of prostaglandin E on the gastrointestinal (GI) tube. The effects of PGE_1 and PGE_2 on the GI mucosa are well documented, such as the reduction in the absorption and the increased hydroelectrolytic secretion in the small bowel [1,2].

PGs are largely involved in the regulation of GI motility. PGE_2, PGI_2 and $PGF_{2\alpha}$, are synthesized by the muscular microsomes in the circular and longitudinal muscle

This paper was presented at the Section of IUPHAR GI Pharmacology Symposium on 'Biochemical pharmacology as an approach to gastrointestinal disorders (basic science to clinical perspectives)', October 12–14, 1995, Pécs, Hungary.

layers of the gut [3] and the endogenous PGs are believed to play a physiological role in the propulsive and non-propulsive movements of the intestine [4–7].

In the small bowel, PGE_2 delays the induction of the subsequent activity front and prolongs the quiescent phase [7,8]. Therefore the diarrhoeagenic effect of PGE_2 cannot be explained by its action alone on small-bowel motility. Moreover, in-vitro experiments do not supply sufficient data concerning the two muscle layers separately.

The effect of PGE_2 was studied mainly on circular muscle strips in samples removed from either the small bowel or the colon. The majority of the results suggests that PGE_2 has a relaxing effect on the circular smooth muscles in the GI tract [6,9,10]. In studies performed on animals or on humans, PGE_2 was found to inhibit colonic motility [11,12]. However, these manometric and electromyographic studies supply information on the movements of the entire gut wall, in which the activity on the circular muscle layer is preponderant [13]. In chronic conditions, the simultaneous effects of PGs on the circular and longitudinal colonic muscle contractions remain almost unknown. Similarly, the mechanisms by which diarrhoea is induced in the different GI pathologies is unclear [14,15].

The aim of our work was to study the effect of different doses of PGE_2 on canine colonic motility in chronic conditions, differentiating and recording simultaneously the longitudinal and circular contractions.

METHODS

Experimental technique

An implantable extraluminal transducer developed in our laboratory was used for measuring simultaneously the circular and the longitudinal movements of the canine colon. The principles of this transducer have been described in detail previously [16].

The detecting unit of the transducer consists of two pairs of lamellae, each pair formed by two lamellae 4 mm in length, placed face-to-face and embedded perpendicularly in a Wheatstone bridge (dimension: 10×10 mm). Strain gauges (CEA – 06 – 062 UW – 120, Micromeasurement Division, USA) were bonded to each lamella. A metal tip (0.5 mm in diameter, 2 mm in length) bonded to the free end of each of the four lamellae makes the contact between the lamellae and the intestinal wall. A constant voltage was supplied to the strain gauges by a 4.5-V DC source. The sensitivity of the transducer was 0.2 mV/0.05 mm. The variation of the voltage was directly proportional to the displacement of the free end of the lamellae. The variation in distance between each pair of lamellae is correlated with the deformation of the intestinal wall in two perpendicular directions. The transducer collects data from a small area of 6×6 mm^2, delimited by the 4 lamellae.

Surgical implantation

After a midventral laparotomy on the dog under general anaesthesia, the transducer is sewn onto the colonic serosa, 10 cm distal to the ileocaecal junction, by four stitches of nylon intestinal thread (3-O). Thus, one pair of lamellae remains on the transverse and the other on the longitudinal axis of the colon. The four tips remain fixed under the serosa, in the muscle layers. The transducer unit is taken to a cannula fixed on the abdominal wall.

Experiments

Experiments were performed on four beagle dogs, of either sex, weighing 15–16 kg each. Recording sessions were performed once a day beginning on the 6th post-operative day. The dogs were fasted for 12 h before each recording session. After connecting the cannula, placed on the abdominal wall, to a polygraphic recorder (Beckman Dynograph Recorder R 611), the mechanical activity of the colon was recorded, measuring the contractions in two perpendicular directions, with the sensitivity set to 0.5 mV/cm and with a cutoff frequency of 30 Hz. The experiments were performed over a period of 4 h, 2 h before (control period) and 2 h after the injection of PGE_2 into the brachial vein over 5 min (prostine E_2) (Dinoproston, Upjohn Laboratories). Three different doses were used (0.1, 1.0 and 10 μg/kg) and each dog underwent two recording sessions with each dose. At the beginning of each experiment, in the control period, the liquid used for the dilution of PGE_2 was injected as control substance, in the same volume as that used for PGE_2 administration.

Analysis

Longitudinal and circular mechanical activities were distinguished during the recordings. According to their duration and distribution in time, two different types of mechanical activity were distinguished: contractile phases and sporadic contractions. Contractile phases were identified, following the definition of Sarna [17], appearing in bursts of contractions at regular intervals, with a mean duration of 7 min. Sporadic contractions which were irregular and independent of the bursts of contractions were identified in the tracing.

In addition to these parameters, we identified contractions with high amplitude which seem to play an important role in segmental and propulsive colonic movements [4,14]. High-amplitude contractions were defined as those in which the amplitude was higher than the highest mean amplitude of all the contractions in each individual tracing [24].

Duration, amplitude and number of contractions were calculated. Comparison was made between data obtained from the control period and data from the period following PGE_2 administration.

The statistical analysis was performed according to the Student's paired test.

RESULTS

Duration of colonic contractions

The duration of contractile phases and of sporadic contractions was measured and calculated for a period of 1 h, and the values before and after PGE_2 administration are shown in Figure 1.

Alterations induced by PGE_2 in the circular and longitudinal muscle movements are entirely different. PGE_2, at each dose used, diminishes the duration of the circular contractions (Figure 1, top). This reduction in the contractile activity time (–38% to –

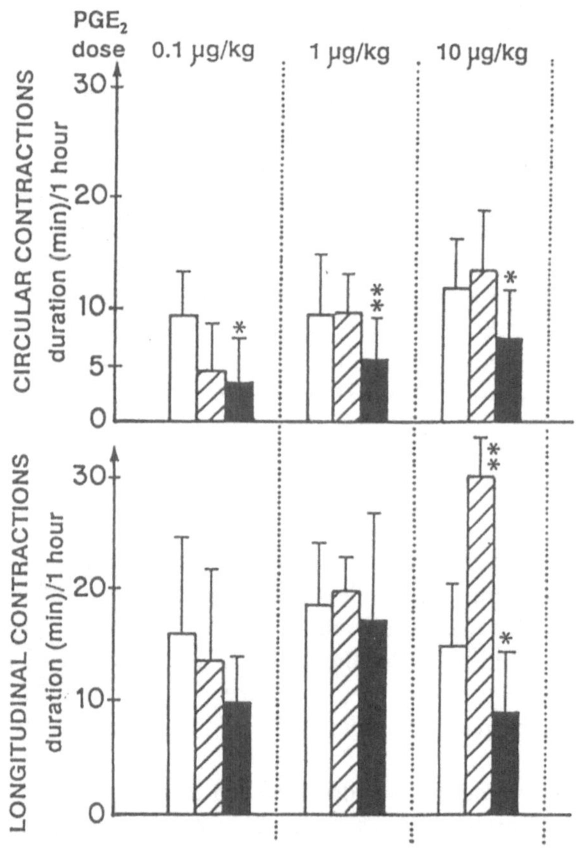

Figure 1. The duration (min) of colonic circular and longitudinal contractions. Values (mean ± SD) represent the total amount of contractile phases and sporadic contractions recorded during 1 h in the control period (open column), and in the first (hatched column) and second hour (solid column) following PGE_2 (0.1, 1.0 and 10 µg/kg) administration. *$p<0.05$; **$p<0.01$

60%) is significant over the 2nd hour following PG administration but it is absent or moderate over the 1st hour after PGE_2 injection.

In comparison, the duration of colonic longitudinal contractions remains unchanged after administration of PGE_2 at doses of 0.1 and 1.0 μg/kg (Figure 1, bottom). However, 10 μg/kg PGE_2 produces an immediate increase (+103%) in the duration of the contractions. This period is followed, in the 2nd hour, by a large reduction in the contractile activity time (–38%).

Amplitude of colonic contractions

The mean amplitude of the contractions, appearing as contractile phases or sporadic contractions, was measured and calculated for a period of 1 h and the values are represented in Figure 2.

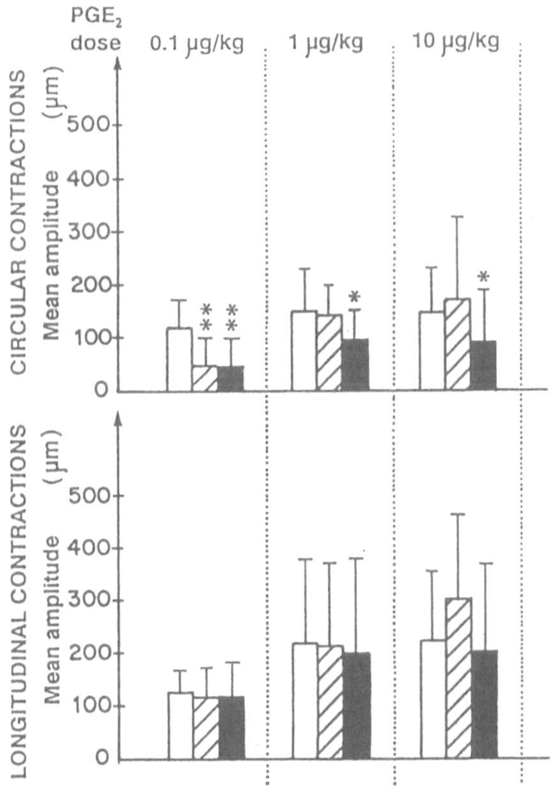

Figure 2. The mean amplitude (μm) of colonic circular and longitudinal contractions. These values (mean ± SD) represent the total amount of contractile phases and sporadic contractions recorded during 1 h in the control period (open column), and in the first (hatched column) and second hour (solid column) of experiments following PGE_2 (0.1, 1.0 and 10 μg/kg) administration. $^{*}p<0.05$; $^{**}p<0.01$

Each dose of PGE_2 administered reduces significantly (–38% to –41%) the amplitude of circular contractions (Figure 2, top). This reduction is present mainly in the 2nd hour following PGE_2 treatment. However, the lowest dose of PGE_2 (0.1 μg/kg) leads to a considerable decrease in the amplitude of contractions (–64%) immediately after PGE_2 administration.

None of the doses of PGE_2 administered changes the amplitude of the longitudinal contractions (Figure 2, bottom).

Duration and number of high-amplitude contractions

Contractions with a high amplitude (giant contractions) are thought to play an important role in the concentric segmentation and in the propulsive motor activity of the colon. The amplitude, the frequency and the duration of these particular contractions are shown in Table 1 during the control period and following PGE_2 infusion. A dose of 0.1 μg/kg PGE_2 reduces significantly the duration (–70%) and the frequency (–98%) of circular high-amplitude contractions. However, 10 μg/kg PGE_2 induces a significant increase (+175%) in the number of longitudinal high-amplitude contractions. Otherwise, the inhibitory effect of PGE_2 on both circular and longitudinal high-amplitude contractions remains moderate.

TABLE 1
High-amplitude contractions of the circular and longitudinal muscles of the colon. Values for amplitude, duration and frequency were obtained in the control period, as well as the percentage changes (%) in the duration and frequency of contractions found after PGE_2 (0.1, 1.0 and 10 μg/kg) administration

		Percentage change after PGE_2		
	Control period	0.1 μg/kg	1 μg/kg	10 μg/kg
Circular contractions				
Amplitude (μm)	266±94			
Duration (min)	0.25±0.05	↓70*	↓40	↓30
Frequency (n/h)	12.3±4.9	↓98*	↓55	↓47
Longitudinal contractions				
Amplitude (μm)	298±157			
Duration (min)	0.47±0.23	↓31	↓19	↓29
Frequency (n/h)	11.2±6.8	↓40	↓26	↑175*

n/h = number of contractions calculated for 1 h period
*$p<0.01$

Rhythm of generation of the colonic contractions

The characteristics of colonic transit are the result of co-ordinated longitudinal and circular muscle contractions. Alterations in this co-ordinated smooth-muscle function, principally in the rhythm of the generation of either type of contraction, results in changes in colonic transit. The rhythm of generation of the longitudinal and circular contractions are influenced differently by PGE_2 (Figure 3). PGE_2 at each dose stimulates rapid or immediate appearance of a premature burst of longitudinal contractions. In the circular muscle, only a high dose (10 μg/kg) of PGE_2 induces premature contractions. Following the PGE_2-induced premature contractions, a long-lasting phase of motor quiescence – compensatory pause – is observed in both types of colonic muscle.

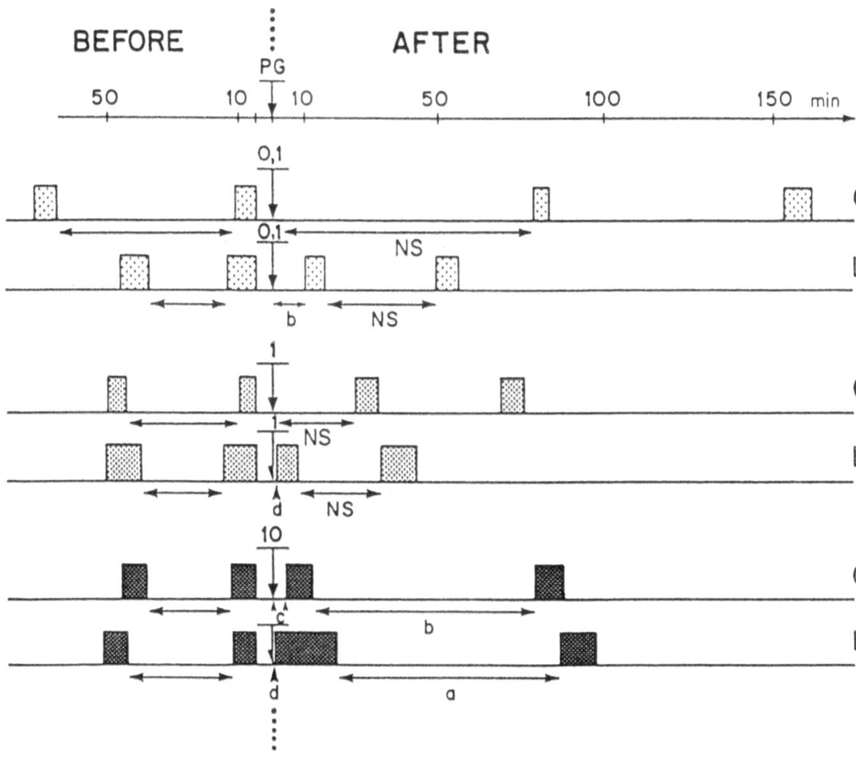

Figure 3. The rhythm of generation (recurrence) of colonic contractions. This scheme represents the distribution of the contractile phases of the circular (C) and the longitudinal (L) contractions in the control state (before) and after PGE_2 (0.1, 1.0 and 10 μg/kg) administration. Arrows (⟷) represent the duration of the quiescence intervals between two consecutive contractile phases. The rhythm of generation of the contractile phases after PGE_2 administration was compared with that of the control state (before PGE_2). a $= p < 0.05$; b $= p < 0.02$; c $= p < 0.01$; d $= p < 0.001$

DISCUSSION

Prostaglandins are thought to play an important role in the modulation of the colonic contractions [2,4,9,11,12]. PGE_2 is synthesized in the gastrointestinal muscle, in both circular and longitudinal layers [13]. In the small bowel, indomethacin, a prostaglandin-synthetase inhibitor, stimulates circular contractions [6] and inhibits longitudinal contractions in vitro [3].

On the other hand, studies on the colon in vitro provide divergent results concerning the effects of PGE_2 on colonic muscle [4,10] but PGE_2 alone has no effect on the isolated and unstimulated colonic muscle cells [9].

Sigmoid manometry on humans has demonstrated an inhibitory effect of PGE_2 on colonic segmental contractions [11] but this technique is unable to detect longitudinal wall movements accurately. EMG recordings in animals suggest the existence of an inhibitory effect of sennoids and PGE_2 on colonic motility [12]. The diarrhoeagenic effect of PGE_2 is still explained by the stimulation of hydroelectrolytic secretion [2] increasing the colonic volume, which is rapidly evacuated when giant migrating contractions appear [18].

However, simultaneous analysis of both longitudinal and circular contractions has never been made before. We used an extraluminal transducer to record the longitudinal and circular motor events of the colon.

According to our results, PGE_2 acts differently on circular and longitudinal colonic contractions. At each dose used, PGE_2 reduces the duration and amplitude of the circular contractions (Figures 1 and 2). The reduction in circular contractile activity involves both the contractile phases and the sporadic contractions. The reduction in the duration and amplitude of the circular contractions is more evident in the 2nd hour following PGE_2 injection and reflects a slow-developing relaxing effect of PGE_2 on the circular muscle.

Regarding the longitudinal contractions, 0.1 and 1.0 μg/kg PGE_2 do not modify the amplitude or the duration of these contractions, but the higher dose (10 μg/kg) of PGE_2 produces an increase in the duration of the longitudinal contractions (Figure 1) and in the number of high-amplitude longitudinal contractions (Table 1). Moreover, these intense longitudinal contractions appear immediately after each dose of PGE_2 in the form of premature bursts of contractions (Figure 3). These intense premature longitudinal contractions may be responsible for the rapid motor events in the colon, rapidly pushing the colonic contents distally and later triggering the mechanism of evacuation.

Regarding the literature, our results provide new information about the complex colonic motor changes induced by PGE_2. Only the relaxing effect of PGE_2 on colonic muscle had been described in previous in-vivo studies [11,12]. The technique used in our experiments revealed the intense longitudinal contractions which appear immediately after PGE_2 administration and which help to explain more clearly the diarrhoeagenic effect related to PGEs.

In previous in-vivo studies, the doses of PGE_2 used to explore colonic motility has varied with the experiments [2,11,12]. The dose when PGE_2 was administered intravenously ranged from 1.6 to 18 μg/kg [2,11]; it was 10 μg/kg via the intra-arterial and 100 μg/kg by the intracolonic route [12]. In our experiments, PGE_2 was infused intravenously, the doses of 1 μg/kg and 10 μg/kg being comparable to those administered in previous studies [2,11]. The smallest dose employed in our experiments has never been used by others; however, this dose is below that necessary to develop a cytoprotective effect in the colonic mucosa [19].

Finally, PGE_2 has different effects on circular and longitudinal contractions. The motor alterations of the circular contractions are unidirectional – relaxation – and are induced dose-independently in our experiments. Longitudinal contractions are also influenced and each dose of PGE_2 produced intense premature longitudinal contractions.

How can we explain the different actions of PGE_2 on the colonic circular and longitudinal muscle contractions? Our results, as well as studies performed in vitro, suggest that different mechanisms are involved in the motor alterations induced by PGE_2. PGs have neurogenic or direct effects on smooth-muscle cells. PGE_2 possesses anticholinergic properties on the intestinal circular muscle [6,9,20] and, in this layer, PGE_2 may provide a post-junctional negative feed-back effect on the excitatory transmission [3,21]. In the intestinal longitudinal muscle, PGE_2 may also interfere with cholinergic transmission [20]. Another mechanism, a progressive and direct cellular effect of PGs, may also exist in the circular muscle layer, limiting the excitability of the myocyte membrane by inducing a decrease in the opening capacity of the calcium channels [6]. There may be two types of PG receptors in the two different layers of colonic muscle. Their potentials or their mechanisms of homologous desensitization could be different in the two layers, explaining the different actions of PGE_2 in the two colonic muscle layers. These differentiated receptor mechanisms may also be used to explain the effects of PGE_2 on gastric [22] and small-bowel motility [13,23].

CONCLUSION

PGE_2 has a regulating effect on colonic motility, even at small doses, and has different actions on the circular and longitudinal colonic contractions. We propose that these separate motor actions of PGE_2 may be an important mechanism in several colonic pathologies producing diarrhoea.

REFERENCES

1. Balint GA, Kiss F, Varkonyi T, Wittmann T, Varro V. Effects of prostaglandin E_2 and $F_{2\alpha}$ on the absorption and portal transport of sugar and on the local intestinal circulation. Prostaglandins. 1979;18:265–8.
2. Milton-Thompson GJ, Cummings JH, Newman A, Billings JA, Misiewicz JJ. Colonic and small intestinal response to intravenous prostaglandin F alpha 2 and E_2 in man. Gut. 1975;16:42–6.
3. Nakahata N, Nakanishi T, Suzuki T. A possible negative feedback control of excitatory transmission via prostaglandins in canine small intestine. Br J Pharmacol. 1980;68:393–8.
4. Eley KG, Bennet A, Stockley HL. The effects of prostaglandins E_1, E_2, F alpha 1 and F alpha 2 on guinea-pig ileal and colonic peristalsis. J Pharm Pharmacol. 1977;29:276–80.

5. Koch KL, Dwyer A, Jeffries GH. Dose–response effects of indomethacin and PGE_2 on electromechanical activity of in vivo rabbit ileum. Am J Physiol. 1986;250:G135–9.
6. Sanders KM. Evidence that prostaglandins are local regulatory agents in canine ileal circular muscle. Am J Physiol. 1984;246:G361–71.
7. Tollstrom T, Hellstrom PM, Yohansson C, Pernow B. Effects of prostaglandins E_2 and F 2 alpha on motility of small intestine in man. Dig Dis Sci. 1988;33:552–7.
8. Konturek SJ, Thor P, Dembinski A, Gustav P. Role of prostaglandins (PGs) in the control of myoelectric activity of the small bowel. Gastroenterology. 1981;80:1197A.
9. Kao HW, Hyman PE, Finn SE, Snale Jr WJ. Effect of prostaglandin E_2 on rabbit colonic smooth muscle cell contraction. Am J Physiol. 1988;255:G807–12.
10. Sanger GJ, Bennett A. Regional differences in the response to prostanoids of circular muscle from guinea-pig isolated intestine. J Pharm Pharmacol. 1980;32:705–8.
11. Hunt RH, Dilawari JB, Misiewicz JJ. The effect of intravenous prostaglandin F alpha 2 and E_2 on the motility of the sigmoid colon. Gut. 1975;16:47–9.
12. Staumont G, Fioramonti J, Frexinos J, Bueno L. Changes in colonic motility induced by sennosides in evidence of a prostaglandin mediation. Gastroenterology. 1988;94:442(A).
13. Sanders KM, Northrup TE. Prostaglandin synthesis by microsomes of circular and longitudinal gastrointestinal muscles. Am J Physiol. 1983;244:G442–8.
14. Kao HW, Zipser RD. Exaggerated prostaglandin production by colonic smooth muscle in rabbit colitis. Dig Dis Sci. 1988;33:697–704.
15. Sharon P, Ligumsky M, Rachmilevitz A, Zor U. Role of prostaglandins in ulcerative colitis. Enhanced production during active disease and inhibition by sulfasalasine. Gastroenterology. 1978;75:638–40.
16. Lambert A, Eloy R, Grenier JF. Transducer for recording electrical and mechanical chronic intestinal activity. J Appl Physiol. 1976;41:942–5.
17. Sarna SK. Myoelectric correlates of motor complexes and contractile activity. Am J Physiol. 1986;250:G213–20.
18. Fioramonti J, Staumont G, Gracia-Villar R, Bueno L. Effects of sennosides on colon motility in dogs. Pharmacology. 1988;36(S1):23–30.
19. Roberts A, Nezamis JE, Lancaster C, Hanchar AJ. Prevention through cytoprotection of clindamycin-induced colitis in hamsters with 16,16-dimethyl PGE_2. Gastroenterology. 1980;78:1245(A).
20. Yagasaki O, Funaki H, Yanagiya I. Contribution of endogenous prostaglandins to excitation of the myenteric plexus of guinea-pig ileum: are adrenergic factors involved? Eur J Pharm. 1984;103:1–8.
21. Milenov K, Rakovska A. The role of prostaglandins in the spontaneous and cholinergic nerve-mediated motility of guinea-pig gastric muscle. Meth Find Exp Clin Pharmacol. 1983;5:121–6.
22. Bennet A, Jarosik C, Sanger GJ, Wilson DE. Antagonism of prostanoid-induced contractions of rat gastric fundus muscle by SC-19220, sodium meclofenamate, indomethacin or trimethoguinol. Br J Pharmacol. 1979;71:169–76.
23. Musch MW, Field M, Miller RJ, Stoff JS. Homologous desensitization to prostaglandins in rabbit ileum. Am J Physiol. 1987;252:G120–7.
24. Karaus M, Sarna SK. Giant migrating contractions during defecation in the dog colon. Gastroenterology. 1987;92:925–33.

Manuscript received 30 Nov. 95.
Accepted for publication 30 Nov. 95.

TS Gaginella et al. (eds.), Biochemical Pharmacology as an Approach to Gastrointestinal Disorders, 115–123

GASTRIC MOTOR EFFECTS OF ENDOTHELINS IN THE LOWER BRAINSTEM OF THE RAT

Z.K. KROWICKI AND P.J. HORNBY
Department of Pharmacology and Experimental Therapeutics, Louisiana State University Medical Center, New Orleans, LA 70112, USA

This paper was first published in: Inflammopharmacology. 1996;4:297–305.

ABSTRACT

To characterize the modulatory effect of endothelin on brainstem control of gastric motor function, endothelin-1 (ET-1) and endothelin-3 (ET-3) were applied to the surface of the dorsal medulla oblongata in α-chloralose and xylazine anaesthetized, artificially ventilated Sprague–Dawley rats, while intragastric pressure and contractility of the pyloric circular and greater curvature longitudinal muscles as well as blood pressure were monitored. Endothelin-1 and ET-3 equipotently (at the same range of doses) increased intragastric pressure and stimulated contractility of the gastric circular muscle as well as increasing arterial blood pressure. All the gastric effects of endothelins were abolished by bilateral vagotomy at the midcervical level. These results demonstrate that endothelins have vagally mediated gastrointestinal effects in the lower brainstem of the rat and support a role for endothelins in gastrointestinal regulation.

Keywords: endothelin, gastric tone, gastric contractility, brainstem

INTRODUCTION

Endothelins (ETs), namely ET-1, ET-2 (vasoactive intestinal contractor) and ET-3, are potent vasoconstrictor peptides with a wide spectrum of both vascular and non-vascular actions in a variety of tissues [1–4]. Among non-mammalian species, the ETs are structurally and functionally related to the sarafotoxins, which are present in the venom of the burrowing asp, *Atractaspis engaddensis* [5]. Endothelin isoforms activate specific receptor subtypes that have been classified as ET_A (selective for ET-1 and ET-2, distributed on the vascular and non-vascular smooth muscle) and ET_B (non-selective, distributed in brain, kidney, vascular endothelium, and on the isolated longitudinal smooth muscle cells of guinea-pig small intestine) [6–8]. The existence of a receptor specific to ET-3 (named ET_C) has been recently demonstrated in cultured endothelial and anterior pituitary cells [9].

The ETs have been mainly considered as modulators of vascular adrenergic [10,11] and non-vascular (e.g. intestinal cholinergic) smooth muscle contractile activity [11–13]. However, there is also a growing body of evidence for a neuromodulatory role of ETs in the central nervous system. The presence of ET immunoreactivity and mRNA

This paper was presented at the Section of IUPHAR GI Pharmacology Symposium on 'Biochemical pharmacology as an approach to gastrointestinal disorders (basic science to clinical perspectives)', October 12–14, 1995, Pécs, Hungary.

in the brain, hypothalamus and pituitary gland of different mammalian species is well accepted [14]. Moreover, numerous autoradiographic studies have documented the presence of ET (mainly ET-1) binding sites in the brainstem nuclei that participate in the regulation of gastrointestinal and cardiovascular function, including the dorsal vagal complex (composed of the nucleus of the solitary tract and the dorsal motor nucleus of the vagus) and rostroventrolateral medulla [4,15–17]. The dorsal motor nucleus of the vagus is the main source of the vagal preganglionic fibres (for review see Reference 18). The proximity of the dorsal vagal complex to the cerebrospinal fluid bathing the fourth cerebral ventricle and its close anatomical association to the area postrema provides routes through which circulating agents may reach specific receptors within the nucleus of the solitary tract and the dorsal motor nucleus of the vagus.

Thus, the primary purpose of this study was to investigate whether ETs, applied to the surface of the dorsal medulla, affect gastric motor function. Since ET-3 was once suggested to be a neural form of ET [2], both ET-1 and ET-3 were used in the experiments.

MATERIALS AND METHODS

Male Sprague–Dawley rats (215–410 g; Charles River Laboratories, Wilmington, MA) were used in the study and all procedures performed were with the approval of the LSUMC Institutional Animal Care and Use Committee. The animals were initially anaesthetized with ketamine and xylazine mixture (im, 50 and 5 mg/kg, respectively) and separate cannulae were placed in left femoral artery and vein. α-Chloralose (80 mg/kg) was administered iv 25 min later. Since ET-1 produces expiratory apnoea in α-chloralose-anaesthetized rats [19], the experiments were performed on artificially ventilated rats (tidal volume 1 ml/100 g; rate 60/min) using a small animal respirator (Kent Scientific Corp., Litchfield, CT). A laparotomy was performed and an intraluminal latex balloon was inserted into the stomach through an incision in the fundus for continuous recording of intragastric pressure. Two small strain gauges were mounted on the surface of the stomach for monitoring of circular smooth muscle contractility of the pyloric region and longitudinal smooth muscle of the greater curvature of the stomach [20]. Heart rate was monitored by a tachograph triggered by the arterial pressure pulse (model 7P4H, Grass Instrument Co., Quincy, MA). In six rats, bilateral vagotomies were performed at the midcervical level in the presence of full surgical anaesthesia. Rectal temperature was maintained between 37.0 and 37.5°C.

Animals were placed in a stereotaxic frame and, after a limited occipital craniotomy, the caudal floor of the fourth ventricle and the surrounding structures of the dorsal medulla oblongata were exposed by incision of the dura mater and the arachnoid membrane. Under visual control through a stereoscopic eyeglass magnifier (Stereomax), 5-μl aliquots of drug solutions and vehicle (0.9% NaCl with 0.1% bovine serum albumin RIA grade) were directly applied to the surface of the fourth ventricle, using a 10-μl Hamilton microsyringe.

Mean arterial pressure was calculated as diastolic pressure plus one-third of the pulse pressure. The area of the response in intragastric pressure for each treatment was calculated using a microcomputer-based imaging system, as described in detail elsewhere [21]. Contractility of the pyloric circular muscle and the fundus longitudinal muscle was calculated as minute motility index (MMI), as described in detail elsewhere [21]. In addition, the peak change in intragastric pressure (maximum difference from baseline), was calculated after application of agents to the dorsal surface of the medulla.

The differences between groups were assessed by one-way repeated measure analysis of variance (ANOVA) followed by the Student–Newman–Keuls test. However, due to the failure of the normality test, the changes in mean blood pressure were evaluated with Kruskal–Wallis one-way ANOVA on ranks with subsequent Dunn's test. Values of $p < 0.05$ were considered statistically significant.

RESULTS

The effects of ET-1 at three doses of 1.6, 16, and 160 pmol and vehicle, applied to the surface of the dorsal medulla, on gastric motor function in α-chloralose and xylazine anaesthetized rats are shown in Figure 1. Endothelin-1 increased intragastric pressure

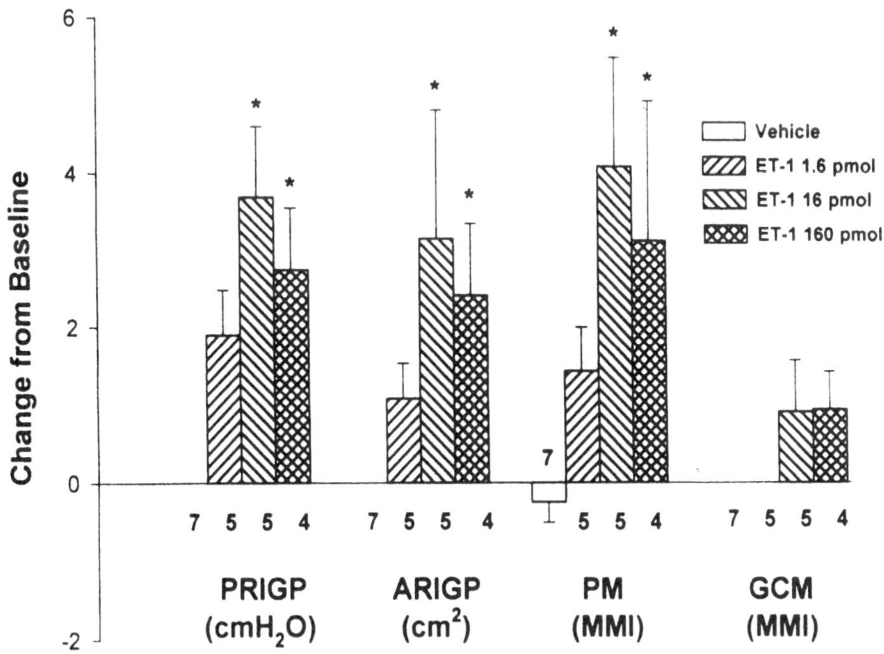

Figure 1. Effects of vehicle or ET-1 (1.6, 16 and 160 pmol), applied to the surface of the dorsal medulla, on intragastric pressure (PRIGP, peak response; ARIGP, area of the response), pyloric circular muscle (PM), and greater curvature longitudinal muscle (GCM) contractility. Data are mean (bar = SE) changes from baseline for number of animals indicated in the histogram. *Statistically significant when compared with the effect of vehicle

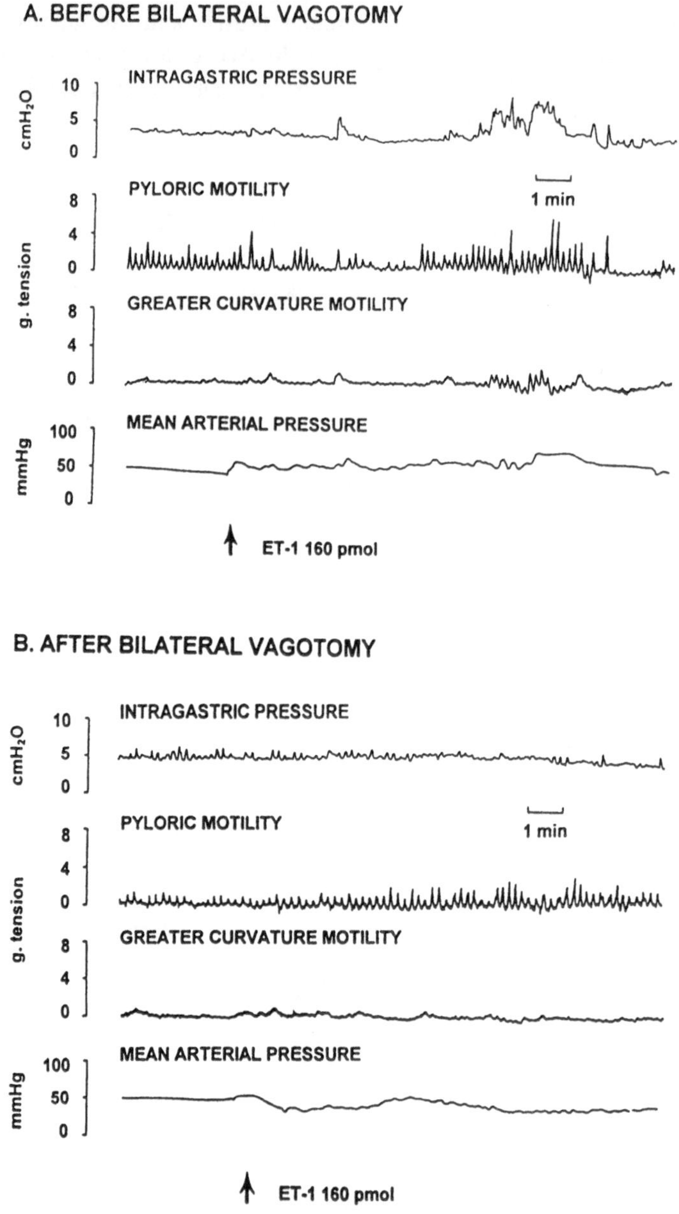

Figure 2. Representative chart recording of one experiment in which ET-1 (160 pmol) was applied to the surface of the dorsal medulla before (A) and after (B) bilateral vagotomy at midcervical level. **A**: ET-1 evoked increases in intragastric pressure, pyloric circular and greater curvature longitudinal muscle contractility, and blood pressure. **B**: After bilateral vagotomy, no discernible gastric responses to ET-1 were noted

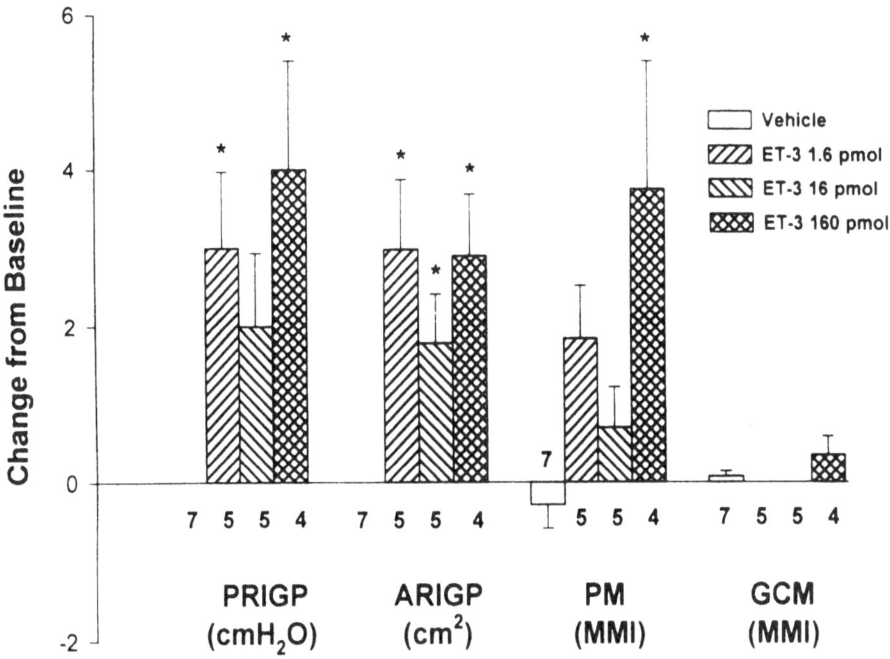

Figure 3. Effects of vehicle or ET-3 (1.6, 16 and 160 pmol), applied to the surface of the dorsal medulla, on intragastric pressure (PRIGP, peak response; ARIGP, area of the response), pyloric circular muscle (PM), and greater curvature longitudinal muscle (GCM) contractility. Data are mean (bar = SE) changes from baseline for number of animals indicated in the histogram. *Statistically significant when compared with the effect of vehicle

(both peak response and area of the response) and stimulated pyloric contractility at doses of 16 and 160 pmol, when compared with the effect of vehicle. However, the changes in greater curvature contractility did not attain statistical significance. Arterial blood pressure increased significantly in response to ET-1 and attained statistical significance at doses of 16 pmol (Δ, 56 ± 13 mmHg, $n = 5$) and 160 pmol (Δ, 63 ± 15 mmHg, $n = 6$) of the peptide when compared with the effect of vehicle ($\Delta = 0$ mmHg, $n = 8$).

A chart recording from a representative experiment in which ET-1 was applied to the surface of the dorsal medulla at a dose of 160 pmol before and after bilateral vagotomy at midcervical level is shown in Figure 2. In this particular animal, a marked increase in intragastric pressure (peak = 4.5 cm H_2O; area of the response = 1.7 cm^2) is accompanied by a slight increase in pyloric motility ($\Delta = 0.4$ MMI) and greater curvature contractility ($\Delta = 1.0$ MMI), and arterial blood pressure ($\Delta = 95$ mmHg; Figure 2A). Gastric motor effects of ET-1 in this rat were completely blocked by bilateral vagotomy (Figure 2B).

The effects of ET-3, applied to the surface of the dorsal medulla at doses of 1.6, 16, and 160 pmol, and vehicle on gastric motor function are shown in Figure 3.

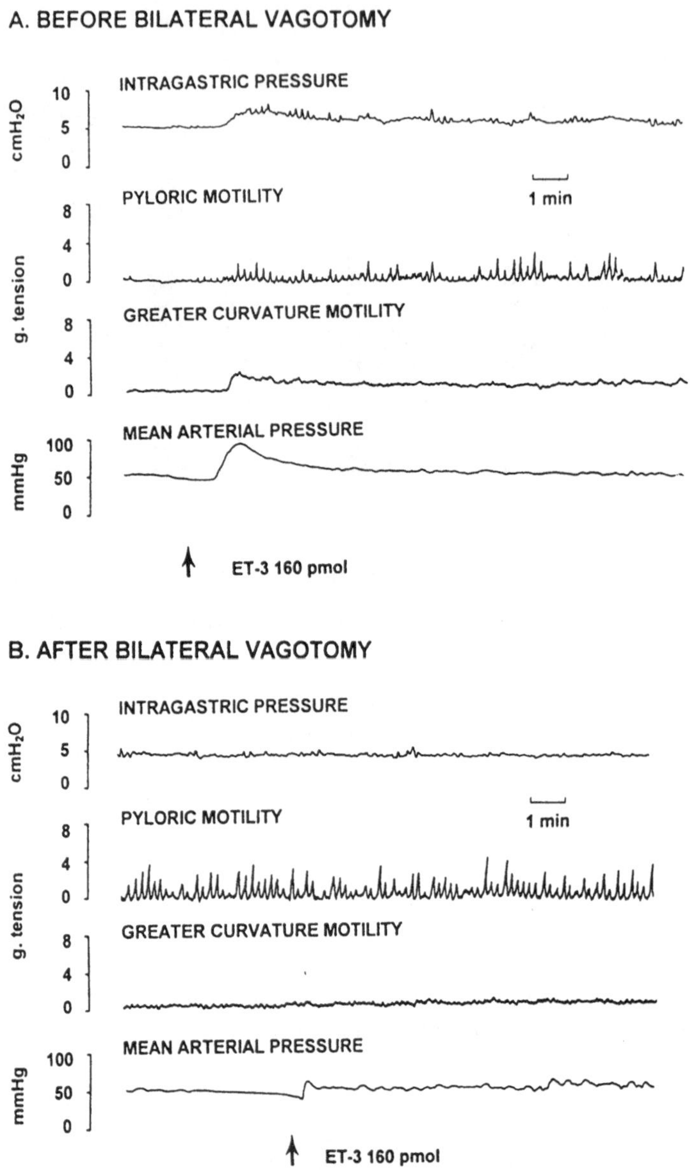

Figure 4. Representative chart recording of 1 experiment in which ET-3 (160 pmol) was applied to the surface of the dorsal medulla before (A) and after (B) bilateral vagotomy at midcervical level. **A**: ET-1 evoked increases in intragastric pressure, pyloric circular and greater curvature longitudinal muscle contractility, and blood pressure. **B**: After bilateral vagotomy, no discernible gastric responses to ET-3 were noted

Endothelin-3 evoked increases in intragastric pressure area of the response at all doses used. However, the increases in pyloric contractility attained statistical significance only at the highest dose of 160 pmol. The changes in greater curvature contractility did not reach statistical significance at any dose of ET-3 used in the study. Arterial blood pressure significantly increased in response to ET-3 at doses of 1.6 pmol (Δ, 30 ± 10 mmHg, $n = 5$) and 160 pmol (Δ, 60 ± 20 mmHg, $n = 3$) when compared with the effect of vehicle ($\Delta = 0$ mmHg, $n = 7$).

Tracings from one experiment in which ET-3 was applied to the surface of the dorsal medulla before and after bilateral vagotomy at the dose of 160 pmol are shown in Figure 4. Increases in gastric tone (peak response = 3.0 cm H_2O; area of the response = 3.8 cm^2), and pyloric contractility ($\Delta = 4$ MMI) were accompanied by an increase in arterial blood pressure ($\Delta = 45$ mmHg; Figure 4A). Bilateral vagotomy completely blocked the gastric motor effects of the peptide (Figure 4B).

DISCUSSION

The major finding of the present study was that ET-1 and ET-3, applied to the surface of the dorsal medulla, increase gastric tone and stimulate gastric contractility in anaesthetized rats in a comparable manner. To our knowledge, this is the first report of central effects of ET on gastric motor function. The most likely brainstem site of action for ET-induced changes in gastric tone and contractility is the dorsal vagal complex; however, these studies are currently under investigation in this laboratory.

Although selective ET receptor subtype antagonists were not used in the study, the fact that ET-1 and ET-3 both evoked changes in gastric motor function of a comparable magnitude at comparable doses of the peptides suggests that these effects are mediated through ET_B receptors. This is because the ET_B receptor possesses similar affinities for all three ET isopeptides [7]. This hypothesis is also supported by the fact that ET_B is the predominant subtype of ET receptor in the brain [7]. Moreover, although no structure–activity studies in medullary nuclei have been reported, the binding characteristics of ET-1 and ET-3 have been shown in the cerebellum [22–24]. In addition, ET-1 and ET-3 are equipotent in stimulating the turnover of inositol phosphates in various regions of the brain [22,25]. Finally, intracisternal administration of ET-1 and ET-3 has similar effects on baroreceptor heart rate reflex parameters in the rat [15].

It is unlikely that the observed changes in gastric motor function were caused by the leakage of the isopeptides to the peripheral circulation. It has been shown that a bolus intravenous injection of 100 pmol of ET-3 did not cause the pattern of cardiovascular changes comparable to those following its intracisternal administration in rats [26].

In our experiments, both ET-1 and ET-3, applied to the surface of the dorsal medulla, increased mean blood pressure. These observations are in line with previous communications which showed marked increases in blood pressure in response to centrally applied ETs [26,27], and a long-lasting vasoconstriction of cerebral blood vessels [28,29]. However, it has also been reported that intracisternal injection of ET-1 or ET-3 at a dose of 25 pmol/kg did not affect heart rate and blood pressure [15] and

ET-1 at doses of 3–10 pmol, applied to the surface of the fourth cerebral ventricle of anaesthetized ventilated rats, decreased mean arterial pressure and heart rate. In the latter communication, the decrease in mean arterial pressure was usually preceded by an increase [30].

The significance of ET in medullary sites controlling autonomic function is not known; however, marked elevation in the plasma levels of ETs and down-regulation of ET receptors in chronic diabetes mellitus may indicate a role of ET not only in the genesis of heart dysfunction [31] but also in the pathogenesis of cardiovascular and gastrointestinal complications in diabetes.

ACKNOWLEDGEMENTS

This work was supported by the Louisiana State University Neuroscience Center of Excellence Incentive Grant to Z.K. Krowicki and, in part, by the National Institute of Diabetes and Digestive and Kidney Diseases Grant DK-42714 to P.J. Hornby.

REFERENCES

1. Yanagisawa M, Kurihara H, Kimura S et al. A novel potent vasoconstrictor peptide produced by vascular endothelial cells. Nature. 1988;332:411–15.
2. Inoue A, Yanagisawa M, Kimura S et al. The human endothelin family: Three structurally and pharmacologically distinct isopeptides predicted by three separate genes. Proc Natl Acad Sci USA. 1989;86:2863–7.
3. Bloch KD, Hong CC, Eddy RL, Shows TB, Quatermouse T. cDNA cloning and chromosomal assignment of the endothelin 2 gene: Vasoactive intestinal contractor peptide is rat endothelin 2. Genomics. 1991;10:236–42.
4. Kohzuki M, Chai SY, Paxinos G et al. Localization and characterization of endothelin receptor binding sites in the rat brain visualized by *in vitro* autoradiography. Neuroscience. 1991;42:245–60.
5. Kloog Y, Ambar I, Sokolovsky M, Kochva E, Wollberg Z, Bdolah A. Sarafotoxin, a novel vasoconstrictor peptide: Phosphoinositide hydrolysis in rat heart and brain. Science. 1988;242:268–70.
6. Arai H, Hori S, Aramori I, Ohkubo H, Nakanishi S. Cloning and expression of cDNA encoding endothelin receptor. Nature. 1990;348:730–2.
7. Sakurai T, Yanagisawa M, Takuwa Y et al. Cloning of a cDNA encoding a non-isopeptide-selective subtype of the endothelin receptor. Nature. 1990;348:732–5.
8. Chijiwara Y, Okabe H, Akiho H, Harada N, Nawata H. Functional endothelin$_A$ receptor on gastric smooth muscle cells. Digestion. 1995;56:171–4.
9. Sakurai T, Yanagisawa M, Masaki T. Molecular characterization of endothelin receptors. Trends Pharmacol Sci. 1992;13:103–8.
10. Wiklund NP, Ohlen A, Cederqvist B. Adrenergic neuromodulation by endothelin in guinea pig pulmonary artery. Neurosci Lett. 1989;101:269–73.
11. Masaki T, Yanagisawa M, Goto K. Physiology and pharmacology of endothelins. Med Res Rev. 1992;12:391–421.
12. Wiklund NP, Wiklund CU, Ohlen A, Gustafsson LE. Cholinergic neuromodulation by endothelin in guinea pig ileum. Neurosci Lett. 1989;101:342–6.
13. Rae GA. Pharmacology of endothelins in the gastrointestinal tract. In: Gaginella TS, ed. Regulatory Mechanisms in Gastrointestinal Function. Boca Raton: CRC Press; 1995:257–75.
14. Polak JM, Terenghi G. Distribution of endothelin, a putative growth promoting peptide, using modern microscopical imaging methods. In: Moody TW, ed. Growth Factors, Peptides, and Receptors. New York: Plenum Press; 1993:3–13.
15. van den Buuse M, Itoh S. Central effects of endothelin on baroreflex of spontaneously hypertensive rats. J Hypertens. 1993;11:379–87.

16. Koseki C, Imai M, Hirata Y, Yanagisawa M, Masaki T. Binding sites for endothelin-1 in rat tissues: An autoradiographic study. J Cardiovasc Pharmacol. 1989;13(Suppl. 5):S153–4.
17. Grisoni E, De Augustin JC, Kalhan SC. Vasoactive intestinal polypeptide causes relaxation of the pyloric sphincter in the rabbit. J Pediatr Surg. 1993;28:1117–20.
18. Krowicki ZK, Hornby PJ. Hindbrain neuroactive substances controlling gastrointestinal function. In: Gaginella TS, ed. Regulatory Mechanisms in Gastrointestinal Function. Boca Raton: CRC Press; 1995:277–319.
19. Fuxe K, Andbjer B, Kalia M, Agnati LF. Centrally administered endothelin-1 produces apnoea in the α-chloralose-anaesthetized male rat. Acta Physiol Scand. 1989;137:157–8.
20. Krowicki ZK, Hornby PJ. Opposing gastric motor responses to TRH and substance P on their microinjection into nucleus raphe obscurus of rats. Am J Physiol. 1993;265:G819–30.
21. Krowicki ZK, Hornby PJ. Serotonin and thyrotropin-releasing hormone do not augment their effects on gastric motility on their microinjection into the nucleus raphe obscurus of the rat. J Pharmacol Exp Ther. 1995;273:499–508.
22. MacCumber MW, Ross CA, Snyder SH. Endothelin in brain: Receptors, mitogenesis, and biosynthesis in glial cells. Proc Natl Acad Sci USA. 1990;87:2359–63.
23. Hiley CR, Jones CR, Pelton JT, Miller RC. Binding of [^{125}I]-endothelin-1 to rat cerebellar homogenates and its interactions with some analogues. Br J Pharmacol. 1990;101:319–24.
24. Schvartz I, Ittoop O, Hazum E. Identification of a single binding protein for endothelin-1 and endothelin-3 in bovine cerebellum membranes. Endocrinology. 1991;128:126–30.
25. Crawford MLA, Hiley CR, Young JM. Characteristics of endothelin-1 and endothelin-3 stimulation of phosphoinositide breakdown differ between regions of guinea-pig and rat brain. Naunyn-Schmiedeberg's Arch Pharmacol. 1990;341:268–71.
26. Kuwaki T, Koshiya N, Takahashi H, Terui N, Kumada M. Modulatory effects of rat endothelin on central cardiovascular control in rats. Jpn J Physiol. 1990;40:97–116.
27. Ouchi Y, Kim S, Souza AC et al. Central effect of endothelin on blood pressure of conscious rats. Am J Physiol. 1989;256:H1747–51.
28. Asano T, Ikegaki I, Satoh SI et al. Endothelin: A potential modulator of cerebral vasospasm. Eur J Pharmacol. 1990;190:365–72.
29. Macrae IM, Robinson M, McAuley M, Reid J, McCulloch J. Effects of intracisternal endothelin-1 injection on blood flow to the lower brain stem. Eur J Pharmacol. 1991;203:85–91.
30. Hashim MA, Tadepalli AS. Hemodynamic responses evoked by endothelin from central cardiovascular neural substrates. Am J Physiol. 1992;262:H1–H9.
31. Patino R, Ibarra J, Molino A, Fernandez-Durango R, Moya J, Fernandez-Cruz A. Increased plasma endothelin in diabetes: An atherosclerosis marker? Diabetologia. 1994;37:333–4.

Manuscript received 3 Nov. 95.
Accepted for publication 5 Nov. 95

TS Gaginella et al. (eds.), Biochemical Pharmacology as an Approach to Gastrointestinal Disorders, 125–130

EFFECTS OF ERYTHROMYCIN ON THE PROPULSIVE MOTILITY OF UPPER GASTROINTESTINAL TRACT IN RATS

O. KARÁDI, B. BÓDIS AND Gy. MÓZSIK*
First Department of Medicine, Medical University of Pécs, Pécs, Hungary
*Correspondence

This paper was first published in: Inflammopharmacology. 1997;5:77–82.

ABSTRACT

The differences between the postprandial mixing or propulsion and the interdigestive motility of the gastrointestinal (GI) tract are already known. Earlier studies showed dose-dependent differences in the effects of erythromycin on interdigestive motility. The various GI side-effects (vomiting, diarrhoea) also suggest that there are different effects of erythromycin on the GI motility. The aim of our study was to examine postprandially the propulsive effects of different doses of erythromycin on the movement of intraluminal contents in the upper GI tract of the rat. The animals were fasted for 24 h before the experiments but water was given freely. The rats received 1.5 ml 1.5% methylcellulose painted with 0.05% phenol-red intragastrically (test solution). Erythromycin (*E. lactobionate*) was given intravenously at doses of 0.05, 0.1, 0.25, 0.5, 1.0 and 5.0 mg/kg 15 min before the administration of a test solution. The animals were sacrificed 20, 60 and 120 min after administration of methylcellulose, when the distance between the front of the painted intraluminal contents and the pylorus was measured and expressed as a percentage of the total length of small intestine. The phenol-red content in the stomach and small intestine was measured spectrophotometrically and the gastric emptying was calculated from the ratio of the measured total and intestinal phenol-red content. Our results showed that the small doses of erythromycin (0.1 and 0.25 mg/kg) accelerated gastric emptying after 20 min but did not change significantly the propulsive motility of upper small intestine; however, large doses of erythromycin (1.0 and 5.0 mg/kg) decreased gastric emptying and upper GI motility after 20 and 60 min. In summary, the prokinetic action of small doses of erythromycin was demonstrated, but its effect-time on GI motility is short and the ratio of the stimulating and inhibitory doses is 1:10.

Keywords: erythromycin, postprandial propulsive motility, gastrointestinal tract

INTRODUCTION

Recently, some studies named erythromycin and the erythromycin-like drugs the new family of the prokinetic agents [1]. The prokinetic action of small doses of erythromycin on gastric emptying and on interdigestive motility, measured by migration motor complexes (MMC) was proved [2]. However, the varied gastrointestinal (GI) side-effects of large doses of erythromycin in clinical practice, such as a vomiting and diarrhoea [6], suggest that erythromycin has different effects on GI motility. Earlier studies also demonstrated the dose-dependent effects of erythromycin on interdigestive motility (MMC) [2]. On the other hand, the pattern of interdigestive motility disappears after a meal because it does not play any role in postprandial motility [3]. The measurement of MMC by manometric methods did not show clearly the efficiency

This paper was presented at the Section of IUPHAR GI Pharmacology Symposium on 'Biochemical pharmacology as an approach to gastrointestinal disorders (basic science to clinical perspectives)', October 12–14, 1995, Pécs, Hungary.

of the propulsive motility on the movement of intraluminal contents. The aim of our study, therefore, was to examine the effects of different doses of erythromycin on the propulsive movement of intraluminal contents in the upper GI tract of the rat.

MATERIALS AND METHODS

The observations were carried out on Sprague–Dawley rats weighing 250–300 g (LATI, Gödöllő, Hungary). The animals were fasted for 24 h before the experiments but they received tap water ad libitum. The experiments were started at 1 pm.

GI motility was examined by the distribution in the GI tract of 1.5 ml of 1.5% methylcellulose (Sigma Chemical Co., St. Louis) intragastrically (ig) administered painted with 0.05% phenol-red (test solution) [4].

Erythromycin (Erythromycin–Lactobionat, Antibiotice S.A.-Iasi, Romania) dissolved in 0.5 ml saline was given intravenously (iv) at doses of 0.05, 0.1, 0.25, 0.5, 1.0 or 5.0 mg/kg 15 min before the ig administration of methylcellulose. Saline (0.5 ml) was given iv to the control group at the same time.

Rats were sacrificed by inhalation of carbon dioxide at 20, 60 and 120 min after methylcellulose administration. The pylorus was clamped and the total GI tract was removed. The distance between the front of the painted intraluminal contents and the pylorus was measured in centimetres and was expressed as a percentage of the total length of the small intestine.

The stomach and small intestine with their contents were homogenized in 20 ml of 0.1 N NaOH for 30 min. Supernatant (7.5 ml) was added to 0.8 ml of 25% trichloroacetic acid. After centrifugation (2400*g*, for 20 min), 2 ml of supernatant were added to 2.5 ml of 0.5 N NaOH. The absorbance of the phenol-red in each sample was measured at a wavelength of 560 nm with a spectrophotometer (Hitachi 124, Japan). Gastric emptying was expressed as a percentage value, as a ratio of the absorbance in the small intestine and the absorbance in the stomach plus small intestine.

Previously, we had studied the metabolism and the absorption of phenol-red content of the test solution in the GI tract. More than 100% of the applied phenol-red was measurable in the GI tract at 60 and 120 min after its ig administration. Phenol-red was not found in the serum, urine and bile after 60 and 120 min in the rats. These results proved that this test solution was a useful tool to measure the distribution of intraluminal contents in the GI tract because the phenol-red is not absorbed from the GI tract and is not digested or involved in the entero-hepatic system in significant quantities. The test solution appeared in the caecum 180 min after its ig administration.

Statistical analysis

The results were calculated as means $\pm$ SEM. The non-paired Student's *t*-test was used for statistical analysis of results. Differences were considered significant when a p value <0.05 was obtained.

RESULTS

At 20, 60 and 120 min, respectively, the control gastric emptying was 55.65±3.05%, 85.9±1.5% and 95±0.9%, and the control values for the distance between the front of painted intraluminal juice and the pylorus were 49.76±2.27%, 78.95±3.67% and 98±1.2%.

Small doses of erythromycin (0.1 and 0.25 mg/kg) significantly accelerated gastric emptying after 20 min, but no significant differences were found after 60 and 120 min (Figures 1 and 2). No significant changes were found in the distances between the front of bulk and the pylorus after 20, 60 or 120 min (Figures 3 and 4).

Large doses of erythromycin (1.0 and 5.0 mg/kg) significantly decreased gastric emptying after 20 min but did not cause significant changes in gastric emptying after 60 or 120 min (Figures 1 and 2). These doses significantly decreased the distance between the front of bulk and the pylorus after 20 and 60 min but not after 120 min (Figures 3 and 4).

DISCUSSION

The erythromycin-induced dose-dependent effects on the propulsive movement of intraluminal contents in the upper GI tract of rats were examined in this study. Earlier studies and clinical observations suggested that different doses of erythromycin have

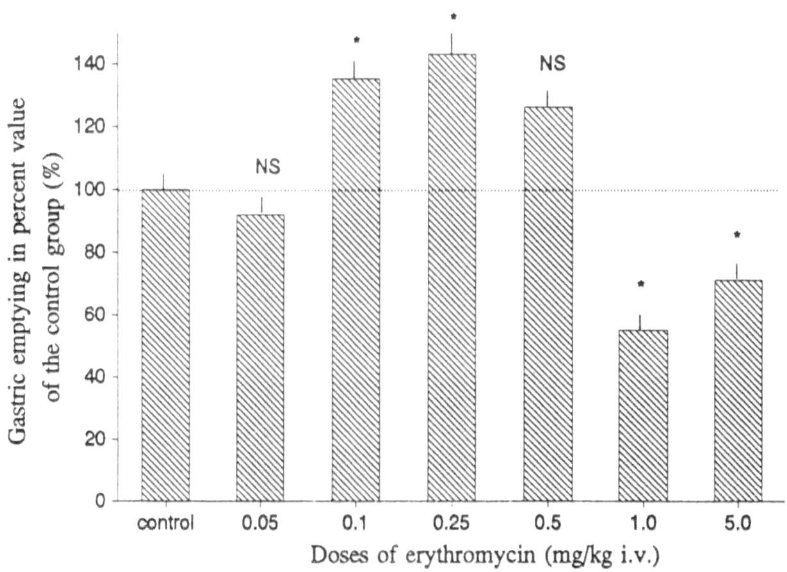

Figure 1. Effect of different doses of erythromycin on gastric emptying after 20 min. The results are expressed as percentage values of the control group (control=100%). (Means±SEM; n=12; NS: not significant; $^{*}p<0.05$)

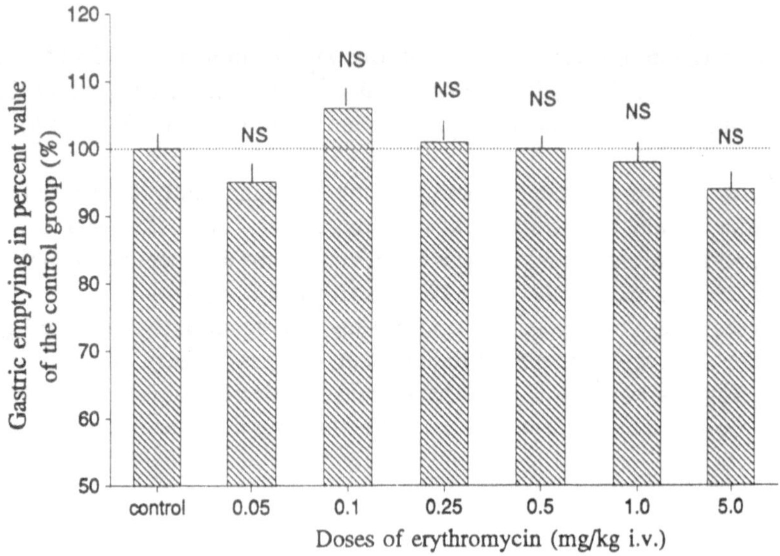

Figure 2. Effect of different doses of erythromycin on gastric emptying after 60 min. The results are expressed as percentage values of the control group (control=100%). (Means ± SEM; n=12; NS: not significant

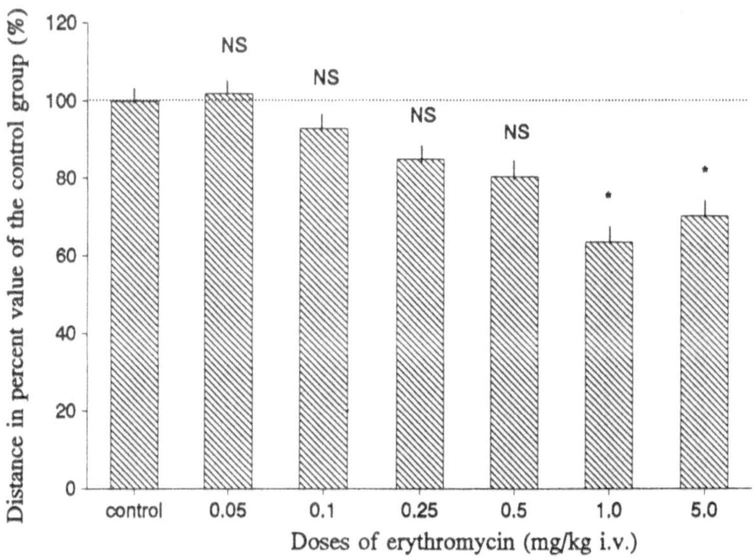

Figure 3. Effect of different doses of erythromycin on the distance between the front of painted intraluminal content and the pylorus after 20 min. The results are expressed as percentage values of the control group (control=100%). (Means ± SEM; n=12; NS: not significant; $^{*}p<0.05$)

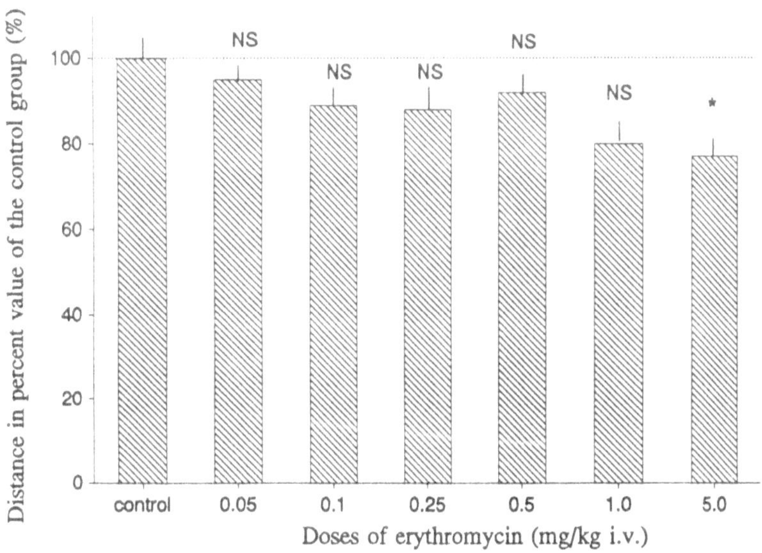

Figure 4. Effect of different doses of erythromycin on the distance between the front of painted intraluminal content and the pylorus after 60 min. The results are expressed as percentage values of the control group (control=100%). (Means ± SEM; n=12; NS: not significant; $^{*}p<0.05$)

different effects on the interdigestive and postprandial GI motility [2,6]. Small doses of erythromycin accelerate gastric emptying after a meal [5] while large doses induce different GI side-effects (vomiting, diarrhoea) [6].

Our results showed that single small doses of erythromycin (0.1 or 0.25 mg/kg) accelerated gastric emptying at 35 min after erythromycin administration (20 min after methylcellulose administration ig) but did not change significantly the distance between the front of bulk and the pylorus. On the other hand, large doses of erythromycin (1.0 and 5.0 mg/kg iv) significantly decreased the gastric emptying 20 min after the administration of the test solution. The distance between the front of the bulk and the pylorus was also decreased in parallel with the inhibition of gastric emptying at 35 and 75 min after administration of 1.0 or 5.0 mg/kg erythromycin. Other studies also demonstrated that microbially ineffective doses of erythromycin inhibited small intestinal motor activity in the fed state while it had no significant effect in the fasted state (using the manometric method) [3].

The stimulatory and inhibitory effects of small and large single iv doses of erythromycin disappeared in the stomach after 20 min and in the small intestine after 60 min. These results suggest that the effect-time of erythromycin in the GI tract is very short. Other studies found that the half-life of iv-administered erythromycin in the circulation is between 30 and 90 min in different species [2,3].

On the other hand, our results showed that the stimulatory and inhibitory effects of erythromycin on GI motility could only be detected in the stomach and upper small intestine. Some studies have proposed that the prokinetic action of small doses of erythromycin is connected with the motilin receptors [1], while the GI side-effects of large doses are independent of the motilin receptors [7]. Motilin receptors are mainly in the upper GI tract, the numbers decreasing aborally in the small intestine [8,9].

In summary, a biphasic motor effect of erythromycin on the postprandial motility of upper GI tract in rats was proved: small doses of erythromycin had a prokinetic effect on the stomach while large doses had an inhibitory effect on upper GI motility after a meal. However, the effect-time of erythromycin, given as a single iv dose, on GI motility was very short and the ratio of stimulating to inhibiting doses was rather small (1:10).

ACKNOWLEDGEMENTS

This study was supported by a grant from the Hungarian National Research Fund (OTKA T-020098).

REFERENCES

1. Weber FH, Richards RD, McCallum RW. Erythromycin: a motilin agonist and gastrointestinal prokinetic agent. Am J Gastroenterol. 1993;88:485–90.
2. Otterson MF, Sarna SK. Gastrointestinal motor effects of erythromycin. Am J Physiol. 1990;259:G355–63.
3. Sarna SK, Soergel KH, Koch TR et al. Gastrointestinal motor effects of erythromycin in humans. Gastroenterology. 1991;101:1488–96.
4. Sütő G, Király Á, Taché Y. Interleukin 1β inhibits gastric emptying in rats: Mediation through prostaglandin and corticotropin-releasing factor. Gastroenterology. 1994;106:1568–75.
5. Urbain JI, Vantrappen G, Janssens J, Van Cutsem E, Peeters T, De Roo M. Intravenous erythromycin dramatically accelerates gastric emptying in gastroparesis diabeticorum and normals and abolishes the emptying discrimination between solids and liquids. J Nucl Med. 1990;31:1490–3.
6. Downey KM, Chaput De Saintonge DM. Gastrointestinal side effects after intravenous erythromycin lactobionate. Br J Clin Pharmacol. 1986;21:295–9.
7. Peeters TL, Depoortere I. Motilin receptor: A model for development of prokinetics. Dig Dis Sci. 1994;39:76–8.
8. Ebert R, Creutzfeldt W. Hormone production: the small intestine and regulatory peptides. In: Caspary WF, ed. Structure and Function of the Small Intestine. Amsterdam: Excerpta Medica; 1987:106–15.
9. Depoortere I, Peeters TL, Vantrappen G. Development of motilin receptors and of motilin- and erythromycin-induced contractility in rabbits. Gastroenterology. 1990;99:652–8

Manuscript received 2 Nov. 95.
Accepted for publication 18 Dec. 95.

TS Gaginella et al. (eds.), Biochemical Pharmacology as an Approach to Gastrointestinal Disorders, 131–139

BICUCULLINE BLOCKS THE INHIBITORY EFFECTS OF SUBSTANCE P BUT NOT VASOACTIVE INTESTINAL POLYPEPTIDE ON GASTRIC MOTOR FUNCTION IN THE NUCLEUS RAPHE OBSCURUS OF THE RAT

Z.K. KROWICKI AND P.J. HORNBY
Department of Pharmacology and Experimental Therapeutics, Louisiana State University Medical Center, New Orleans, LA 70112, USA

This paper was first published in: Inflammopharmacology. 1997;5:57–65.

ABSTRACT

We have shown previously that substance P (SP) and vasoactive intestinal polypeptide (VIP), microinjected into the caudal nucleus raphe obscurus (nROb) of the rat decreases intragastric pressure via vagally mediated pathways. Since γ-aminobutyric acid (GABA) is a transmitter of interneurons innervating non-adrenergic, non-cholinergic pathways that modulate gastric peristalsis, we tested the hypothesis that peripheral GABA is a mediator of inhibitory effects of SP and VIP in the nROb on gastric motor function. Substance P (135 pmol) or VIP (100 pmol) were microinjected into the nROb of the same α-chloralose-anaesthetized rats before and 60 min after peripheral administration of bicuculline methiodide (0.4 mg/kg sc), a $GABA_A$ receptor antagonist. As expected, both SP and VIP, microinjected into the nROb, evoked marked decreases in intragastric pressure before bicuculline. However, the gastric motor effects of SP, but not VIP, were abolished by bicuculline. Therefore we conclude that SP-evoked gastric relaxation in the nROb is mediated through a peripheral GABA-ergic pathway.

Keywords: γ-aminobutyric acid, bicuculline, substance P, vasoactive intestinal polypeptide, gastric tone, gastric motility, brainstem, nucleus raphe obscurus

The nucleus raphe obscurus (nROb) in the caudal medulla oblongata has recently emerged as an important structure involved in the brain control of gastric functions [1–4]. This raphe nucleus maintains direct anatomic and functional connections with the dorsal motor nucleus of the vagus (DMV) [1,5], a major site of origin of vagal gastric preganglionic fibres (for review see Reference 6). Substance P (SP)-immunoreactivity is present in both cells [7] and fibres [8] of the raphe nuclei along with SP receptor immunoreactivity [9] and tachykinin binding sites [10]. Substance P microinjected into the nROb of the rat decreases intragastric pressure and tends to inhibit gastric motility via a vagally mediated pathway [11]. Moreover, gastric inhibition caused by microinjection of SP into the nROb is mediated by central [12] and peripheral nitric oxide (NO)-containing pathways [13].

Vasoactive intestinal polypeptide (VIP)-positive fibres have been found in the dorsal vagal complex [14–16] and raphe nuclei [16]. Preliminary data show that microinjection of VIP into the nROb at doses of 1–100 pmol dose-dependently decreases

This paper was presented at the Section of IUPHAR GI Pharmacology Symposium on 'Biochemical pharmacology as an approach to gastrointestinal disorders (basic science to clinical perspectives)', October 12–14, 1995, Pécs, Hungary.

intragastric pressure and inhibits contractility of gastric smooth muscle [17].

Recent studies revealed that, in the enteric nervous system, γ-aminobutyric acid (GABA) is a transmitter of interneurons innervating not only excitatory (cholinergic) but also inhibitory (non-adrenergic, non-cholinergic; NANC) pathways [18,19] that modulate intestinal peristalsis and gastric acid secretion [20]. Although a majority of evidence supports NO as a NANC inhibitory neurotransmitter in the vagus nerve and vagally mediated relaxation of the stomach is dependent on NO [21–25], other transmitters are also involved. Specifically, a recent study by Krantis and Glasgow demonstrated that NO-mediated relaxations of the gastro-duodenum are targeted by GABA [26] and VIP-induced relaxations of the antrum are mediated by NO [27].

It was therefore the primary purpose of this study to investigate the involvement of peripheral GABA in mediating the inhibitory gastric motor effects of SP and VIP in the nROb.

MATERIALS AND METHODS

Male Sprague–Dawley rats (180–380 g; Charles River Laboratories, Wilmington, MA) were used in the study and all procedures were performed with the approval of the LSUMC Institutional Animal Care and Use Committee. The animals were initially anaesthetized with ketamine and xylazine mixture (im, 50 and 5 mg/kg, respectively) and separate cannulae were placed in the left femoral artery and vein. Afterwards, α-chloralose (80 mg/kg iv) was administered and a tracheotomy performed to ease respiration. After laparotomy, an intraluminal latex balloon was inserted into the stomach through an incision in the fundus for continuous recording of intragastric pressure. Two small strain gauges were mounted on the surface of the stomach for monitoring of circular smooth muscle contractility of the pyloric region and longitudinal smooth muscle of the greater curvature of the stomach [28]. Rectal temperature was maintained between 37.0 and 37.5°C.

Animals were placed in a stereotaxic frame and the dorsal surface of a medulla and obex were exposed by an occipital craniotomy. Five-barrelled glass micropipettes (FHC, Brunswick, ME; 20 µm total external tip diameter) were used in all experiments. The micropipette tip was stereotaxically placed in the nROb (co-ordinates: 0.7 mm rostral to the obex, 0.0 mm lateral from the midline, and 1.3 down from the surface of the brain at the level of the obex). All microinjections (vehicle, agents and 1% pontamine sky blue) were delivered in a volume of 30 nl (30 psi) using a pneumatic pico-pump model PV 830 (World Precision Instruments, New Haven, CT). At the end of each experiment the animals were perfused transcardially, and the brains were removed for later histological determination of the injection sites, as described in detail elsewhere [2].

Substance P (Bachem California, Torrance, CA) was dissolved in 0.9% saline containing 0.2% ascorbic acid (as an antioxidant); VIP (American Peptide Co., Sunnyvale, CA) was dissolved in 0.9% saline with 0.01% bovine serum albumin. The doses of SP and VIP were chosen to produce submaximal gastric responses on the basis of our previous study using a range of doses [11,17]. Bicuculline methiodide (BMI, 0.4

mg/kg sc), a $GABA_A$ receptor antagonist, or vehicle (0.9% saline) were administered 60 min before repeat microinjections of vehicle, SP and VIP into the nROb.

The area of the response in intragastric pressure for each treatment was calculated using a microcomputer-based imaging system, as described in detail elsewhere [28]. In addition, the peak change in intragastric pressure relative to preinjection levels was calculated. Contractility of the pyloric circular muscle and the fundus longitudinal muscle was expressed as minute motility index (MMI), as described in detail elsewhere [28].

The differences between groups were assessed by one-way repeated measures analysis of variance (ANOVA) followed by Student–Newman–Keuls test. However, due to the failure of the normality test, the changes in greater curvature contractility in response to VIP treatment were evaluated with Friedman repeated measures ANOVA on ranks. Values of $p < 0.05$ were considered statistically significant.

RESULTS

Figure 1 shows the effects of SP (135 pmol) microinjected into the nROb before and after BMI on intragastric pressure, expressed as both peak change from the baseline and the area of the response, as well as on pyloric and greater curvature contractility. Microinjection of SP into the nROb elicited a significant decrease in both peak and total area of the response of intragastric pressure when compared with the effect of vehicle. Pyloric, but not greater curvature, contractility was also significantly reduced. Repeated microinjections of SP into the nROb in the same animals 60 min after administration of BMI resulted in small changes in intragastric pressure and pyloric motility that did not differ from the effect of vehicle.

Chart recordings from a representative experiment where SP (135 pmol) was microinjected into the nROb before and after BMI are shown in Figure 2. In this particular animal, BMI completely blocked the inhibitory effect of SP on gastric motor function.

Figure 3 illustrates the effect of VIP (100 pmol) microinjected into the nROb before and after BMI on intragastric pressure and gastric contractility. Microinjection of VIP into the nROb significantly decreased intragastric pressure and pyloric motility. Repeated microinjection of VIP (100 pmol) into the nROb 60 min after peripheral administration of BMI did not influence the effect of peptide on intragastric pressure. The inhibitory effect of VIP in the nROb on the contractility of pyloric smooth muscle did not attain statistical significance when compared with the effect of vehicle; however, the changes in pyloric contractility in response to VIP before and after BMI did not differ from each other.

Figure 4 shows a chart recording from a representative experiment which illustrates that after microinjection of VIP (100 pmol) into the nROb there was a decrease in intragastric pressure and inhibition of pyloric contractility. The inhibitory effect of VIP on intragastric pressure was even more evident when repeated after peripheral administration of BMI.

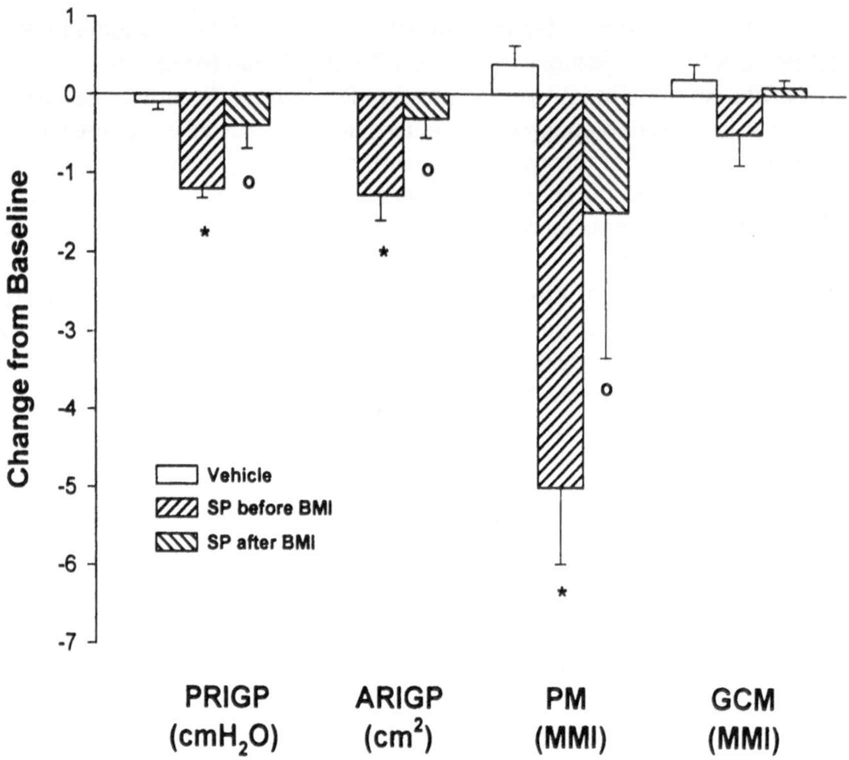

Figure 1. Effects of vehicle or SP (135 pmol), microinjected into the nROb before and after bicuculline methiodide (BMI), on intragastric pressure (PRIGP, peak response; ARIGP, area of the response), pyloric circular muscle (PM), and greater curvature longitudinal muscle (GCM) contractility. Data are mean (bar = SE) changes from baseline for number of animals indicated in the histogram. *Statistically significant when compared with the effect of vehicle; °Statistically significant when compared with the effect of SP

DISCUSSION

In the present paper, we confirm that SP and VIP in the nROb have inhibitory effects on gastric motor function in α-chloralose-anaesthetized rats [11,17] and show that the central inhibitory effect of SP (but not VIP) on intragastric pressure and circular muscle contractility in the pyloric region of the stomach is mediated via peripheral $GABA_A$ receptors.

We have reported previously that neither atropine, VIP-antagonist nor NO synthase inhibitor alone could abolish the inhibitory effect of SP in the nROb on gastric tone and contractility [13]. However, as we have shown in this study, blockade of $GABA_A$ receptors is sufficient alone to prevent the gastric motor effects of SP in the nROb.

There is ample evidence that the GABA is a neurotransmitter in the enteric nervous system [18,29,30]. GABA has been localized within nerve bundles innervating the circular muscle layer of the gastrointestinal tract [18,31–33]. Also, GABA receptors are

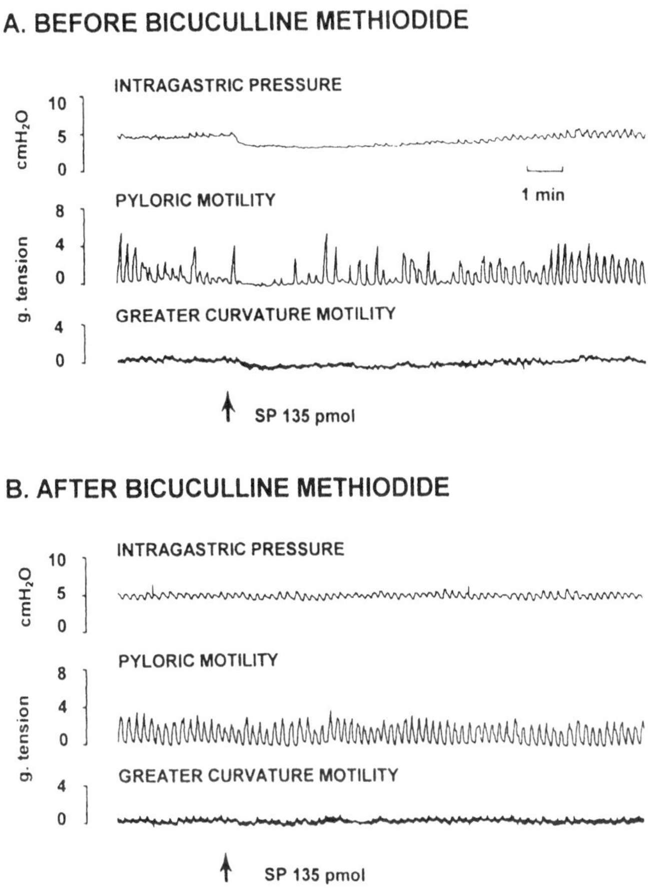

Figure 2. Representative chart recording of one experiment in which SP (135 pmol) was microinjected into the nROb before (**A**) and after (**B**) bicuculline methiodide (BMI). **A**: SP evoked a decrease in intragastric pressure and pyloric circular muscle contractility. **B**: after BMI, no discernible gastric responses to SP were noted

present on myenteric nerves and in this way GABA modulates the motor innervation of the gastrointestinal tract [29,34]. GABA is believed to control the motility of the gastrointestinal tract through cholinergic neurons [30,35] and central GABAergic mechanism [36,37]. Nonetheless, little is known regarding the mechanism of GABA action in the control of gastric motor function. At low concentration, GABA was considered to bind to high-affinity $GABA_A$ receptor on the cholinergic neurons, causing the release of acetylcholine that evoked contraction of the smooth muscle. At high concentrations ($>10^{-10}$ mol/L), GABA binds to both high affinity $GABA_A$ receptors on the cholinergic neurons and low affinity $GABA_A$ receptors on the smooth muscle, resulting in its contraction [18]. However, GABA also inhibits both release of

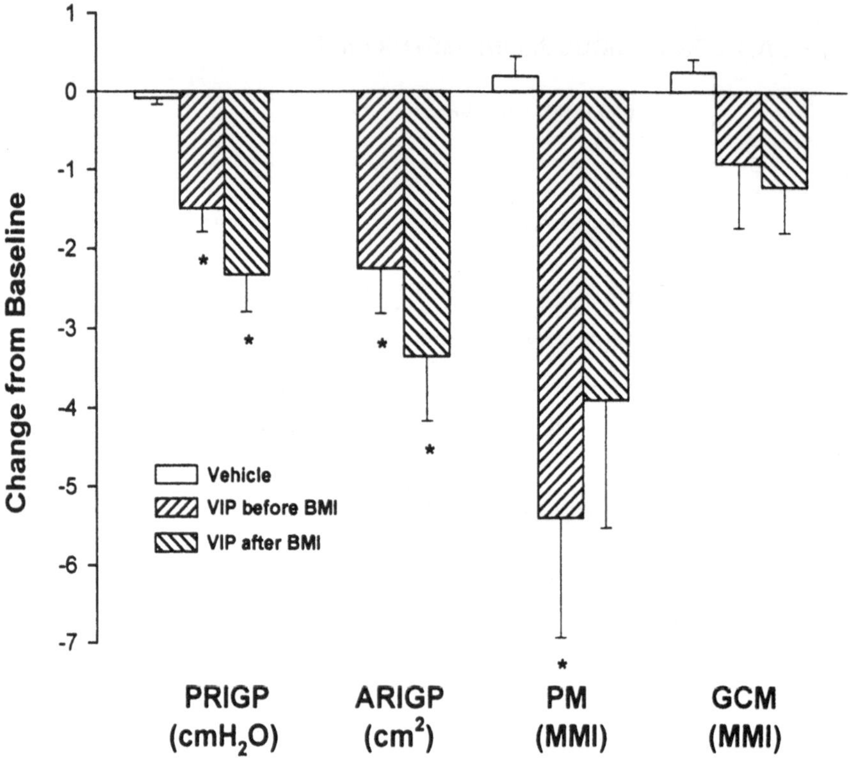

Figure 3. Effects of vehicle or VIP (100 pmol), microinjected into the nROb before and after peripheral administration of bicuculline methiodide (BMI), on intragastric pressure (PRIGP, peak response; ARIGP, area of the response), pyloric circular muscle (PM), and greater curvature longitudinal muscle (GCM) contractility. Data are mean (bar = SE) changes from baseline for number of animals indicated in the histogram. *Statistically significant when compared with the effect of vehicle

acetylcholine and intestinal smooth muscle contractions evoked by electrical stimulation. This inhibitory effect of GABA is not antagonized by bicuculline or picrotoxin and is, therefore, not mediated through $GABA_A$ receptors [38]. Thus, $GABA_B$ receptors of the enteric nervous system are believed to be responsible for the presynaptic inhibition of cholinergic excitatory neurons resulting in gastrointestinal relaxation [39]. It has been shown that both cholinergic and adrenergic receptors are involved in the postsynaptic regulation of GABA release. Specifically, acetylcholine inhibits K^+-evoked release of [^{3}H]GABA from the isolated small intestine [40].

Krantis and co-workers [41] have recently demonstrated that the blockade of $GABA_A$ receptors significantly reduces or even abolishes antral relaxations in the anaesthetized rat in a manner similar to the effect of a NO synthase inhibitor and NO-mediated relaxations of the gastroduodenum are targeted by GABA [26]. Therefore, we

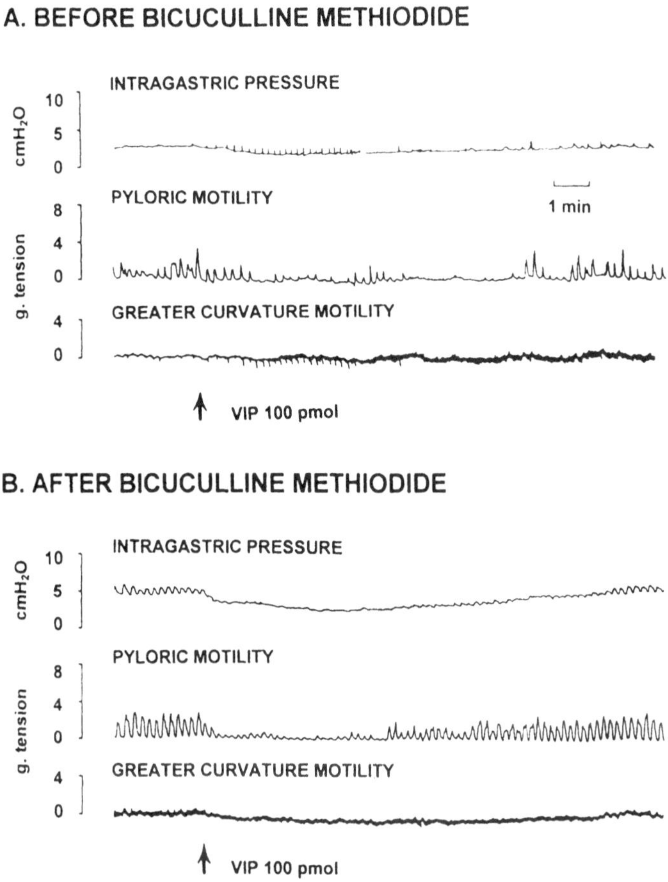

Figure 4. Representative chart recording of one experiment in which VIP (100 pmol) was microinjected into the nROb before (**A**) and after (**B**) bicuculline methiodide (BMI). **A**: VIP evoked a decrease in intragastric pressure and inhibited pyloric muscle contractility. **B**: BMI did not change gastric relaxation in response to VIP

conclude that SP in the nROb must activate NO pathways that are dependent on $GABA_A$ receptor activation as well as presynaptic inhibition of acetylcholine. The peripheral pathways and mechanism of VIP in the nROb-induced gastric relaxation is not elucidated by the present study. Since relaxant activity occurring in the rat gastroduodenum in vivo can be distinguished by its dependence upon either NO (A-GABAergic mediated) or adenosine 5′-triphosphate (ATP) [41], it is possible that VIP mediated in the nROb gastric relaxation involves ATP. Further experiments are needed to test this hypothesis. Nonetheless, we hope that our communication adds a new scope to the understanding of the involvement of GABA in vagally mediated gastric relaxation.

ACKNOWLEDGEMENTS

This work was supported by the National Institute of Diabetes and Digestive and Kidney Diseases, Grant DK-42714 to P.J. Hornby and, in part, by the Louisiana State University Neuroscience Center of Excellence Incentive Grant to Z.K. Krowicki.

REFERENCES

1. Hornby PJ, Rossiter C, White RL, Norman WP, Gillis RA. Caudal medullary raphe neurons modulate gastric motility via projections to the dorsal nucleus of the vagus in the cat. Am J Physiol. 1990;258:G637–47.
2. Krowicki ZK, Hornby PJ. Serotonin microinjected into the nucleus raphe obscurus increases intragastric pressure in the rat via a vagally mediated pathway. J Pharmacol Exp Ther. 1993;265:468–76.
3. McCann MJ, Hermann GE, Rogers RC. Nucleus raphe obscurus (nRO) influences vagal control of gastric motility in rats. Brain Res. 1989;486:181–4.
4. White RL Jr, Rossiter CD, Hornby PJ, Harmon JW, Kasbekar DK, Gillis RA. Excitation of neurons in the medullary raphe increases gastric acid and pepsin production in cats. Am J Physiol. 1991;260:G91–6.
5. Rogers RC, Kita H, Butcher LL, Novin D. Afferent projections to the dorsal motor nucleus of the vagus, a horseradish peroxidase histochemical study. Brain Res Bull. 1980;5:365–73.
6. Krowicki ZK, Hornby PJ. Hindbrain neuroactive substances controlling gastrointestinal function. In: Gaginella TS, ed. Regulatory Mechanisms in Gastrointestinal Function. Boca Raton: CRC Press, Inc.; 1995:277–319.
7. Kachidian P, Poulat P, Marlier L, Privat A. Immunohistochemical evidence for the coexistence of substance P, thyrotropin-releasing hormone, GABA, methionine-enkephalin, and leucine-enkephalin in the serotonergic neurons of the caudal raphe nuclei – a dual labeling in rat. J Neurosci Res. 1991;30:521–30.
8. Hornby PJ, Ruiz C. Hindbrain substance P afferents to the gastric region of the nucleus raphe obscurus of rats. Gastroenterology. 1993;104:A522.
9. Nakaya Y, Kaneko T, Shigemoto RN, Mizuno N. Immunohistochemical localization of substance P receptor in the central nervous system of the adult rat. J Comp Neurol. 1994;347:249–74.
10. Mantyh PW, Gates T, Mantyh CR, Maggio JE. Autoradiographic localization and characterization of tachykinin receptor binding sites in rat brain and peripheral tissues. J Neurosci. 1989;9:258–79.
11. Krowicki ZK, Hornby PJ. Opposing gastric motor responses to TRH and substance P on their microinjection into nucleus raphe obscurus of rats. Am J Physiol. 1993;265:G819–30.
12. Krowicki ZK, Hornby PJ. The inhibitory effect of substance P on gastric motor function in the nucleus raphe obscurus is mediated via nitric oxide in the dorsal vagal complex. J Auton Nerv Syst. [In press].
13. Krowicki ZK, Hornby PJ. Nitric oxide synthase inhibition reduces the effect of substance P microinjected into the nucleus raphe obscurus on intragastric pressure in the rat. Soc Neurosci Abstr. 1993;19:960.
14. Palkovits M, Leranth C, Eiden LE, Rotsztejn W, Williams TH. Intrinsic vasoactive intestinal polypeptide (VIP)-containing neurons in the baroreceptor nucleus of the solitary tract in the rat. Brain Res. 1982;244:351–5.
15. Sims KB, Hoffman DL, Said SI, Zimmerman EA. Vasoactive intestinal polypeptide (VIP) in mouse and rat brain: An immunocytochemical study. Brain Res. 1980;186:165–83.
16. Roberts GW, Woodhams PL, Bryant MG, Crow TJ, Bloom SR, Polak JM. VIP in the rat brain: Evidence for a major pathway linking the amygdala and hypothalamus via the stria terminalis. Histochemistry. 1980;65:103–19.
17. Krowicki ZK, Arimura A, Hornby PJ. Opposing gastric motor responses to vasoactive intestinal polypeptide (VIP) and pituitary adenylate cyclase-activating polypeptide (PACAP) on their microinjection into nucleus raphe obscurus (nRO) of the rat. Acta Neurobiol Exp. 1995;55(Suppl.):Abstract 57.
18. Tsai LH, Tsai W, Wu JY. Action of myenteric GABAergic neurons in the guinea pig stomach. Neurochem Int. 1993;23:187–93.

19. Nichols K, Staines W, Wu J-Y, Krantis A. Immunopositive GABAergic neural sites display nitric oxide synthase-related NADPH diaphorase activity in the human colon. J Auton Nerv Syst. 1995;50:253–62.
20. Erdo SL, Bowery NG. GABAergic Mechanisms in the Mammalian Periphery. New York: Raven Press; 1986.
21. Allescher H-D, Daniel EE. Role of NO in pyloric, antral, and duodenal motility and its interaction with other inhibitory mediators. Dig Dis Sci. 1994;39:73S–5S.
22. Barbier AJ, Lefebvre RA. Involvement of the L-arginine:nitric oxide pathway in nonadrenergic noncholinergic relaxation of the cat gastric fundus. J Pharmacol Exp Ther. 1993;266:172–8.
23. Martinez V, Jiminez M, Gonalons E, Vergara P. Mechanism of action of CCK in avian gastroduodenal motility: Evidence for nitric oxide involvement. Am J Physiol. 1993;265:G842–50.
24. Rodriguez-Membrilla A, Martinez V, Jiminez M, Gonalons E, Vergara P. Is nitric oxide the final mediator regulating the migrating myoelectric complex cycle? Am J Physiol. 1995;268:G207–14.
25. Meulemans AL, Helsen LF, Schuurkes JA. Role of NO in vagally-mediated relaxations of guinea-pig stomach. Naunyn Schmiedebergs Arch Pharmacol. 1993;347:225–30.
26. Krantis A, Glasgow I. Relaxations of the rat gastroduodenum in vivo occur within distinct patterns and utilise different transmitters. Gastroenterology. 1995;108:A632.
27. Krantis A, Glasgow I. Interplay of VIP, NO and GABAergic mechanisms in relaxations of the rat antrum *in vivo*. Gastroenterology. 1995;108:A631.
28. Krowicki ZK, Hornby PJ. Serotonin and thyrotropin-releasing hormone do not augment their effects on gastric motility on their microinjection into the nucleus raphe obscurus of the rat. J Pharmacol Exp Ther. 1995;273:499–508.
29. Kaplita PV, Waters DH, Triggle DJ. Gamma-aminobutyric acid action in guinea-pig ileal myenteric plexus. Eur J Pharmacol. 1982;79:43–51.
30. Taniyama K, Saito N, Miki Y, Tanaka C. Enteric gamma-aminobutyric acid-containing neurons and the relevance to motility of the cat colon. Gastroenterology. 1987;93:519–25.
31. Krantis A. Selective uptake of gamma-[^{3}H]aminobutyric acid by neural elements and vascular nerves of the rat intestinal submucosa. Neurosci Lett. 1990;109:1–6.
32. Krantis A, Webb T. Autoradiographic localization of [^{3}H]gamma-aminobutyric acid in neuronal elements of the rat gastric antrum and intestine. J Auton Nerv Syst. 1989;29:41–8.
33. Krantis A, Tufts K, Morris GP. [^{3}H]GABA uptake and GABA localization in mucosal endocrine cells of the rat stomach and colon. J Auton Nerv Syst. 1994;47:225–32.
34. Kerr DIB, Ong J. GABAergic mechanisms in the gut. Their role in the regulation of gut motility. In: Erdo SL, Bowery NG, eds. GABAergic Mechanisms in the Mammalian Periphery. New York: Raven Press; 1986:153–74.
35. Tanaka C. Gamma-aminobutyric acid in peripheral tissues. Life Sci. 1985;37:2221–35.
36. Greenwood B, DiMicco JA. Activation of the hypothalamic dorsomedial nucleus stimulates intestinal motility in rats. Am J Physiol. 1995;268:G514–21.
37. Sivarao DV, Krowicki ZK, Hornby PJ. Microinjection of bicuculline methiodide into the nucleus ambiguus and the nucleus raphe obscurus increases intragastric pressure in rats. Gastroenterology. 1995;108:A1007.
38. Kleinrok A, Kilbinger H. Gamma-aminobutyric acid and cholinergic transmission in the guinea-pig ileum. Naunyn-Schmiedeberg's Arch Pharmacol. 1983;322:216–20.
39. Ong J, Kerr DIB. $GABA_A$- and $GABA_B$-receptor-mediated modification of intestinal motility. Eur J Pharmacol. 1983;86:9–17.
40. Hashimoto S, Tanaka C, Taniyama K. Presynaptic muscarinic and α-adrenoreceptor-mediated regulation of GABA release from myenteric neurones of the guinea-pig small intestine. Br J Pharmacol. 1986;89:787–92.
41. Krantis A, Glasgow I, Johnson F. Within the multiple inhibitory innervations of the rat gastroduodenum, GABAergic neurones target nitric oxide (NO) related motor pathways. Gastroenterology. 1995;108:A632

Manuscript received 3 Nov. 95.
Accepted for publication 9 Nov. 95.

TS Gaginella et al. (eds.), Biochemical Pharmacology as an Approach to Gastrointestinal Disorders, 141–167

PATHOLOGICAL BASIS AND CLINICAL ASPECTS OF OESOPHAGEAL MOTOR DISORDERS

J. LONOVICS[1*] AND L. SIMON[2]
[1]First Department of Medicine, Albert Szent-Györgyi Medical University, Szeged;
[2]Division of Gastroenterology, Szekszárd County Hospital, Szekszárd, Hungary
*Correspondence

ABSTRACT

Among oesophageal motility disorders gastro-oesophageal reflux disease (GORD) affects a substantial number of population, whereas other motility disturbances including achalasia, hypertensive lower oesophageal sphincter, diffuse oesophageal spasm, and nutracker oesophagus occur relatively rarely. GORD is a complex motility disorder affecting the upper gut, which results in a pathologic reflux of gastric and intestinal contents to the oesophagus. Hypomotility changes involve both the oesophagus and the lower oesophageal sphincter (LOS), as well as the stomach. Pharmacologic basis of oesophageal motility disorder is not clearly understood, an improper release of acetylcholine or a vagally-mediated noncholinergic nonadrenergic inhibitory mechanism (candidate neurotransmitters are vasoactive intestinal peptide (VIP) and nitric oxide (NO)) is suspected. Failure of the motility defense mechanisms and tissue resistance of the oesophagus will lead to the development of symptoms and morphological alterations, e.g. reflux oesophagitis. In the development of atypical symptoms such as non-cardiac chest pain and respiratory complications, local factors, aspiration of the refluxed material and a vagally mediated coronary or bronchial spasm may be involved. Achalasia or cardiospasm is characterized by lack of relaxation of the LOS and loss of peristalsis in the lower two-thirds of the oesophagus. Motility disorder is caused mainly be denervation of postganglionic non-cholinergic non-adrenergic inhibitory neurons, resulting in a marked impairment of both acetylcholine and VIP or NO release. On the contrary, hypertensive LOS is characterized by increasing resting LOS pressure associated with normal sphincter relaxation and oesophageal peristalsis. In diffuse oesophageal spasm simultaneous or repetitive non-propagating contractions are recorded, while in nutcracker oesophagus manometry shows a pattern of high-amplitude but peristaltic contractions. In spastic motility disorders neural dysfunction may involve both afferent (sensory) and efferent fibres resulting in exaggerated response of the oesophagus to cholinergic stimulation. Nonspecific oesophageal motility disorders are associated with broad spectrum of manometric abnormalities including frequent nontransmitted contractions, retrograde contractions, low amplitude contractions, prolonged duration of peristaltic waves, and isolated incomplete LOS relaxation and their clinical significance is yet unknown.

Keywords: oesophageal motor disorders, gastro-oesophageal reflux disease, achalasia, diffuse oesophageal spasm, nutcracker oesophagus

INTRODUCTION

During the past two decades, there has been remarkable progress in methodology for the study of oesophageal motility in experimental animals, as well as in humans. Experimental studies have revealed basic mechanisms involved in the control of motor function of the oesophagus, while application of precise intraluminal pressure measurements, radiological techniques, particularly cineradiography and radionuclide

This paper was presented at the Section of IUPHAR GI Pharmacology Symposium on 'Biochemical pharmacology as an approach to gastrointestinal disorders (basic science to clinical perspectives)', October 12–14, 1995, Pécs, Hungary.

scintigraphy have expanded our understanding of oesophageal motility disorders and their relationships with symptoms. Unfortunately, research in this area has been hampered by the inability to gather pathological specimens of muscle and nerves in diseases that are not life threatening. Many tools are available now for evaluating oesophageal function to assist in the diagnosis of patients with oesophageal motility disorders; however, to provide adequate treatment, understanding of the pathophysiological bases of these disorders is of the utmost importance.

NORMAL MOTILITY PATTERN OF THE OESOPHAGUS

Normal motility pattern of the oesophagus represents a peristaltic movement, which is propagating distally and, by reaching the lower oesophageal sphincter (LOS), induces relaxation. Peristaltic reflex, which results in an aborally propagating oesophageal muscle contraction, is initiated by swallowing or by intraluminal distension. Peristalsis, a co-ordinated propulsive movement of the circular and longitudinal muscles, consists of a contraction front, which is preceeded by a relaxation that propels the bolus in an aboral direction. The contraction front consists of a contraction of circular muscle and relaxation of longitudinal muscle behind the bolus, whereas receptive relaxation is the result of contraction of the longitudinal muscle and relaxation of the circular muscle. The tonically contracted ring of circular muscle that forms the LOS relaxes in response to swallowing. This relaxation is followed by a transient contraction, also called hypercontraction [1–4].

Neurohumoral control of oesophageal peristalsis

Peristaltic movement of the oesophagus is controlled by a complex neural mechanism, which is modulated by peptidergic and hormonal effects. Neural regulation is exercised at three levels:

1. The enteric nervous system (ENS), composed of the myenteric and submucosal plexuses;
2. The extrinsic preganglionic parasympathetic motor neurons that synapse with secondary (postganglionic) nerve cells in the myenteric plexus, the postganglionic sympathetic nerves, passing from the superior cervical ganglion in some species and from cervical and thoracic, as well as celiac ganglia, in others, which terminate in the myenteric and submucous plexus and in relation to blood vessels;
3. The central nervous system through the autonomic nervous system's parasympathetic and sympathetic connections.

Afferents arising in the oesophagus enter the ENS ganglia, the sympathetic prevertebral ganglia and the CNS via the vagus and sympathetic nerves. The system also receives extra-intestinal input through gastrointestinal hormones and neuropeptides. All this information is integrated into commands that act through the smooth muscle cell activity to produce the motility pattern described above [1,5–7].

The terminal motor innervation to the smooth muscle of the oesophagus arises from cell bodies in the myenteric ganglia, making them postganglionic nerves [8,9]. Numerous non-peptide and potential peptide neurotransmitters have been identified in axons coursing through the smooth muscle [10–15]. To date, two non-peptide substances, acetylcholine and nitric oxide (NO), are the only proven neurotransmitters released from these neurons, which play a basic role in the development of oesophageal peristalsis [3,16–23]. These mediators may act directly on smooth muscle cell membranes or their effect may be transferred by interstitial cells of Cajal, which are located between neurons and smooth muscle and make gap junctions with adjacent smooth muscle cells.

Peristaltic reflex may be elicited by swallowing (primary peristalsis) or by oesophageal distension (secondary peristalsis). The swallowing centre plays an important role in the initiation of oesophageal peristalsis, while its organization into a progressing front of contraction depends entirely on a programming mechanism within the oesophagus [24–27]. The electrophysiological events in the smooth muscle of the oesophagus that underlie peristaltic contractions in vivo are well described [28,29]. Both swallowing and vagal nerve stimulation result in a prompt hyperpolarization of the circular smooth muscle membrane potential along the length of the smooth muscle oesophagus. This hyperpolarization is followed by a transient depolarization of the plasma membrane that is associated with a burst of smooth muscle spike potentials, which result in oesophageal contraction. The progressive nature of the peristaltic contraction depends, therefore, on the timing of the depolarization and spike potentials. The timing of these excitatory events appears, in turn, to be determined by the preceding membrane hyperpolarization.

There is strong evidence that membrane hyperpolarization, which elicits delayed contractions ('off contraction' or an 'off response') following a latency period is induced by NO synthesized in the non-adrenergic non-cholinergic (NANC) nerves within the myenteric plexus [16,17,30–32], since inhibitors of NO synthesis attenuate the nerve-induced hyperpolarization, the depolarization, and the off contraction in a dose-dependent manner. In the membrane depolarization and generation of peristaltic contractions, the cholinergic pathway plays a role since atropine decreases the amplitude of peristaltic contractions produced by swallowing, vagal stimulation or intrinsic nerve stimulation [3,20–23]. Earlier studies suggested that cholinergic nerve activity is responsible for controlling the timing of peristalsis in the proximal portion of the smooth muscle oesophagus [22,23]. Neither the timing nor the progression of these off contractions, at any level of the smooth muscle oesophagus, was changed, however after muscarinic receptor blockade by atropine, whereas inhibitors of NO synthesis shortened the time between swallowing and the appearance of peristaltic contractions, and resulted in nearly simultaneous contractions [19]. These results indicate that NO, produced in response to nerve stimulation, plays an important role in the genesis and the timing of the off contraction [16,17]. Oesophageal peristalsis, therefore, is the result of an NO-induced event that programs the appearance of acetylcholine-evoked spike potentials. The cellular mechanisms that underlie nerve-induced hyperpolarization of the circular oesophageal smooth muscle are debated. One body of evidence supports the hypothesis that both intrinsic nerve stimulation and exogenous NO hyperpolarize the plasma membrane by increasing potassium ion conductance [34–37]. Other evidence supports the hypothesis that intrinsic nerve stimulation results in a decrease in chloride ion conductance [38]. Smooth muscle spike potentials result in the opening of plasma membrane calcium channels and the inward movement of calcium ions. This by raising the free cytosolic calcium ion concentration, activates the contractile machinery and produces contraction of the circular muscle. The off contraction of circular oesophageal muscle depends upon this mechanism and upon the extracellular calcium [39,40]. Thus, the depolarization and spike potentials are the electrophysiological correlates of the off contractions.

The basic motility pattern of the oesophagus is modulated by extrinsic innervation as well as by CNS. Parasympathetic innervation is predominantly stimulatory, whereas sympathetic innervation is inhibitory [1].

Neurohumoral control of the lower oesophageal sphincter

LOS is a tonically contracted muscle ring located at the distal end of the oesophagus. The increased tone of the LOS depends mainly upon the intracellular pool of calcium, since depletion of intracellular calcium stores in the absence of extracellular calcium leads to the loss of LOS tone. This tone may be modulated both by neural and hormonal influences. Cholinergic and sympathetic nerves supplying this region are both excitatory [24,41–43]. Gastrin, substance P and motilin all increase the tone of the sphincter [44–46], while the effect of dopamine is inhibitory [47]. The prostaglandins have been postulated as participants in the determination of LOS pressure [48] and, certainly, many prostanoids can affect the sphincter. They are thought to be responsible for the low sphincter tone that occurs in the presence of experimentally induced oesophagitis.

The relaxation of the sphincter induced by swallowing and by other manoeuvres, such as oesophageal distention, clearly neurogenic. Axons of the postganglionic inhibitory neurons terminate within the circular muscle of the LOS where they release an inhibitory neurotransmitter, almost certainly NO, that mediates LOS relaxation [16,17,19,31]. The electrophysiological correlate of LOS relaxation, whether caused by swallowing, vagal nerve stimulation or electrical stimulation of intrinsic nerves, is hyperpolarization of the smooth muscle membrane [28,49,50]. This hyperpolarization differs somewhat from that recorded from neighbouring oesophageal muscle in that it is not followed by membrane depolarization.

At least two neuropeptides, VIP and calcitonin gene-related peptide, have also been proposed as neurotransmitters that may mediate LOS relaxation in response to nerve stimulation, but their physiological roles have not yet been established [11,12,51,52].

There are other bioactive substances capable of relaxing the LOS, but many of them are not yet demonstrated in oesophageal innervation. Some may act through oesophageal inhibitory innervation as paracrine or endocrine agents. These include cholecystokinin, somatostatin, glucagon, some prostaglandins, dopamine, the female sex hormones, secretin, neurotensin and gastric inhibitory peptide [1,47,53–55].

GASTRO-OESOPHAGEAL REFLUX DISEASE

Gastro-oesophageal reflux disease (GORD) and reflux oesophagitis are broad terms used to describe pathological events related to the exposure of the oesophagus or oropharynx to gastric content. Simple gastro-oesophageal reflux occurs physiologically but, due to effective oesophageal clearance activity, the oesophagus–gastric juice exposure time is rather short and does not result in morphological damage or clinical symptoms. In sharp contrast, GORD involves more frequent (pathological) reflux which may lead to the development of endoscopically observable damage to oesophageal tissue (reflux oesophagitis etc.) and characteristic clinical symptoms (heartburn etc.). Although simple gastro-oesophageal reflux, GORD and reflux oesophagitis can be regarded as lying on a continuum, these terms should not be confused with each other. GORD is considered to be a separate clinical entity, caused by a complex motility disorder of the oesophagus and LOS (and sometimes the stomach), whereas reflux oesophagitis is simply one of the morphological consequences of GORD [56].

The clinical picture presented by the patient with GORD is highly variable. The majority of patients with GORD have occasional or chronic but mild symptoms, such as heartburn, with no objective evidence of the disorder and these patients rarely seek medical assistance. The other group of patients who do seek physician's help have more troublesome and frequent symptoms and will evidence some degree of objective pathology on examination. Finally, a group of patients described as 'the tip of the iceberg' have chronic persistent symptoms, associated with serious complications [57].

It seems that symptoms of GORD affect a large proportion of the population. However, proper statistical information on the epidemiology of GORD and reflux oesophagitis is limited for the reasons described above.

Pathogenesis of GORD

GORD is the result of disturbed motility of oesophagus and LOS, which enables gastric or intestinal contents to reflux into the oesophagus. Motility disorder affects mainly the LOS, although impaired oesophageal clearance or delayed gastric emptying may also contribute to the development of pathological reflux. GORD, therefore, is a multifactorial disease whose initiating event is a true motility disorder that leads to the reflux of gastric contents into the oesophageal lumen. Reflux oesophagitis and symptoms develop in susceptible persons due to prolonged contact between oesophageal epithelium and noxious substances in the refluxate. In healthy subjects, there is a three-tiered defence system, including antireflux barrier, luminal clearance mechanisms, and tissue resistance, which protects oesophagus against noxious gastric content. Failure of the *defence mechanisms* described above allows gastric and intestinal contents (*offence mechanisms*) to reflux into the oesophagus and leads to the development of symptoms and morphological alterations.

Defence mechanisms

Antireflux barriers: These barriers, which protect the oesophagus by limiting the frequency and volume of refluxate entering the lumen, include the LOS, the intra-abdominal segment of the oesophagus, the diaphragmatic crura, the phrenoesophageal ligament, the mucosal rosette, and the acute angle of His [58]. The major antireflux barrier is the high-pressure zone of approximately 10–30 mmHg at the gastro-oesophageal junction. The high-pressure zone is generated predominantly by contraction of the LOS. In resting states, the high-pressure zone due to LOS contraction creates a barrier to the transfer of acid–pepsin from stomach to oesophagus. However, since reflux occurs in everyone, the LOS is an imperfect barrier. In healthy subjects, this imperfection is due to phenomenon known as transient LOS relaxation (TLOSR). In GORD, the antireflux barrier may become insufficient by three mechanisms:

1. Increase in the frequency of TLOSRs (spontaneous reflux) is the main mechanism that leads to pathological reflux into the oesophagus. TLOSRs are spontaneous non-swallow-initiated events that permit reflux by obliterating the high-pressure zone by way of a vagally mediated NANC mechanism; the candidate neurotransmitters are VIP or NO [59,60]. The increased frequency of reflux noted after meals is probably the result of gastric distention, inducing more frequent TLOSRs permitting gas to be vented from the stomach. In healthy individuals the entry of reflux into the oesophagus is almost immediately followed by an increase or no change in the contractility of the oesophageal body that may inhibit acid reflux into the oesophagus. In GORD patients the contraction of the oesophagus decreases in response to the reflux, favouring the rise of the acid in the oesophageal body during TLOSRs, which suggests that GORD may ensue at least in part from a failure in the excitatory (cholinergic) pathway [61].
2. Stress reflux results from a transient increase in intra-abdominal pressure that creates enough force to overcome the poor squeeze of the otherwise competent LOS [62,63].
3. Free reflux can occur any time when LOS tone is low or absent. The mechanisms responsible for impaired LOS contractility have not yet been established. LOS incompetence could be a primary neuromuscular defect or, alternatively, a secondary defect, i.e. the result and not the cause of reflux oesophagitis [64,65].

Hiatus hernia: The relationship between sliding hiatus hernia and GORD remains controversial. Once considered synonymous, now they clearly are not. Most subjects with hernias do not have reflux oesophagitis, while most subjects with oesophagitis, particularly when severe, do have hernias, suggesting that sliding hernias may be the consequence, rather than the cause, of reflux oesophagitis [66–70].

Luminal clearance mechanism: The second tier in oesophageal defence against reflux damage is luminal clearance. In healthy individuals, pH in the oesophagus is rapidly normalized after acid reflux. Two components account for this effect: neutralization by saliva and clearance by oesophageal peristalsis. In patients with GORD, abnormalities in clearance mechanisms, peristaltic dysfunctions (impairment of both primary and secondary peristalsis) and reduced salivary flow have all been demonstrated [56,57,71]. It is very important to emphasize that, during sleep, oesophageal clearance is virtually inoperative. Thus, due to prolonged acid–oesophagus contact time, the oesophageal mucosa is completely unprotected at night [72,73].

Tissue resistance: This is a group of oesophageal structure/functions that interact to prevent or minimize epithelial damage from noxious luminal contents [71]. They are subdivided into pre-epithelial (mucus–unstirred water layer–bicarbonate complex) epithelial (membranes and intercellular junctions, bicarbonate secretion and ability to extrude H^+ ions), and postepithelial (blood flow) defences. Tissue resistance in the oesophagus is weaker than that in the stomach. Therefore, these defence mechanisms are unable to protect oesophageal mucosa when pathological reflux occurs.

Offence mechanisms

Composition and potency of refluxate: The substances found in the stomach that can contribute to the noxious quality of the refluxate include: hydrochloric acid, pepsin, bile salts and pancreatic enzymes. The overwhelming majority of subjects with GORD secrete acid and have acidic refluxate. Although oesophagitis is more frequent in acid hypersecretory states, such as Zollinger–Ellison syndrome, hyperacidity itself does not necessarily lead to the development of reflux oesophagitis unless oesophageal defences are impaired. The main problem in GORD is that, due to disturbed motility, acid occurs in the wrong place, that is in the oesophagus where resistance to acid is limited. Neutral or alkaline reflux is rather rare and mainly occurs in postgastrectomy patients or persons who have atrophic gastritis or pernicious anaemia, where the major injurious agents are deconjugated bile salts and pancreatic enzymes [74].

Clinical manifestations

Oesophageal symptoms

1. Heartburn: the most common symptom, characterized by retrosternal burning and discomfort or pain, which is exacerbated by hydrogen ions or by spicy or fried food.

2. Waterbrash: heartburn with bitter taste and sensation of excess mucus secretion in the pharynx.

3. Dysphagia: difficulty in swallowing.

4. Odynophagia: pain in swallowing; occurs mainly in patients with severe erosive (infectious) oesophagitis.

5. Globus: 'lump in the throat' sensation induced by high acid reflux.

6. Belching: noisy voiding of gas from the stomach through the mouth [72,75].

Non-oesophageal signs and symptoms

1. Non-cardiac chest pain is an angina-like pain caused by acid stimulation of pain receptors or acid-induced spasm of the oesophagus. In ischaemic heart disease, real coronary spasm may be induced by reflux oesophagitis through a vagal reflex arch.

2. Respiratory complications: Regurgitation and aspiration is a sensation of fluid in the pharynx or airways, associated with choking or cough. Aspiration may cause apnoea and sudden death in infants. In adults, respiratory tract involvement (asthma with wheezing and dry coughing, pneumonitis, nocturnal choking, morning hoarseness) is due to acid stimulation in damaged mucosa that elicits bronchoconstriction directly or by a vagal route [72,75,76].

Patients with GORD can present with a variety of symptoms, described above, that may range from mild and intermittent to severe and persistent. Neither the type of symptom nor their severity correlates well with the degree of injury to the oesophagus. Just as reflux symptoms vary widely among patients, the course of the disease is also variable. In some patients, symptoms may remit spontaneously without treatment. In others, symptoms may be intractable despite treatment, and complications may develop. It is important to emphasize that serious complications, including Barrett's oesophagus, strictures, bleeding etc., may develop even in those patients who are relatively asymptomatic [72,75].

Complications of GORD

Stricture

Repetitive, prolonged exposure to acid refluxate can cause transmural inflammation and consequent fibrosis of the oesophageal wall with loss of compliance and/or development of frank stricture in approximately 10% of patients with severe GORD [72]. The risk of stricture formation is increased in patients with Barrett's oesophagus or with oesophageal motor dysfunction.

Haemorrhage

Insidious blood loss is more common in GORD than frank haemorrhage. It results from either diffuse ulcerative oesophagitis or, more often, from a single penetrating ulcer. It is generally associated with inflamed hiatus hernia or Barrett's oesophagitis.

Perforation

This is a rare complication in GORD, generally occuring in patients with severe oesophagitis associated with Zollinger–Ellison syndrome or Barrett's oesophagus.

Barrett's oesophagus

Barrett's oesophagus can be a serious complication of GORD because of its malignant potential. In this condition, the normal squamous epithelial cell lining of the oesophagus is replaced by metaplastic columnar-type epithelium during cell regeneration initiated when the oesophagus is injured by reflux. The incidence of adenocarcinoma in patients with Barrett's oesophagus is estimated to be 30–40 times higher than in the general population. In addition, Barrett's oesophagus is frequently associated with stricture or ulcer [72,77,78].

Oesophageal cancer

Barrett's metaplasia and chronic reflux oesophagitis have been implicated as contributing to an increased risk of oesophageal adenocarcinoma. Nearly all patients with adenocarcinoma have Barrett's metaplasia. Therefore, screening endoscopy for the early detection of dysplasia in Barrett's metaplasia is highly recommended since it may identify malignant transformation at a stage that will permit curative resection in time [77].

Diagnostic studies

Barium studies

Oesophagography yields little information in mild cases of GORD. However, in moderate to severe cases, it may detect thickened oesophageal folds and strictures. Radiography can also demonstrate the presence and size of a hiatus hernia and screen for oesophageal, stomach and duodenal abnormalities [68].

Endoscopy and biopsy

Endoscopy is a very accurate diagnostic tool when GORD is associated with reflux oesophagitis and can be conveniently performed as an outpatient procedure [79]. Diagnostic accuracy of endoscopy can be improved by histological examination of a biopsy specimen. Tissue biopsy is also required to confirm Barrett's oesophagus, which is suggested macroscopically by reddened tongues of columnar epithelium extending up the oesophagus. Endoscopy also permits staging of GORD based on objective findings. Among different classifications of reflux oesophagitis, the Savary–Miller classification is the most widely accepted. Reflux oesophagitis is divided into four categories:

Stage I: Linear erosions that remain solitary;

Stage II: Confluent erosions, occupying a considerable part of the circumference but not yet circular;

Stage III: Circular erosions and/or ulcerations, occupying the whole of the circumference;

Stage IV: Deep ulcerations resulting in peptic stricture and associated with fibrous atrophy or endobrachyoesophagus.

In approximately 30–50% of cases of GORD, no macroscopic changes are detected by endoscopy; this is often described as Stage 0.

Continuous intraoesophageal pH monitoring

Due to its superb specificity, 24-h monitoring of oesophageal pH levels 5 cm above the oesophagogastric junction has become increasingly accepted as a major method for diagnosis of GORD [72]. Reflux can be evaluated at near-physiological conditions because the patient is supplied with portable equipment and is permitted to sleep, drink and eat. It provides information on number, severity and timing of reflux episodes (evaluation is based upon rapid computerized data analysis which allows generation of different scoring systems to describe pathological reflux, e.g. the DeMeester score) and the success of treatment. In addition, abnormal continuous pH monitoring results have been used to confirm reflux as a cause of pulmonary symptoms and of angina-like pain [80].

Acid infusion testing

Based on a proven correlation between oesophageal acid infusion and oesophagitis symptoms and the provocation of heartburn, the Bernstein acid infusion test helps to determine whether symptoms originate in the oesophagus.

Radionuclide scintiscanning

Radionuclide techniques have been developed for evaluating reflux, gastric emptying and oesophageal function [80–82]. The technique is not as sensitive as acid reflux testing; however, it is more reliable in detecting reflux than barium studies and is the simplest way to demonstrate pulmonary aspiration which is otherwise difficult to assess [83]. Oesophageal transit and clearance can also be measured by scintigraphy.

Oesophageal manometry

Manometry measures basal pressure at the LOS and the body of the oesophagus. Sphincter relaxation, after-contraction and peristalsis are assessed by measurements taken after liquid is swallowed [84]. Manometry is not part of routine evaluation. Nevertheless, manometry can be important, notably in averting the performance of inappropriate antireflux surgery and in identifying associated or unassociated abnormalities in oesophageal motility [72].

Medical management

The goals of treatment in GORD are to relieve subjective complaint, to heal oesophagitis and to prevent recurrence. These goals may be achieved by reducing exposure of the oesophagus to acid. Although acid exposure of the oesophagus can be reduced surgically, the vast majority of patients should initially be managed medically. Medical management can be separated into two categories: (a) lifestyle modifications and (b) drug therapy. Both therapies work to either reduce the noxious potency of the refluxate or increase the effectiveness of oesophageal defences (i.e. antireflux barrier, clearance mechanisms, epithelial resistance). Although GORD is considered to be pirmarily a motility disorder, historically, reduction of the potency of acidic refluxate first became the therapy of choice. Prokinetic agents that are capable of stimulating oesophageal clearance and gastric emptying, as well as increasing the tone of LOS, were introduced later.

Lifestyle changes

Initial therapy should include simple lifestyle modifications that can produce meaningful long-term results in mild or even moderate cases. Desirable lifestyle modifications include: at least a 6-inch elevation of the head of the bed, dietary modifications (low-fat diet, small-size meals), avoidance of irritants (citrus juices, tomato products, coffee, tea, alcohol, peppermint etc.), weight loss if overweight, avoidance of bending and clothing that constricts, and avoidance of medication that inhibits motility or relaxes LOS (anticholinergics, sedatives, tranquilizers, theophylline, prostaglandins, calcium channel blockers etc.). Patients should be advised not to lie down after meals and to decrease or stop smoking and alcohol consumption [85–87].

Drug therapy

Antacids and alginates: Antacids or antacid–alginate combinations are often the first choice in managing mild to moderate symptoms in GORD since they provide quick symptomatic relief in most patients [84,88,89]. However, neither of these substances promotes histological evidence of healing.

Histamine H_2-receptor antagonists: In clinical practice, H_2-receptor antagonists, including cimetidine, ranitidine, nizatidine and famotidine, have gained the greatest acceptance in the treatment of GORD because of their potency to achieve effective acid neutralization when properly applied [84]. Dosing of H_2-receptor antagonists in GORD strikingly differs from that in ulcer disease. In ulcer disease, night-time administration is usually appropriate in most patients; however, in GORD, 24-h acid neutralization (i.e. maintenance of the pH at a level consistently above the critical threshold of 4) is required. In proper dose-distribution (two or four times daily), H_2-blockers not only provide fast symptom relief but also promote significant healing in reflux oesophagitis [90].

Proton pump inhibitors: Proton pump inhibitors (omeprazole, lansoprazole and pantoprazole) which block the H^+/K^+ pump within the parietal cell have recently been added to the armamentarium of GORD treatment. Because of its potent inhibition of acid production, omeprazole has proved outstandingly successful in treating even severe resistant cases of reflux oesophagitis. Results of several clinical trials [91,92] show omeprazole to be superior to ranitidine for short-term treatment of GORD, with endoscopic evidence of healing in 88–96% of patients after an eight-week course. Indications for its use appear to be erosive or more severe ulcerative complications of GORD.

Prokinetic drugs: These include metoclopramide, domperidone and cisapride. Through varying mechanisms and to varying degrees, they increase LOS tone, accelerate gastric emptying and improve oesophageal clearance. Although all of them provide significant symptomatic relief in the various forms of GORD, with the exception of cisapride, they failed to achieve significant histological and endoscopic improvement. In a double-blind trial, cisapride (10 mg qid), which stimulates $5HT_4$ receptors at the level of the myenteric plexus, proved to be equivalent to ranitidine (150 mg bid) in improving objective findings [93]. Therefore, cisapride monotherapy has been approved in the treatment of milder forms of reflux oesophagitis. Cisapride, which provides a causative therapy in GORD, has increasingly been recommended in combination with both H_2-blockers and proton pump inhibitors. Erythromycin, a macrolide antibiotic, has been shown to initiate migrating motor complexes through the stimulation of motilin receptors and is considered to be the first member of a new prokinetic family (members are called motilides). Erythromycin has been used to promote gastric emptying in patients with diabetic gastroparesis [94]; however, elucidation of the prokinetic activity of the other synthetic motilide analogues awaits future studies.

Sucralfate: Sucralfate, a polysaccharide sulphate that has long been used as an antiulcer drug, has been tried in GORD. Surprisingly, it failed to achieve improvement in stage I or stage II oesophagitis but it exerted a significant healing effect in stage III oesophagitis.

Maintenance therapy: Recurrence of symptoms of GORD is common; up to one third of patients may relapse within six months. Therefore, maintenance therapy (often life-long) may be required. Maintenance treatment with a conventional dose of H_2-blockers is often disappointing. However, high-dose therapy with these drugs does lower the relapse rate. There is evidence that cisapride also prevents relapses, and the use of this prokinetic drug for maintenance therapy seems to be promising. In severe relapse, however, it is often necessary to opt for maintenance treatment with omeprazole or other proton pump inhibitors [84,87,90–93].

Dilatation of peptic strictures

Peptic strictures in the oesophagus can generally be easily dilated. Several endoscopic techniques are available, that can be performed on an outpatient basis with a significant success rate. It should be emphasized that, following a successful dilatation of a stricture, its cause, namely pathological reflux, must also be treated.

Surgical intervention

Patients requiring surgery represent a relatively small percentage of patients with GORD. Intractable symptoms or rapid relapse when therapy is discontinued suggests the need for surgery in this group. Patients with complications of GORD should also be evaluated for surgery. Surgery, such as the Nissen fundoplication or Belsey procedure, is indicated in patients with persistent chest pain, bleeding, chronic aspiration, intractable asthma, stricture formation or dysplastic Barrett's oesophagus. Some patients object strongly to the idea of long-term medication; they prefer an operation. A gradual increase in the demand for antireflux surgery has already been seen, especially in young patients, and a further increase can be expected when a laparoscopic surgical approach becomes readily available.

ACHALASIA

Achalasia, or cardiospasm, was the first motor disorder of the oesophagus to be recognized clinically [95]. In this disease, there is a double defect in oesophageal function. The LOS does not appropriately relax, offering resistance to the flow of liquids and solid materials from the oesophagus into the stomach. In addition, there is a loss of peristalsis in the lower two thirds of the smooth muscle portion of the oesophagus. Therefore, both the outflow tract and the pumping mechanism of the oesophagus are abnormal in achalasia.

Achalasia usually presents in persons between 25 and 60 years of age but onset in childhood is also well documented [96]. Most studies find that men and women are affected equally. Achalasia is uncommon but not rare. A study from the British Isles estimated a prevalence of 10 cases of achalasia per 100 000 population [97].

Pathophysiology

Abnormalities in both muscle and nerve components can be detected in achalasia, although the neural lesion is thought to be of primary importance. Three major neuroanatomical changes have been described:

1. Loss of ganglion cells within the myenteric plexus;

2. Degeneration of the vagus nerve; and

3. Qualitative as well as quantitative changes in the dorsal motor nucleus of the vagus.

Of these three findings, the loss of ganglion cells is best substantiated. Along with the destruction of ganglion cells, there is a reduction in nerve fibres within the wall of the oesophagus in achalasia [98,99].

It has been postulated that postganglionic neurons that mediate LOS relaxation are selectively damaged in achalasia. Immunohistochemical studies have demonstrated a marked reduction in VIP staining in neurons as well as a reduction in the concentration of VIP in the lower oesophagus of achalasia patients [100]. In view of the potent smooth-muscle-relaxing effects of VIP, this could account for the incomplete relaxation of the LOS characteristic of achalasia. Because peristalsis in the smooth-muscle portion of the oesophagus is triggered by an initial phase of inhibition by NANC postganglionic neurons, selective destruction of these inhibitory neurons in achalasia could conceivably explain aperistalsis as well [101].

Neurophysiological studies have confirmed the presence of denervation of the smooth-muscle segment of the oesophagus in patients with achalasia. Muscle strips from the circular layer of the oesophageal body in achalasia contract if directly stimulated by acetylcholine but not in response to ganglionic stimulation by nicotine. Similarly, strips from the LOS do not relax in response to ganglionic stimulation in achalasia patients but they do in normal controls [102]. Further evidence of denervation is shown by the exaggerated response of the oesophageal body and the LOS to a sympathetic acetylcholine, mecholyl [103,104]. This heightened response has been interpreted as evidence of denervation hypersensitivity. While pathological damage to inhibitory neurons is well documented, recent studies have suggested that postganglionic cholinergic stimulatory fibres to the LOS may be spared in achalasia. The LOS pressure in achalasia increases after administration of the acetylcholinesterase inhibitor, edrophonium, and decreases after administration of the muscarinic antagonist, atropine [105].

Clinical features

Cardinal symptoms of achalasia include dysphagia, regurgitation and chest pain which are associated with weight loss and severe bronchopulmonary complications.

Dysphagia

All patients have solid food dysphagia, with the majority of patients usually having variable degrees of liquid dysphagia [96,106]. The onset of dysphagia is usually gradual, beginning with solids but including liquids intermittently. Patients may report the use of specific manoeuvres, e.g. certain postural manoeuvres, slow deliberate swallowing, use of liquid or carbonated beverages etc., to improve oesophageal emptying [106].

Regurgitation

Regurgitation of undigested food in the oesophagus is a common complaint, occurring in 60–90% of patients with achalasia [106,107]. The material brought up is often recognized as food that has been eaten many hours previously. Typically, patients note food or saliva backing up in the mouth while they are asleep. Regurgitated food and saliva may end up on the pillowcase or sometimes in the trachea, producing severe bouts of coughing or choking [108].

Chest pain

Chest pain is reported by one third to one half of patients with achalasia and tends to improve with the course of the disease [96,106]. Chest pain is often precipitated by eating, can awaken the patient at night, and may be so severe that it is confused with chest pain evoked by ischaemic heart disease.

Heartburn

Between 25% and 45% of patients with achalasia may complain of symptoms compatible with heartburn [96,106]. The pyrosis, however, is not caused by acid reflux but rather results from the production of lactic acid by bacterial fermentation of retained food in the oesophagus [109]. This explains why heartburn in achalasia is not improved by antacids or H_2 antagonists.

Weight loss

Weight loss is very common and usually increases with the duration of the disease. It may be the best historic parameter for assessing the severity of achalasia and usually correlates with the degree of oesophageal emptying before and after treatment [106].

Bronchopulmonary complications

Approximately 10% of achalasia patients may have significant bronchopulmonary complications as a result of regurgitation of material from the oesophagus [110]. Patients with oesophageal symptoms of long duration may actually come to medical attention because of pulmonary complications. Organisms involved most commonly are aerobic and anaerobic oropharyngeal flora, which are aspirated, leading to bronchitis, bronchial pneumonia or lung abscess.

Diagnostic approach

Achalasia is suspected from characteristic symptoms and the diagnosis is usually not difficult. Early cases, however, may be misdiagnosed if the diagnosis is based mainly upon radiographic studies, which at this time, fails to reveal oesophageal dilatation or marked distortion of the LOS.

Radiographic studies

Radiographic studies are the primary screening test in patients with achalasia. Plain film may outline the widened mediastinum as well as pulmonary infiltrates in long-standing achalasia. The barium swallow may reveal the dilated oesophagus, the lack of peristalsis and the LOS relaxation.

Endoscopy

Endoscopic examination is always required to exclude neoplastic processes. Typical endoscopic findings include dilatation and atony of the oesophageal body with normal mucosa. The LOS does not open with air insufflation; however, the instrument should easily pass through the sphincter into the stomach with gentle pressure.

Oesophageal manometry

The diagnosis of achalasia should always be established by oesophageal manometry. This is particularly important if radiographs are normal or inconclusive. Four manometric features are characteristics of achalasia: absence of peristalsis in the distal smooth muscle segment of the oesophageal body, incomplete or abnormal LOS relaxation, elevated LOS pressure, and elevated intraoesophageal pressures relative to the gastric baseline [111].

Radionuclide studies

Radiolabelled liquid or solid test meal studies show an adynamic pattern because the material lies in the atonic oesophagus. A similar finding may be seen in malignant obstruction. Therefore, these tests lack the specificity of manometry and have not been widely used.

Treatment

Due to the irreversible nature of neural lesions, treatment is directed at palliation of the symptoms and prevention of complications. This is mainly accomplished by reducing LOS pressure by three modalities: drug therapy, forceful dilatation and surgical myotomy.

Pharmacotherapy

A number of drugs acting on LOS smooth muscle have been tried with inconsistent results. The most experience has been reported with isosorbide dinitrate and the calcium channel blocker, nifedipine [112–114].

The sublingual use of isosorbide dinitrate, 5–10 mg before meals, has been shown to decrease mean resting LOS pressure, the relaxation lasting at least 90 min. Long-term therapy for up to 19 months results in marked relief of dysphagia [112]. After 20 mg nifedipine sublingually, LOS pressure was reduced by 30–40% [113,114]. In placebo-controlled clinical studies, excellent results have been reported with long-term nifedipine administration by Italian groups [115,116]. However, results from other groups showed only minimal clinical improvement [117,118].

Two new treatment modalities have been applied recently. Low-frequency transcutaneous electric nerve stimulation (TENS) has been shown to alleviate the dysphagia in achalasia patients probably by releasing VIP [119]. A preliminary report demonstrated that endoscopic intrasphincteric injection of botulinum toxin totally relieved symptoms and markedly improved objective markers of delayed emptying in 80% of achalasia patients for up to 6 months [120].

Since the results of pharmacotherapy are inconsistent, the mainstay of therapy remains oesophageal dilatation and surgical myotomy. Gastroenterologists should be aware of this fact and, if an initial trial of pharmacotherapy fails to induce convincing improvement, endoscopic dilatation and/or surgical myotomy should be indicated before the development of a marked oesophageal dilatation and severe bronchopulmonary complications.

SPASTIC MOTILITY DISORDERS OF THE DISTAL OESOPHAGUS

In addition to GORD and achalasia, a variety of new oesophageal motility disorders have been recognized, particularly in patients with non-cardiac chest pain syndromes. Manometric patterns of these disorders are characterized by normal peristalsis intermittently interrupted by simultaneous contractions, high-amplitude or long-duration waves, or dysfunction of the LOS. There has been great confusion in the literature as to whether these manometric abnormalities represent separate distinct entities or variations of diffuse oesophageal spasm. It seems appropriate to accept the latter possibility. According to this concept, diffuse oesophageal spasm has recently been split into four categories: diffuse oesophageal spasm, nutcracker oesophagus, hypertensive LOS and a group of non-specific oesophageal motility disorders [121–124]. It was suggested that these manometric disorders should be grouped under the general term spastic motility disorders of the distal oesophagus [125].

Pathophysiology

The most striking gross change reported in the spastic motility disorders of the oesophagus is diffuse muscular thickening, mainly of the lower two thirds of the oesophagus [126,127]. However, there are well-documented cases of these motility disorders in which thickening was not found at thoracotomy [128].

Little specific evidence of neuropathology has been reported. In contrast to achalasia, loss of ganglion cells in the intramural plexus has not been demonstrated in these disorders. However, some patients with diffuse oesophageal spasm have exhibited changes in the vagus nerve which were much more diffuse than those reported for patients with achalasia [127].

Despite little evidence of neuropathology, physiological studies suggest that there may be some neural dysfunction. In these disorders, the oesophagus is particularly sensitive to cholinergic stimulation, which produces an exaggeration of abnormal manometric findings in many patients [129–131]. An impaired NANC inhibitory neural mechanism and an imbalance between excitatory and inhibitory innervation was also suggested to play a role in the development of the motility changes seen in these spastic disorders. However, some of the motor abnormalities described above are also seen in healthy subjects in response to edrophonium chloride, a cholinesterase inhibitor, and even to normal physiological stimuli [132–134].

Increasing evidence indicates that central nervous system processing could participate and produce some of these spastic manometric abnormalities. Psychologically stressful interviews may produce simultaneous and repetitive contractions in normal subjects that resemble the described contraction abnormalities [135]. Perception of these manometric abnormalities, however, differs strikingly between normal subjects and patients suffering from psychiatric disorders, particularly anxiety disorders, panic attacks, depression or somatization disorders [136].

A model has recently been proposed to explain the possible role of the central nervous system in the interaction between the motility disorders and pain perception, that is, in symptom development [111,125]. According to this model, the location of pathology (disease locus) is not known but appears to include both a motor component and a sensory component. These two limbs may not be involved equally in all cases and can be stimulated independently by various manoeuvres. Balloon distension studies have been shown to reproduce pain at low distending volumes without noticeable motor changes in these patients [137], while, in others, high distending volumes did not provoke any subjective complaints. This evidence for lower visceral pain thresholds suggests that a sensory disorder may play an important role in pathological pain perception in some patients. In this model, the oesophageal contraction abnormalities may only be markers or epiphenomena for the disease and may only occasionally provoke the sensory limb.

Manometric features

The manometric features of the spastic motility disorders are restricted to the smooth-muscle portion of the oesophagus, particularly the distal segment proximal to the LOS. The motility findings of these disorders are discussed as if they were separate entities so as to emphasize specific manometric features and their prevalence. However, this segregation may be artificial because the spastic motility disorders are quite variable, changing patterns from day to day and even from hour to hour.

Diffuse oesophageal spasm

The clinical syndrome of diffuse oesophageal spasm was first described by Hamilton Osgood in 1889 [see Reference 138]. Characteristic manometric findings in diffuse oesophageal spasm include simultaneous contractions, repetitive contractions, high-amplitude contractions, contractions of prolonged duration, and abnormalities of the LOS, which consist of incomplete sphincter relaxation or hypertensive sphincters [125]. Simultaneous waves, usually in the distal oesophagus, are mixed with normal peristaltic sequences, showing that the oesophagus has not completely lost its ability to produce propagating contractions and thereby suggesting a partial or intermittent effect [111].

Nutcracker oesophagus

In 1977, Brand and associates reported that 41% of non-cardiac chest pain patients with abnormal oesophageal manometry showed a pattern of high-amplitude peristaltic contractions [123]. Two years later, Benjamin and colleagues confirmed these observations and coined the term nutcracker oesophagus [139]. Nutcracker oesophagus is a descriptive term for the manometric findings in a patient with chest pain or dysphagia characterized by average distal oesophageal peristaltic pressures greater than two standard deviations above a well-documented normal range. The average peristaltic pressure (mean of 10 wet swallows) may exceed 180 mmHg. These extremely strong peristaltic waves can be shown to respond appropriately to pharmacological agents that attenuate oesophageal contractions, such as atropine, or nitrates.

Hypertensive lower oesophageal sphincter

The presence of an excessively high resting LOS was first described in 1960 by Code and colleagues at the Mayo Clinic [140]. Although many of these patients had other oesophageal motility abnormalities (particularly diffuse oesophageal spasm), approximately 50% showed only isolated abnormalities of the LOS, characterized by increased resting LOS pressures associated with normal sphincter relaxation and normal peristalsis. A subsequent report also found excessively large and prolonged contractions of the sphincter after relaxation, a phenomenon called hypercontracting sphincter [141].

Non-specific oesophageal motility disorders

Oesophageal contraction patterns that are outside the range of normal findings but that do not readily fit into the previously described categories have been classified into the general category of non-specific oesophageal motility disorders. These miscellaneous manometric abnormalities include frequent non-transmitted contractions, retrograde contractions, low-amplitude contractions, prolonged duration peristaltic waves and isolated incomplete LOS relaxation [142].

Clinical features

Spastic disorders of the oesophagus appear at any age; the mean age of presentation is approximately 40 years. In contrast to achalasia, a female predominance seems to be present in most studies [122,143]. The cardinal symptoms of spastic oesophageal motility disorders are dysphagia and chest pain. Patients often present with a combination of both symptoms. The prevalence of chest pain is constant across the various spastic disorders but the prevalence and severity of dysphagia increase as patients have more manometric features consistent with classic diffuse oesophageal spasm [143].

Dysphagia

Dysphagia for liquids and solids is present in 30–60% of patients with spastic motility disorders [122,143]. The symptom is intermittent in nature, varying on a daily basis from mild to very severe, and there may be periods of relatively normal swallowing. Dysphagia is usually not progressive or severe enough to interfere markedly with eating or to produce weight loss.

Chest pain

Intermittent anterior chest discomfort is reported by 80–90% of patients with spastic motility disorders [122,143]. Chest pain is usually described as squeezing, is substernal in location, and may radiate into the back, neck, jaw or arms, making it sometimes indistinguishable from angina. Pain episodes may last from minutes to hours. Relief of symptoms may require narcotics or nitroglycerin, further confusing the distinction between oesophageal and cardiac pain.

The mechanism producing pain in these spastic motility disorders is poorly understood. A popular hypothesis is that oesophageal motility disorders produce chest pain as a result of high intramural oesophageal tension that inhibits blood flow for a critical time period [130]. However, the arterial blood supply to the oesophagus is extensive [144] and it is unlikely that oesophageal blood flow could be critically compromised by local contractions. Furthermore, chest pain improvement does not predictably correlate with amplitude reduction of contractions by pharmacotherapy [145] or surgical myotomy [146]. Since the relationship between chest pain and motor abnormalities does not appear to be causal, an altered pain perception with a lower visceral pain threshold may play an important role in symptom development.

Heartburn

Heartburn is present in as many as 20% of patients with spastic motility disorders [143]. Some of them may concurrently have GORD [123,147] or acid reflux may be the primary cause of their motility disorders [148].

Diagnosis

Although spastic motility disorders are defined by oesophageal manometry, the intermittent nature of these abnormalities frequently requires the use of other oesophageal tests, which include: radiological studies, endoscopy, radionuclide studies, different provocative tests with intravenous edrophonium chloride [149], and balloon distension [137], 24-h pH and motility testing [125].

Medical treatment

The most important step in patients with chest pain and spastic motility disorders is to be as certain as possible of its distinction from angina pectoris.

Having excluded ischaemic heart disease, nitrates, calcium-channel blocking agents and psychotropic drugs may be tried. Symptomatic improvement and a manometric response to nitroglycerin has been reported [150]. However, no controlled studies with nitrates are available in patients with spastic oesophageal motility disorders.

A dramatic dose–response effect on oesophageal contractions has been reported in patients with nutcracker oesophagus with nifedipine therapy [151] but double-blind placebo-controlled studies with calcium-channel blockers have been disappointing [145].

A double-blind placebo-controlled study has provided evidence that anxiolytic or antidepressant agents may alter visceral pain perception and may evoke significant symptom relief [152].

Oesophageal dilatation

In selected cases with spastic motility disorders, oesophageal dilatation may promote transient symptom relief from dysphagia or chest pain [153].

Surgical myotomy

If dysphagia becomes so severe that weight loss is observed or if pain is unbearable, surgical relief, usually Heller myotomy, should be considered [146].

REFERENCES

1. Conklin JL, Christensen J. Motor function of the pharynx and esophagus. In: Johnson LR, ed. Physiology of the Gastrointestinal Tract. New York: Raven Press; 1994:903–28.
2. Humphries TJ, Castell DO. Pressure profile of esophageal peristalsis in normal humans as measured by direct intraesophageal transducers. Am J Dig Dis. 1977;22:641–5.
3. Dodds WJ, Christensen J, Dent J, Wood JD, Arndorfer RC. Esophageal contractions induced by vagal stimulation in the opossum. Am J Physiol. 1978;235:E392–E401.
4. Sugarbaker DJ, Rattan S, Goyal RK. Swallowing induces sequential activation of esophageal smooth muscle during peristalsis. Am J Physiol. 1984;247:G515–19.
5. Baumgartner MG, Lange W. Adrenergic innervation of the oesophagus in the cat (Felis domestica) and rhesus monkey (Macacus rhesus). Z Zellforsch. 1969;95:529–45.
6. Geboes K, Desmet V. Histology of the esophagus. Front Gastrointest Res. 1978;3:1–17.
7. Jacobowitz D, Nemir P. The autonomic innervation of the esophagus of the dog. J Thorac Cardiovasc Surg. 1969;58:678–84.
8. Gabella G. Innervation of the gastrointestinal tract. Int Rev Cytol. 1979;59:129–93.
9. Furness JB, Costa M. The enteric nervous system. Edinburgh: Churchill Livingstone; 1986.
10. Christensen J, Rick GA, Robinson BA, Stiles MJ, Wix MA. The arrangement of the myenteric plexus throughout the gastrointestinal tract of the opossum. Gastroenterology. 1983;85:890–9.
11. Alumets J, Fahrenkrug J, Hákanson R, Schaffalitsky de Muckadell OB, Sundler F, Uddman R. A rich VIP nerve supply characteristic of sphincters. Nature. 1979;280:155–6.
12. Christensen J, Williams TH, Jew J, O'Dorisio TM. Distribution of vasoactive intestinal polypeptide-immunoreactive structures in the opossum esophagus. Gastroenterology. 1987;92:1007–18.
13. Singaram C, Sengupta A, Sugarbaker DJ, Goyal RK. Peptidergic innervation of the human esophageal smooth muscle. Gastroenterology. 1991;101:1256–63.
14. Wattchow DA, Furness JB, Costa M, O'Bryen PE, Peacock M. Distribution of neuropeptides in the human esophagus. Gastroenterology. 1987;93:1363–71.
15. Rodrigo J, Polak JM, Fernandez I, Ghatei MA, Muldberry P, Bloom SR. Calcitonin gene-related peptide immunoreactive sensory and motor nerves of the rat, cat, and monkey esophagus. Gastroenterology. 1985;88:444–51.
16. Murray J, Du C, Ledlow A, Bates JN, Conklin JL. Nitric oxide: mediator of nonadrenergic noncholinergic responses of oppossum esophageal muscle. Am J Physiol. 1991;261:G401–6.

17. Du C, Murray J, Bates J, Conklin JL. Nitric oxide: mediator of nonadrenergic hyperpolarization of opossum esophageal muscle. Am J Physiol. 1991;261:G1012–16.
18. Knudsen MA, Svane D, Tottrup A. Importance of the L-arginine-nitric oxide pathway in NANC nerve function in the opossum esophageal body. Dig Dis Sci. 1991;9:365–70.
19. Yamato S, Spechler SJ, Goyal RK. Role of nitric oxide in esophageal peristalsis in the opossum, Gastroenterology. 1992;103:197–204.
20. Dodds WJ, Christensen J, Dent J, Wood JD, Arndorfer RC. Pharmacological investigation of primary peristalsis in smooth muscle portion of opossum esophagus. Am J Physiol. 1979;237:E561–6.
21. Dodds WJ, Dent J, Hogan WJ, Arndorfer RC. The effect of atropine on esophageal motor function in man. Gastroenterology. 1978;74:1028.
22. Crist J, Gidda JS, Goyal RK. Intramural mechanisms of esophageal peristalsis: roles of cholinergic and noncholinergic nerves. Proc Natl Acad Sci USA. 1984;81:3595–9.
23. Blank EL, Greenwood B, Dodds WJ. Cholinergic control of smooth muscle peristalsis in the cat esophagus. Am J Physiol. 1989;257:G517–23.
24. Kravitz JJ, Snape WJ, Cohen S. Effect of thoracic vagotomy and vagal stimulation on esophageal function. Am J Physiol. 1966;238:233–8.
25. Ryan JP, Snape WJ, Cohen S. Influence of vagal cooling on esophageal function. Am J. Physiol. 1977;232:159–64.
26. Christensen J. Pharmacologic identification of the lower esophageal sphincter. J Clin Invest. 1970;49:681–91.
27. Christensen J, Lund GF. Esophageal responses to distention and electrical stimulation. J Clin Invest. 1969;48:408–19.
28. Rattan S, Gidda JS, Goyal RK. Membrane potential and mechanical responses to vagal stimulation and swallowing. Gastroenterology. 1983;85:922–8.
29. Sugarbaker DJ, Rattan S, Goyal RK. Mechanical and electrical activity of esophageal smooth muscle during peristalsis. Am J Physiol. 1984;246:G145–50.
30. Murray J, Bates JN, Conklin JL. Nerve-mediated nitric oxide production by the opossum lower esophageal sphincter. Dig Dis Sci. 1994 [in press].
31. Tottrup A, Svane D, Forman A. Nitric oxide mediating NANC inhibition in opossum lower esophageal sphincter. Am J Physiol. 1991;260:G385–9.
32. Christink F, Jury J, Cayabyab F, Daniel EE. Nitric oxide may be the final mediator of non-adrenergic, non-cholinergic inhibitory junction potentials in the gut. Can J Physiol Pharmacol. 1991;69:1448–58.
33. Crist J, Gidda JS, Goyal RK. Characteristics of 'on' and 'off' contractions in esophageal circular muscle in vitro. Am J Physiol. 1984;264:G137–44.
34. Kannan MS, Jager LP, Daniel EE. Electrical properties of smooth muscle cell membrane of opossum esophagus. Am J Physiol. 1985;248:G342–6.
35. Jury J, Jager LP, Daniel EE. Unusual potassium channels mediate nonadrenergic nerve mediated inhibition in opossum esophagus. Can J Physiol Pharmacol. 1985;63:107–12.
36. Sims SM, Vivaudo MB, Hillemeier C, Biancani P, Walsh JV, Singer JJ. Membrane currents and cholinergic regulation of K^+ current in esophageal smooth muscle cells. Am J Physiol. 1990;258:G794–802.
37. Du C, Conklin JL. Inhibitory junction potentials in the opossum esophageal circular muscle of cGMP as an intracellular mediator. Gastroenterology. 1990;98:A347.
38. Crist JR, He XD, Goyal RK. Chloride-mediated inhibitory junction potentials in opossum esophageal circular muscle. Am J Physiol. 1991;261:G752–62.
39. DeCarle DJ, Christensen J, Szabo AC, Templeman DC, McKinley DR. Calcium dependence of neuromuscular events in eosphageal smooth muscle of the opossum. Am J Physiol. 1983;232:E547–52.
40. Biancani P, Hillemeier C, Bitar KN, Maklouf G. Contraction mediated by Ca^{2+} influx in esophageal muscle and Ca^{2+} release in the LES. Am J Physiol. 1987;253:G760–6.
41. Dodds WJ, Stef JJ, Stewart ET, Hogan WJ, Arndorfer RC, Cohen EB. Responses of feline esophagus to cervical vagal stimulation. Am J Physiol. 1978;235:E63–73.
42. Christensen J, Daniel EE. Effects of some autonomic drugs on circular esophageal smooth muscle. J Pharmacol Exp Ther. 1968;159:243–9.
43. Behar J, Kerstein M, Biancani P. Neural control of lower esophageal sphincter (LES) closure. Gastroenterology. 1977;72:1029.
44. Behar J, Biancani P. Effect of cholecystokinin-octapeptide on lower esophageal sphincter. Gastroenterology. 1977;73:57–61.
45. Reynolds JC, Ouyang A, Cohen S. A lower esophageal sphincter reflex involving substance P. Am J Physiol. 1984;246:G346–54.

46. Gutierrez JG, Thanik KD, Chey WY, Yajima H. The effect of motilin on the lower esophageal sphincter of the opossum, Am J Dig Dis. 1977;22:402–5.
47. Rattan S, Goyal RK. Effect of dopamine on the esophageal smooth muscle in vivo. Gastroenterology. 1976;70:377–81.
48. Daniel EE, Crankshaw J, Sarna S. Prostaglandins and tetrodotoxin-intensive relaxation of opossum lower esophageal sphincter. Am J Physiol. 1979;235:E153–72.
49. Zelcer E, Weisbrodt NW. Electrical and mechanical activity of the lower esophageal sphincter in the cat. Am J Physiol. 1984;246:G243–7.
50. Daniel EE, Taylor GS, Holman ME. The myogenic basis of active tension in the lower esophageal sphincter. Gastroenterology. 1976;70:874.
51. Rattan S, Gonella P, Goyal RK. Inhibitory effect of calcitonin gene-related peptide and calcitonin in opossum esophageal smooth muscle. Gastroenterology. 1988; 94:284–93.
52. Goyal RK, Rattan S, Said SI. VIP as a possible neurotransmitter of non-cholinergic, non-adrenergic inhibitory neurons. Nature. 1980;288:378–80.
53. Fischer RS, Dimarinio AJ, Cohen S. Mechanism of cholecystokinin inhibition of lower esophageal sphincter pressure. Am J Physiol. 1975;228:1469–73.
54. Bybee EE, Brown FC, Georges LP, Castell DO, McGuigan JE. Somatostatin effects on lower esophageal sphincter function. Am J Physiol. 1979;237:E77–81.
55. Jaffer SS, Makhlouf GM, Schorr BA, Zfass AM. Nature and kinetics of inhibition of lower esophageal sphincter by glucagon. Gastroenterology. 1974;67:42–6.
56. Nebel OT, Fornes MF, Castell DO. Symptomatic gastroesophageal reflux: Incidence and precipitating factors. Am J Dig Dis. 1976;21:953–6.
57. Castell DO. Introduction to pathophysiology of gastroesophageal reflux. In: Castell DO, Wu WC, Ott DJ, eds. Gastroesophageal Reflux Disease: Pathogenesis, Diagnosis, Therapy. Mt Kisco, NY: Futura Publishing Co., Inc.; 1985:3–9.
58. Heine KJ, Mittal RK. Crural diaphragm and lower esophageal sphincter as antireflux barriers. Viewpoints Dig Dis. 1991;23:1.
59. Tottrup A, Svane D, Forman A. Nitric oxide mediating NANC inhibition in opossum lower esophageal sphincter. Am J Physiol. 1991;23:1.
60. Martin CJ, Patrikios J, Dent J. Abolition of gas reflux and transient lower eosphageal sphincter relaxation by vagal blockade in the dog. Gastroenterology. 1986;91:890.
61. Janssens J, Sifrim D, Lerut A. Esophageal motility disorders: a pathophysiological concept. Gastroenterology. 1995;108:A621.
62. Dodds WJ, Dent J, Hogan WJ et al. Mechanisms of gastroesophageal reflux in patients with reflux esophagitis. N Engl J Med. 1982;307:1547–52.
63. Ott DJ, Katz PO, Wu WC. Anti-reflux barriers. In: Castell DO, Wu WC, Ott DJ, eds. Gastroesophageal Reflux Disease: Pathogenesis, Diagnosis Therapy. Mt Kisco, NY: Futura Publishing Co., Inc; 1985:35–54.
64. Higgs RH, Castell DO, Eastwood GL. Studies on the mechanism of esophagitis-induced lower esophageal sphincter hypotension in cats. Gastroenterology. 1976;71:51.
65. Biancani P, Barwick K, Selling J, McCallum R. Effects of acute experimental esophagitis on mechanical properties of the lower esophageal sphincter. Gastroenterology. 1984;87:8.
66. Kramer P. Does a sliding hiatus hernia constitute a distinct clinical entity? Gastroenterology. 1969;57:442.
67. Wright RA, Hurwitz AL. Relationship of hiatal hernia to endoscopically proved reflux esophagitis. Dig Dis Sci. 1979;24:311–13.
68. Ott DJ, Wu WC, Gelfand DW. Reflux esophagitis revisited: Prospective analysis of radiologic accuracy. Gastrointest Radiol. 1981;6:1–7.
69. Cohen S, Harris ID. Does hiatus hernia affect competence of the gastroesophageal sphincter? N Engl J Med. 1971;284:1053–7.
70. Mittal RK, Lange RC, McGallum RW. Identification and mechanism of delayed esophageal acid clearance in subjects with hiatus hernia. Gastroenterology. 1987;92:130–5.
71. Orlando RC. Reflux esophagitis. In: Yamada T, ed. Textbook of Gastroenterology. Philadelphia: JB Lippincott; 1992:1123–47.
72. Hogan WJ, Dodds WJ. Gastroesophageal reflux disease (reflux esophagitis). In: Sleisinger MH, Fordtran JS, eds. Gastrointestinal Disease: Pathophysiology, Diagnosis, Management. 4th edn. Philadelphia: WB Saunders; 1989:594–619.
73. Kahrilas PJ, Dodds WJ, Hogan WJ, Arndorfer RC, Reece A. Esophageal peristaltic dysfunction in peptic esophagitis. Gastroenterology. 1986;91:897–904.

74. Dubois A. Role of gastric factors in the pathogenesis of gastroesophageal reflux: Emptying, acid and pepsin, bile reflux. In: Castell DO, Wu WC, Ott DJ, eds. Gastroesophageal Reflux Disease: Pathogenesis, Diagnosis, Therapy. Mt. Kisco, NY: Futura Publishing Co., Inc.: 1985:81–97.
75. Soll AH. Duodenal ulcer and drug therapy. In: Sleisinger MH, Fordtran JS, eds. Gastrointestinal Disease: Pathophysiology, Diagnosis, Management. 4th edn. Philadelphia: WB Saunders; 1989:814–79.
76. Mansfield LE, Hameister AA, Spaulding HS, Smith NJ, Glab N. The role of vagus nerve in airway narrowing caused by intraesophageal hydrochloric acid provocation and esophageal distension. Ann Allergy. 1981;47:431–4.
77. Cameron AJ, Ott BJ, Payne WS. The incidence of adenocarcinoma in columnar-lined (Barrett's) esophagus. N Engl J Med. 1985;313(14):857–9.
78. Spechler SJ, Robbins AH, Rubins HB et al. Adenocarcinoma and Barrett's esophagus: An overrated risk? Gastroenterology. 1984;87:927–33.
79. Cotton PB, Shorvon PJ. Analysis of endoscopy and radiography in the diagnosis, follow-up and treatment of peptic ulcer disease. Clin Gastroenterol. 1984;13:383–403.
80. Ravich WJ. The pH probe in the evaluation of gastroesophageal reflux disease. In: Castell DO, Wu WC, Ott DJ, eds. Gastroesophageal Reflux Disease: Pathogenesis, Diagnosis, Therapy. Mt. Kisco, NY: Futura Publishing Co., Inc.: 1985:167–84.
81. Rudd TG, Christie DL. Demonstration of gastroesophageal reflux in children by radionuclide gastroesophagography. Radiology. 1979;131:483–6.
82. Heyman S. Esophageal scintigraphy (milk scans) in infants and children with gastroesophageal reflux. Radiology. 1982;144:891–3.
83. Cowan RJ. Gastroesophageal scintigraphy. In: Castell DO, Wu WC, Ott DJ, eds. Gastroesophageal Reflux Disease: Pathogenesis, Diagnosis, Therapy. Mt. Kisco, NY: Futura Publishing Co., Inc.: 1985:185–207.
84. Waterfall WE, Craven MA, Allen CJ. Gastroesophageal reflux: Clinical presentations, diagnosis and management. Can Med Assoc J. 1986;135:1101–9.
85. Jamieson GG, Duranceau A. Gastroesophageal Reflux. Philadelphia: WB Saunders; 1988:112–21.
86. Castell DO. Overview of treatment of gastroesophageal reflux disease. In: Castell DO, Wu WC, Ott DJ, eds. Gastroesophageal Reflux Disease: Pathogenesis, Diagnosis, Therapy. Mt. Kisco, NY: Futura Publishing Co., Inc.: 1985:211–20.
87. Pace F, Bianchi Porro G. Medical treatment of reflux oesophagitis: Review of traditional therapies and omeprazole. Ital J Gastroenterol. 1988;20(Suppl):23–9.
88. McEvoy GK. AHFS Drug Information 92. Bethesda, MD: American Society of Hospital Pharmacists; 1992:1708–10.
89. Chevrel B. A comparative crossover study on the treatment of heartburn and epigastric pain: Liquid Gaviscon and a magnesium–aluminium antacid gel. J Int Med Res. 1980;8:300–3.
90. Sontag SJ. The medical management of reflux esophagitis: Role of antacids and acid inhibition. Gastroenterol Clin N Am. 1990;19:683–712.
91. Klinkenberg-Knol EC et al. Double-blind multicentre comparison of omeprazole and ranitidine in the treatment of reflux oesophagitis. Lancet. 1987;1:349–51.
92. Vantrappen G, Rutgeerts L, Schurman P, Coenegrachts J-L. Omeprazole (40 mg) is superior to ranitidine in short-term treatment of ulcerative reflux esophagitis. Dig Dis Sci. 1988;33:523–9.
93. Janisch JD, Huttermann W, Bouzo MH. Cisapride versus ranitidine in the treatment of reflux esophagitis. Hepatogastroenterology. 1988;35:125–7.
94. Jansen J, Peeters TL, Vantrappen G et al. Improvement of gastric emptying in diabetic gastroparesis by erythromycin. N Engl J Med. 1990;322:1028–31.
95. Willis T. Pharmacutice rationalis sive diatribe de medicamentorum operationibus in human corpore. London, Hagac. Comitis: A Leers; 1974.
96. Kahrilas PJ, Kishle SM, Helm JF et al. Comparison of pseudoachalasia and achalasia. Am J Med. 1987;82:439.
97. Mayberry JF, Atkinson M. Variations in the prevalence of achalasia in Great Britain and Ireland: an epidemiological study based on hospital admissions. Q J Med. 1987;237:67.
98. Lendrum FC. Anatomic features of the cardiac orifice of the stomach with special reference to cardiospasm. Arch Intern Med. 1937;59:474.
99. Cassella RR, Brown AL Jr, Sayre GP, Ellis F Jr. Achalasia of the esophagus: pathologic and etiologic considerations. Ann Surg. 1964;160:474.
100. Aggestrup S, Uddman R, Sundler F et al. Lack of vasoactive intestinal peptide nerves in esophageal achalasia. Gastroenterology. 1983;84:924.
101. Kimura K. The nature of idiopathic esophagus dilatation. Jpn J Gastroenterol. 1929;1:199.

102. Misiewicz JJ, Wallace SL, Anthony PP, Gummer JW. Achalasia of the cardia: pharmacology and histopathology of isolated cardiac sphincteric muscle from patients with and without achalasia. Q J Med. 1969;38:17.
103. Kramer P, Ingelfinger FJ. Esophageal sensitivity to Mecholyl in cardiospasm. Gastroenterology. 1951;19:242.
104. Heitmann P, Espinoza J, Csendes A. Physiology of the distal esophagus in achalasia. Scand J Gastroenterol. 1969;4:1.
105. Holloway RH, Dodds WJ, Helms JF et al. Integrity of cholinergic innervation of the lower esophageal sphincter in achalasia. Gastroenterology. 1986;90:924.
106. Wong RKH, Johnson LF. Achalasia. In: Castell DO, Johnson LF, eds. Esophageal Function in Health and Disease. New York: Elsevier Biomedical; 1983:99.
107. Olsen AM, Holman CB, Anderson HA. Diagnosis of cardiospasm. Dis Chest. 1953;23:477.
108. Stacher G, Kiss A, Wiesnagrotzki S et al. Oesophageal and gastric motility disorders in patients categorized as having primary anorexia nervosa. Gut. 1986;27:1120.
109. Smart HL, Foster PN, Evans DF et al. Twenty-four hour oesophageal acidity in achalasia before and after pneumatic dilatation. Gut. 1987;28:883.
110. Vantrappen G, Hellmans J, Deloof W et al. Treatment of achalasia with pneumatic dilatation. Gut. 1987;28:883.
111. Castell JA. The computer in the motility laboratory. In: Castell DO, Richter JE, Dalton CB, eds. Esophageal Motility Testing. Amsterdam: Elsevier; 1987:91.
112. Gelfand M, Rozen P, Keren S, Gilat T. Effect of nitrates on LOS pressure in achalasia: a potential therapeutic aid. Gut. 1981;22:312.
113. Gelfand M, Rozen P, Gilat T. Isosorbide dinitrate and nifedipine treatment of achalasia: a clinical, manometric and radionuclide evaluation. Gastroenterology. 1982;83:963.
114. Traube M, Hongo M, Magyar L, McCallum RW. Effects of nifedipine in achalasia and in patients with high-amplitude peristaltic esophageal contractions. J Am Med Assoc. 1984;252:1733.
115. Coccia G, Bortolotti M, Michetti P, Dodero M. Prospective clinical and manometric study comparing penumatic dilatations and sublingual nifedipine in the treatment of oesophageal achalasia. Gut. 1991;32:604.
116. Coccia G, Bortolotti M, Michetti P, Dodero M. Return of peristalsis after nifedipine therapy in patients with idiopathic esophageal achalasia. Am J Gastroenterol. 1992;87:1705.
117. Traube M, Dubovik S, Lange RC, McCallum RW. The role of nifedipine therapy in achalasia: results of a randomized double-blind, placebo-controlled study. Am J Gastroenterol. 1989;84:1259.
118. Triadafilopoulos G, Aaronson M, Sackel S, Burakoff R. Medical treatment of esophageal achalasia. Double-blind crossover study with oral nifedipine, verapamil, and placebo. Dig Dis Sci. 1991;36:260.
119. Guelrud M, Rossiter A, Souney PF, Sulbaran M. Transcutaneous electrical nerve stimulation decreases lower esophageal sphincter pressure in patients with achalasia. Dig Dis Sci. 1991;36:1029.
120. Pasricha PJ, Ravich WJ, Hendrix TR, Kalloo AN. Treatment of achalasia with intrasphinteric injections of botulinum toxin – results of a pilot study. Gastroenterology. 1993;104:A168.
121. Richter JE, Castell DO. Diffuse esophageal spasm: a reappraisal. Ann Intern Med. 1984;100:242.
122. Katz PO, Dalton CB, Richter JE et al. Esophageal testing in patients with non-cardiac chest pain and/or dysphagia. Ann Intern Med. 1987;106:593.
123. Brand DL, Martin D, Pope CE. Esophageal manometrics in patients with angina-like chest pain. Am J Dig Dis. 1977;22:300.
124. Traube M, Abibi R, McCallum RW. High amplitude peristaltic esophageal contractions associated with chest pain. J Am Med Assoc. 1983;250:2655.
125. Richter JE. Motility disorders of the esophagus. In: Yamada T, ed. Textbook of Gastroenterology. Philadelphia: JB Lippincott Company; 1995:1174–213.
126. Gillies M, Nicks R, Skyring A. Clinical, manometric and pathologic studies in diffuse esophageal spasm. Br Med J. 1967;2:527.
127. Ferguson TB, Woodbury JD, Roper CL, Burford TH. Giant muscular hypertrophy of the esophagus. Ann Thorac Surg. 1969;8:209.
128. Ellis FH, Olsen AM, Schlegel JF, Code CF. Surgical treatment of esophageal hypermotility disturbances. J Am Med Assoc. 1964;188:862.
129. Kramer P, Fleshler B, McNally E, Harris LD. Oesophageal sensitivity to Mecholyl in symptomatic diffuse spasm. Gut. 1967;8:120.
130. Mellow M. Symptomatic diffuse esophageal spasm. Manometric follow-up and response to cholinergic stimulation and cholinesterase inhibition. Gastroenterology. 1977;73:237.
131. Nostrant TT, Saves J, Haber T. Betanechol increases the diagnostic yield in patients with esophageal chest pain. Gastroenterology. 1986;91:1141.

132. Richter JE, Hackshaw BT, Wu WC, Castell DO. Edrophonium: a useful provocative test for esophageal chest pain. Ann Intern Med. 1985;103:14.
133. Alban-Davies H, Kaye MD, Rhodes J. Diagnosis of oesophageal spasm by ergometrine provocation. Gut. 1982;23:89.
134. Richter JE, Wu WC, Johns DN et al. Esophageal manometry in 95 healthy adult volunteers. Dig Dis Sci. 1987;32:583.
135. Rubin J, Nagler R, Spiro HM, Pilot ML. Measuring the effect of emotions on esophageal motility. Psychosom Med. 1962;24:170.
136. Clouse RE, Lustman PJ. Psychiatric illness and contraction abnormalities of the esophagus. N Engl J Med. 1983;309:1337.
137. Richter JE, Barish CF, Castell DO. Abnormal sensory perception in patients with esophageal chest pain. Gastroenterology. 1986;91:845.
138. Keshavarzian A, Iber FL, Ferguson Y. Esophageal manometry and radionuclide emptying in chronic alcoholics. Gastroenterology. 1987;92:751.
139. Benjamin SB, Gerhardt DC, Castell DO. High amplitude, peristaltic esophageal contractions associated with chest pain and/or dysphagia. Gastroenterology. 1979;77:478.
140. Code CF, Schlegel JF, Kelly ML. Hypertensive gastroesophageal sphincter. Proc Mayo Clin. 1960;35:391.
141. Garett JM, Godwin DH. Gastroesophageal hypercontracting sphincter. J Am Med Assoc. 1969;208:992.
142. Aliperti G, Clouse RE. Incomplete lower esophageal sphincter relaxation in subjects with peristalsis: prevalence and clinical outcome. Am J Gastroenterol. 1991;86:609.
143. Reidel WL, Clouse RE. Variations in clinical presentations of patients with contraction abnormalities. Dig Dis Sci. 1985;30:1065.
144. Lieberman-Meffert DM, Luescher U, Neff U et al. Esophagectomy without thoracotomy: is there a risk of intramediastinal bleeding. Ann Surg. 1987;206:184.
145. Richter JE, Dalton CB, Bradley LA, Castell DO. Oral nifedipine in the treatment of non-cardiac chest pain in patients with the nutcracker esophagus. Gastroenterology. 1987;93:21.
146. Ellis FH, Crozier RE, Shea JA. Long esophagomyotomy for diffuse esophageal spasm and related disorders. In: Siewart JR, Holscher AH, eds. Diseases of the Esophagus. Pathophysiology, Diagnosis, Conservative and Surgical Treatment. New York: Springer-Verlag; 1988:913.
147. Ott DJ, Richter JE, Wu WC et al. Radiologic and manometric correlation in 'nutcracker esophagus'. Am J Roentgenol. 1986;692:1986.
148. Swamy N. Esophageal spasm: clinical and manometric response to nitroglycerin and long-acting nitrates. Gastroenterology. 1977;72:23.
149. Lee CA, Reynolds JC, Ouyang A, Cohen S. Esophageal chest pain: value of high-dose provocative testing with edrophonium chloride in patients with normal esophageal manometries. Dig Dis Sci. 1987;32:682.
150. Orlando RC, Bozymski EM. Clinical and manometric effects of nitroglycerin in diffuse esophageal spasm. N Engl J Med. 1973;289:23.
151. Richter JE, Spurling TJ, Cordova CM, Castell DO. Effects of oral calcium channel blocker, diltiazen, on esophageal contractions. Dig Dis Sci. 1984;29:649.
152. Ghillebert G, Janssens J, Vantrappen G et al. Ambulatory 24-hour intraesophageal pH and pressure recordings vs provocation tests in the diagnosis of chest pain of esophageal origin. Gut. 1990;31:738.
153. Winters C, Artnak EJ, Benjamin SB et al. Esophageal bougienage in symptomatic patients with the nutcracker esophagus. J Am Med Assoc. 1984;252:3630.

Manuscript received 25 Nov. 95.
Accepted for publication 25 Nov. 95.

Section III–IV

BIOCHEMICAL–PHARMACOLOGICAL MECHANISMS IN NEURAL AND HORMONAL NORMAL AND PATHOLOGICAL REACTIONS INVOLVED IN GI FUNCTIONS

TS Gaginella et al. (eds.), Biochemical Pharmacology as an Approach to Gastrointestinal Disorders, 171–185

DISTRIBUTION OF MUSCARINIC RECEPTOR mRNAs IN THE STOMACHS OF NORMAL OR IMMOBILIZED RATS

B. HUNYADY[1,3], É. MEZEY[2], K. PACAK[2], Gy. HARTA[2] AND M. PALKOVITS[1*]
[1]National Institute of Mental Health; [2]National Institute of Neurological Disorders and Stroke, NIH, Bethesda, MD, USA; [3]First Department of Medicine, Medical University of Pécs, Pécs, Hungary
*Correspondence

This paper was first published in: Inflammopharmacology. 1996;4:399–413.

ABSTRACT

Five subtypes of cholinergic muscarinic receptors (M1–M5) have been cloned and characterized by pharmacological and molecular biological methods during the past decade. The M3 subtype was demonstrated in acid-secreting cells, both by functional measurements and binding assays, while the M1 subtype is reported in the intramural ganglionic cells. In the present study, the distribution of M1–M5 mRNAs was mapped by in-situ hybridization histochemistry. Sections (12-μm thick, frozen) from different parts of the stomachs from control or immobilized (3 h immobilization on two consecutive days) rats were hybridized with [^{35}S]UTP labelled ribonucleotides (400–500 nucleotides each) directed to mRNAs of the M1–M5 subtypes. M1 and M3 mRNAs were present in different locations and in different densities in the rat stomach; however, there was a complete lack in detection of mRNAs of the M2, M4 or M5 subtypes. M1 mRNA was found over the enteric ganglionic cells and over some deep epithelial and tunica propria cells of the prepyloric area. No labelling was seen over the epithelial cells of the fundic mucosa. The distribution of M1 mRNA was not changed by immobilization. M3 mRNA was detected over a portion of parietal cells (immunolabelled using a monoclonal antibody) of fundic mucosa and over smooth muscle cells of the tunica muscularis. A large number of tunica propria cells and some enteric ganglions were also labelled for M3 subtype. Weak labelling was seen over the surface mucous cells. The density of the labelling was increased in stressed rats, particularly over the tunica propria cells. These data complete earlier observations obtained by pharmacological and radio ligand binding assays on M1 and M3 subtypes in the rat stomach and support the existence of a non-epithelial, non-neuronal cell regulatory system in the GI tract.

Keywords: acetylcholine, muscarinic acetylcholine receptor, stomach, immobilization, in-situ hybridization histochemistry, immunohistochemistry, messenger RNA, rat

INTRODUCTION

Acetylcholine (ACh) released by enteric neurons has a crucial role in the regulation of gastric secretion and motility [1]. Binding sites for ACh have been classified traditionally on the basis of actions of cholinergic agonists as muscarinic acetylcholine receptors (mAChRs) or nicotinic acetylcholine receptors. Muscarinic receptors were initially demonstrated by pharmacological methods in the autonomic effector cells (innervated by parasympathetic neurons) and in the central nervous system [2].

This paper was presented at the Section of IUPHAR GI Pharmacology Symposium on 'Biochemical pharmacology as an approach to gastrointestinal disorders (basic science to clinical perspectives)', October 12–14, 1995, Pécs, Hungary.

TABLE 1

Classification of muscarinic acetylcholine receptors based on pharmacological properties and cloned cDNA sequences

	M1	M2	M3	M4	M5
Previously used name	Neural M_1 $M_{1\alpha}$, A	Cardiac M_2 $M_{2\alpha}$, M_{2A}, C	Glandular M_2 Smooth muscle M_2 $M_{2\beta}$, M_{2B}, B	M_2	
'Selective' agonist	McNA-343 Xanomeline [60] L-689,660 AF 102B	Carbachol Bethanechol BM5	Carbachol Bethanechol L-689,660	BM5	
'Selective' antagonist	Pirenzepine Telenzepine Dicyclomine UH-AH 37 BM5 4-DAMP	Methoctramine AF-DX 116 AF-DX 384 AQ-RA 741 Himbacine Pancuronium Stercuronium Gallamine	Hexahydrosila– difenidol, p-fluorohexa- hydrosiladifenidol UH-AH 37 BM5 4-DAMP LG 50643 NPC-14695	AF-DX 384	
Sequence name	*m1*	*m2*	*m3*	*m4*	*m5*
Previously used sequence name	mAChR I M1, HM_1	mAChR II M2, HM_2	mAChR III M4, HM_4	mAChR IV M3, HM_3	
Site of first cloning	Porcine brain	Porcine heart	Rat brain	Rat brain	Rat brain
Number of amino acids	460	466	589/590	478/479	531/532

Abbreviations: BM5: *N*-methyl-*N*-(methyl-4-pyrrolidino-2-butynyl) acetamide [54]; UH-AH 37: 6-chloro-5,10-dihydro-5-[(1-methyl-4-piperidinyl)acetyl]-11H-dibenzo-[b,e][1,4]diazepine-11-one hydrochloride [55]; AF-DX 116: 11,2-(diethylamino)methyl-1-piperidinyl acetyl-5,11-dihydro-6H-pyrido-2,3-b 1,4-benzodiazepine-6-one [56]; AF-DX 384: (+–)-5,11-dihydro-11-([(2-(2-[(dipropylamino)methyl]-1-piperidinyl)ethyl)amino]carbonyl)-H-pyrido(2,2-b)(1,4)benzodiazepine-6-one [37]; 4-DAMP: diphenyl-acetoxy-4-methylpiperidine methiodide [56]; L-689,660: 1-azabicyclo[2,2,2]octane,3-(6chloropyrazinyl) maleate [57]; NPC-14695: 3-(4-benzyl-piperazinyl)-1-1-cyclobutyl-1-hydroxy-1-phenyl-2-propane-one [58]; AQ-RA 741: 11-[[4-[4-(diethylamino)butyl]-1-piperidinyl]acetyl]-5,11-dihydro-6H-pyridol[2,3-b][1,4]benzodiazepine-6-one [59]

Nicotinic receptors are located in the neuromuscular junction (in the striated muscles) and in the autonomic ganglia [3].

Using muscarinic agonists and antagonists, three subtypes of mAChRs (M1–M3) have been characterized in the gut, as detailed below [4]. In an attempt to reduce the still existing confusion in terminology of mAChRs, we applied the nomenclature of Hulme et al. [5] (Table 1).

Binding sites at acid-secreting parietal cells, demonstrated by Ecknauer et al. [6], Black and Shankley [7] and Soll and Berglindh [8], were later characterized as M3 subtypes in the rat, human and rabbit [9–12]. Based on ^{3}H-labelled quinuclidinyl benzilate (a muscarinic antagonist) binding, Culp et al. also claimed muscarinic receptors in mucous and chief cells [13] without further subclassification. Muscarinic receptors were also reported in cells involved in the regulation of gastric secretion, i.e. M1 subtypes in G cells (secreting gastrin) [14] and D cells (producing the antisecretory mediator, somatostatin) [14,15], but M3 subtypes (M2 in the terminology of the cited authors) in enterochromaffin-like/mucosal mast cells (producing histamine) [16–19]. ACh is also the ligand on the smooth muscles of the gut and a transmitter in the enteric ganglia [20]. Both M3 (smooth muscle M2, glandular M2) and M2 (cardiac M2) subtypes are suggested in the smooth muscles of the gut by Ladinsky et al. [21], Hanack and Pfeiffer [22] and Bellido et al. [23]. In the enteric ganglia, M1 excitatory receptors are present in the perikaria of cholinergic, noradrenergic and non-cholinergic non-adrenergic postsynaptic neurons and interneurons, while M3 receptors (called M2 by the terminology of the cited authors) were characterized on both presynaptic and prejunctional nerve endings [24–26]. However, Soejima et al. [27] argued for the presence of presynaptic M1 receptor involvement in the agonist-mediated enhancement of acetylcholine release evoked by electrical stimulation instead of autoinhibition by M3 receptor stimulation. Dietrich and Kilbinger [28] reported M1 prejunctional receptors in the circular smooth muscle of the guinea-pig ileum.

Molecular sequences of five mAChRs (m1–m5) have been published so far [29–34] (Table 1). Pharmacological properties of cloned and native mAChRs have been compared by transfecting the receptor cDNAs into different cell lines [35–38]. In this model, mAChR-coupled intracellular events were also extensively investigated [39–45] (Table 2). Maeda et al. [46] confirmed the existence of M1 and M3 mRNAs in exocrine glands and M2 and M3 mRNAs in smooth muscles by blot hybridization technique. In a previous study, using oligonucleotide probes for in-situ hybridization histochemistry (ISHH), Mezey and Palkovits [47] were not able to detect the messenger RNA (mRNA) of any of mAChRs in epithelial cells (including parietal cells) of the gastric mucosa. In contrast, very consistent labelling for certain mAChR subtypes was found in the non-epithelial cells of the tunica propria in the gut wall. Although the intensity of the signal in these cells might have been amplified by a series of chemical interactions, it was confirmed to be specific [48]. In the present study, we decided to try to repeat these unexpected results using highly sensitive ribonucleotide probes in the ISHH protocol. We also planned to investigate stress-related changes in the mAChR mRNA expression using immobilized rats. Immobilization is one of the most consistently ulcerogenic stressors in the stomach [49].

TABLE 2
Postreceptor events coupled to expressed muscarinic receptors*

Sequence name	m1	m2	m3	m4	m5
PI response	Stimulates	No effect	Stimulates	No effect	Stimulates
cAMP response	Stimulates	Inhibits	Stimulates	Inhibits	Stimulates
Arachidonic acid response	Stimulates	No effect	Stimulates	No effect	Not tested
Ca^{2+}-dependent K^+ channel in A9 and NG-108 cells	Opens	No effect	Opens	No effect	Not tested
M-current in NG-108 cells	Inhibits	No effect	Inhibits	No effect	Not tested
Ca^{2+}-independent current in Xenopus oocytes	None	Stimulates	None	Stimulates	Not tested

*Based on studies by Bonner [34]

MATERIALS AND METHODS

Animals and tissue handling

Adult male Sprague–Dawley rats (250–300 g) were used, five animals in both the control and immobilized groups. The animals were kept under standard laboratory conditions. Food (pellets) and tap water were allowed ad libitum. In order to produce gastric and duodenal erosions, five animals were stressed by immobilization. This procedure consisted of taping the limbs of the animals to a metal frame for 3 h twice, on two consecutive days. At the end of the second immobilization, the animals were sacrificed by decapitation under pentobarbital anaesthesia (80 mg/kg pentobarbital sodium ip). No immobilization procedure was carried out on control animals. They were sacrificed by the same decapitation method.

Stomachs of the animals were rapidly removed, opened at the fornix, washed out by 1 × phosphate buffered saline (PBS) and immediately frozen on dry ice. Frozen sections (12 μm thick) were cut on a cryostat for both immunohistochemistry (IHC) and ISHH. The sections were thaw-mounted and air-dried at 37°C onto silanized slides, frozen and stored at –80°C until used. Parallel-treated and hybridized rat brain sections were used as positive controls.

In-situ hybridization histochemistry (ISHH)

We used the ISHH procedure described by Young [50] and modified by Bradley et al. [51]. In brief, still-frozen sections were fixed in 4% formaldehyde in 1 × PBS (pH 7.4) fixative for 10 min at 20°C, and treated subsequently with 0.25% acetic anhydride in 0.1 mol/L triethanolamine-HCl (pH 8.0) over a 10-min period to reduce non-specific hybridization of the probe. Then, the sections were rinsed in 0.3 mol/L NaCl–0.03 mol/L sodium citrate solution, dehydrated in ethanol, delipidated with chloroform for 5 min, rinsed in ethanol and air dried. Sections were hybridized overnight at 55°C with 0.8–1 × 10^6 cpm/section labelled probes (described next) in a humid chamber. Non-specifically hybridized probes were washed out, then the sections were dried, dipped into NTB3 nuclear track emulsion (Eastman Kodak, Rochester) and stored desiccated for 28 days at 4°C, when they were developed using Kodak Dektol at 15°C. Non-immunolabelled sections were counter-stained with Giemsa solution (Sigma). Finally, the sections were washed, dried and mounted by Cytoseal 60 mounting medium (Stephens Scientific).

[^{35}S]UTP-labelled riboprobes were prepared by SP6 RNA polymerase according to the Maxiscript kit (AMBION) using the following templates kindly given by Dr Tom Bonner: nucleotides 820–1194 of rat M1 cDNA (gene bank accession number M16406), 728–1285 of human M2 cDNA (M16404), 1559–2244 of rat M3 cDNA (M16408), 654–1195 of rat M4 cDNA (M16409), and 1206–1758 of rat M5 cDNA (M22926). We did not possess a cDNA template for the rat M2 receptor, but this shows a 98% homology with the human M2 receptor cDNA.

Immunohistochemistry (IHC)

Additionally, some sections were immunostained for the proton pump (known to be exclusively present in parietal cells in the gastrointestinal system) by a mouse monoclonal antibody, a kind gift of Dr Adam Smolka [52], before the ISHH procedure. Sections from the freezer were fixed with the above fixative and conditions. To decrease non-specific staining, fixed sections were pretreated for 30 min at 20°C in a blocking solution containing 1% normal donkey serum (the host species of the secondary antibody) and 0.6% Triton X-100 in 1 × PBS (pH 7.4). After several rinses in PBS, the primary antibody, diluted 1:1000 in the blocking solution, was applied to the sections for 1 h at 20°C. After repeated washes in PBS, the sections were incubated in a Cy3-red fluorescent conjugated anti-mouse IgG (made in donkey, Jackson ImmunoResearch) secondary antibody in a dilution of 1:1000 in the blocking solution for 1 h at 20°C. Immunofluorescent labelling was viewed with a Leitz Dialux 20 fluorescent microscope both before and after the ISHH procedure. Negative controls included stainings with non-immune mouse IgG or serum, and leaving out the primary or secondary antibodies. ISHH protocol started on the immunostained sections at the dehydration stage.

RESULTS

M1 and M3 mRNAs were present in different locations and in different densities in the rat stomach (Table 3). By contrast, there was a lack in detection of mRNAs of the M2, M4 or M5 subtypes, although all of our riboprobes (including the M2 riboprobe made using the human template) did label the mAChR mRNAs in the control rat brain sections, with the known distribution [46,53].

TABLE 3
Distribution of M1 and M3 muscarinic receptor subtype mRNAs in different cell types in the stomach of control or immobilized rats

	Control rats		Immobilized rats	
	M1 mRNA	M3 mRNA	M1 mRNA	M3 mRNA
Enteric ganglia	+++	+	+++(0)	+(0)
Smooth muscle cells	–	++	–	++(0)
Tunica propria cells	+	+	+(0)	++(↑)
Epithelial cells				
Parietal cells	–	++	–	+++(↑)
Chief cells	–	++(?)	–	++(0)
Mucous cells	–	?	–	?
Endocrine cells	++	?	++(0)	?

–, not expressed; +/++/+++, density of mRNA expression; 0, not changed; ↑, increased; ?, insufficient data.

No labelling for M1 mRNA was seen in the fundic epithelium, including mucous cells, proton pump immunoreactive parietal cells and chief cells (Figure 1). For every visualized enteric ganglion, a relatively large number (5–8%) of deep epithelial cells in the prepyloric area of the stomach (where parietal and chief cells are rare) and some tunica propria cells were labelled for M1 mRNA (Figure 2). The distribution and density of M1 mRNA were not affected by immobilization, although the immobilization provoked deep erosions on the stomach mucosa.

M3 mRNA was detected unevenly in the epithelial cells of the parietal-cell-rich fundic portion of the stomach mucosa (Figure 3). In the subsequent study, where parietal cells were additionally immunostained, we were able to colocalize the M3 mRNA to a portion (20–25%) of parietal cells (Figure 4). The other portion of proton pump immunoreactive cells was negative for M3 mRNA. We also found labelled non-parietal epithelial cells over the bases of gastric glands in the fundic mucosa (Figure 3). These cells can be considered as chief cells based on their shape and position. The number of labelled cells has characteristically decreased in the prepyloric area (where parietal and chief cells are rare). The signal for M3 mRNA in the mucin-secreting cell

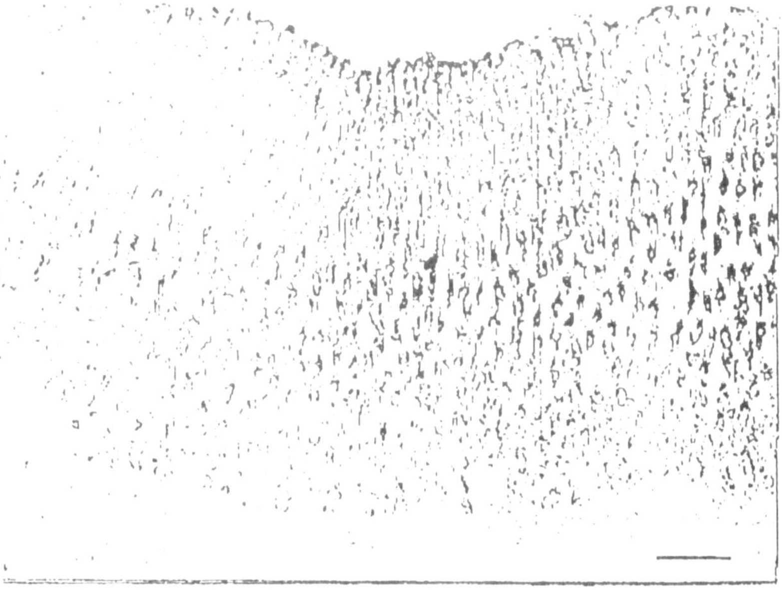

Figure 1. M1 receptor mRNA was not detectable in the fundic epithelium of rat stomach. Vertical section. Bright field photograph. Bar scale: 100 μm

layer was very weak, if any (Figure 3). Furthermore, we were able to demonstrate M3 mRNA in a large number of certainly not epithelial cells in the tunica propria of rat stomach (Figures 3 and 6). Smooth muscle cells of the tunica muscularis were also positive for M3 subtype (Figure 5). Moreover, M3 mRNA was found in some enteric ganglia (not shown).

Both the intensity of the M3 subtype labelling in epithelial and tunica propria cells and the number of labelled cells markedly increased in stressed rats (Figure 6), characteristically in the middle and lower part, and in the tunica propria of fundic (oxyntic) mucosa.

DISCUSSION

In the present study, we completed our previous results on expression of mAChR mRNAs in the rat stomach [47]. In addition to the large number of tunica propria cells found by labelled oligonucleotide probes for both M1 and M3 mRNAs, in this study, using ribonucleotide probes, we were able to detect mAChR mRNAs in epithelial and smooth muscle cells of the gastric mucosa. Recent success in demonstration of mAChR mRNAs can be explained by the modified hybridization protocol, both the improved sensitivity of ribonucleotide probes and the reduced artificial signal amplification in some tunica propria cells [48]. Nevertheless, demonstration of both

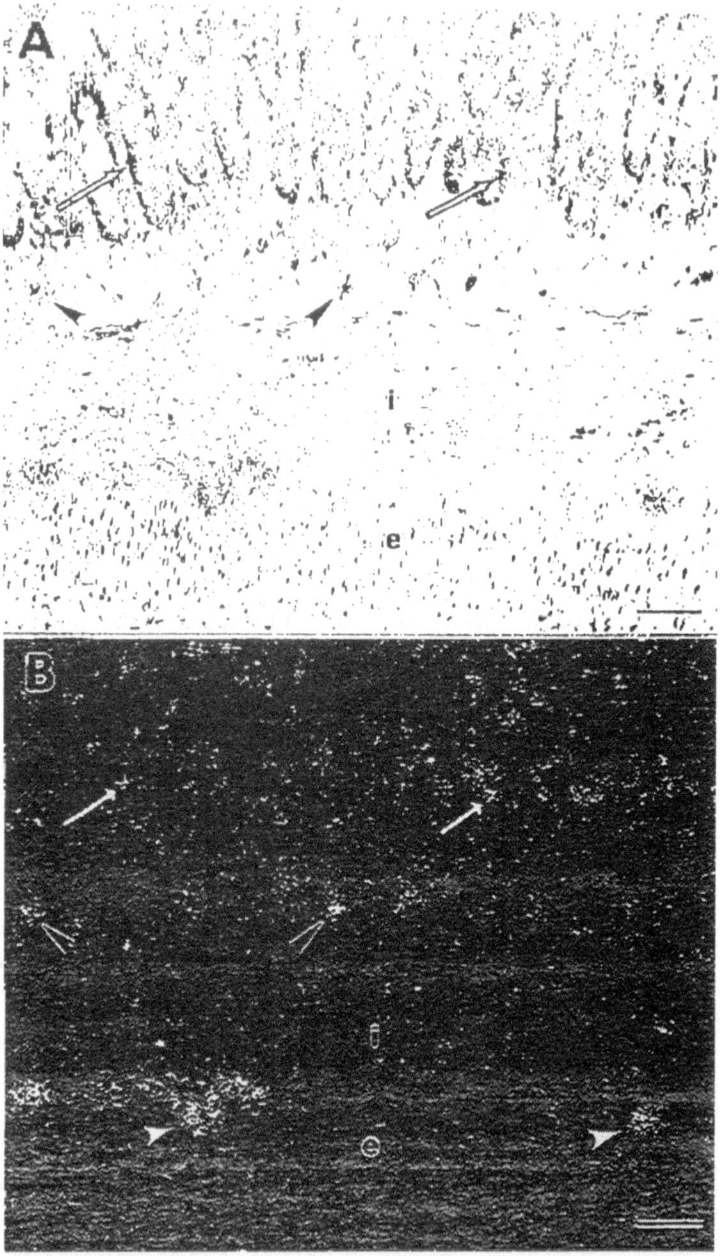

Figure 2. M1 receptor mRNA-labelled epithelial cells (blank arrows) located in the antral mucosa are probably gastrin-producing G cells. Myenteric ganglia (blank arrowheads) between the internal (i) and external (e) muscular layer, and some tunica propria cells (arrowheads) were also labelled for M1 mRNA. Vertical section. A = bright field, B = dark field photographs of the same area. Bar scales: 50 μm

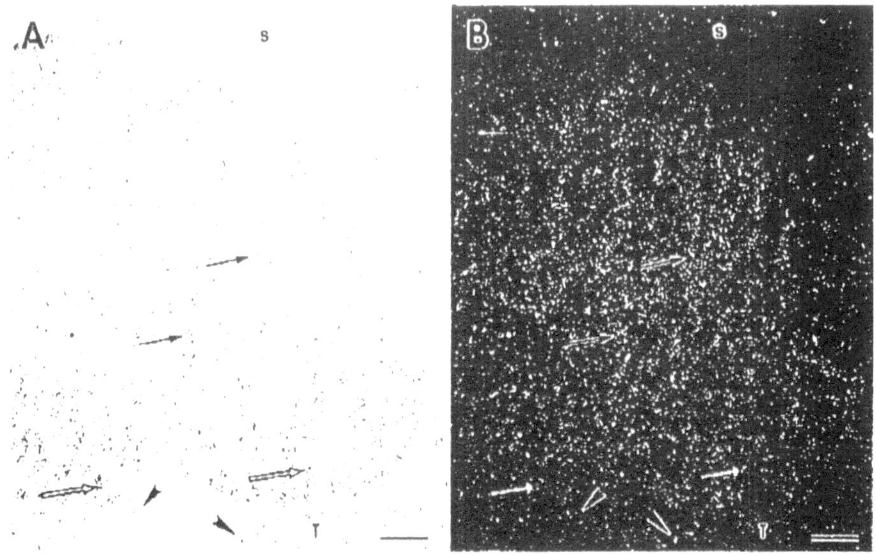

Figure 3. M3 receptor mRNA in different cell types of the fundic (oxyntic) glands of rat stomach. Very low or no signal over the surface layer(s). Uneven distribution of the signal over the parietal-cell-rich middle part (arrows) and chief-cell-rich deep part (blank arrows) of gastric glands. Vertical section. A = bright field, B = dark field photographs of the same area. Bar scales: 100 μm

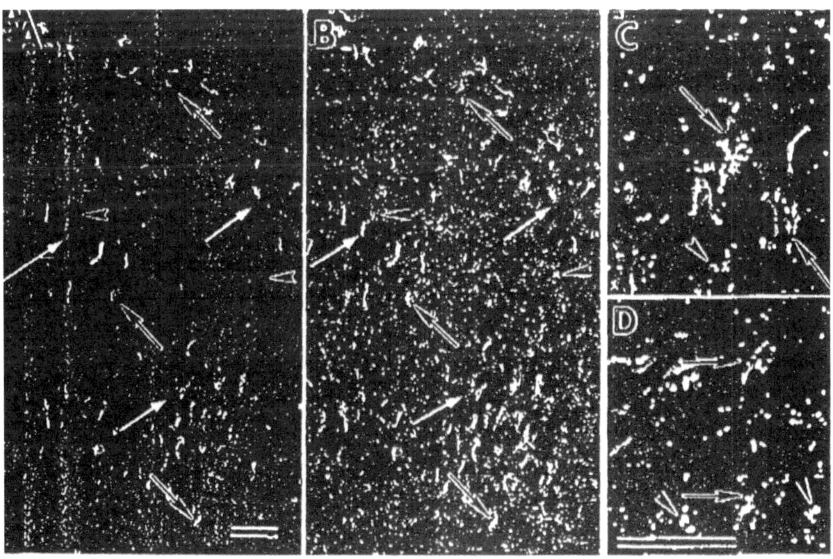

Figure 4. M3 receptor mRNA-labelled proton-pump immunoreactive parietal cells (arrows), and non-immunoreactive epithelial or tunica propria cells (arrowheads). A high proportion of parietal cells did not express the M3-receptor mRNA (blank arrows). A = photograph of the fluorescent field, filtered in the emission spectrum of CY3-red, where the proton pump immunoreactive parietal cells are visible (blank arrows). B, C and D = summarized photographs of both the fluorescent fields and the dark fields, where additionally bright greys of the mRNA signal are visible (arrowheads). Tangential section. Bar scales: 25 μm

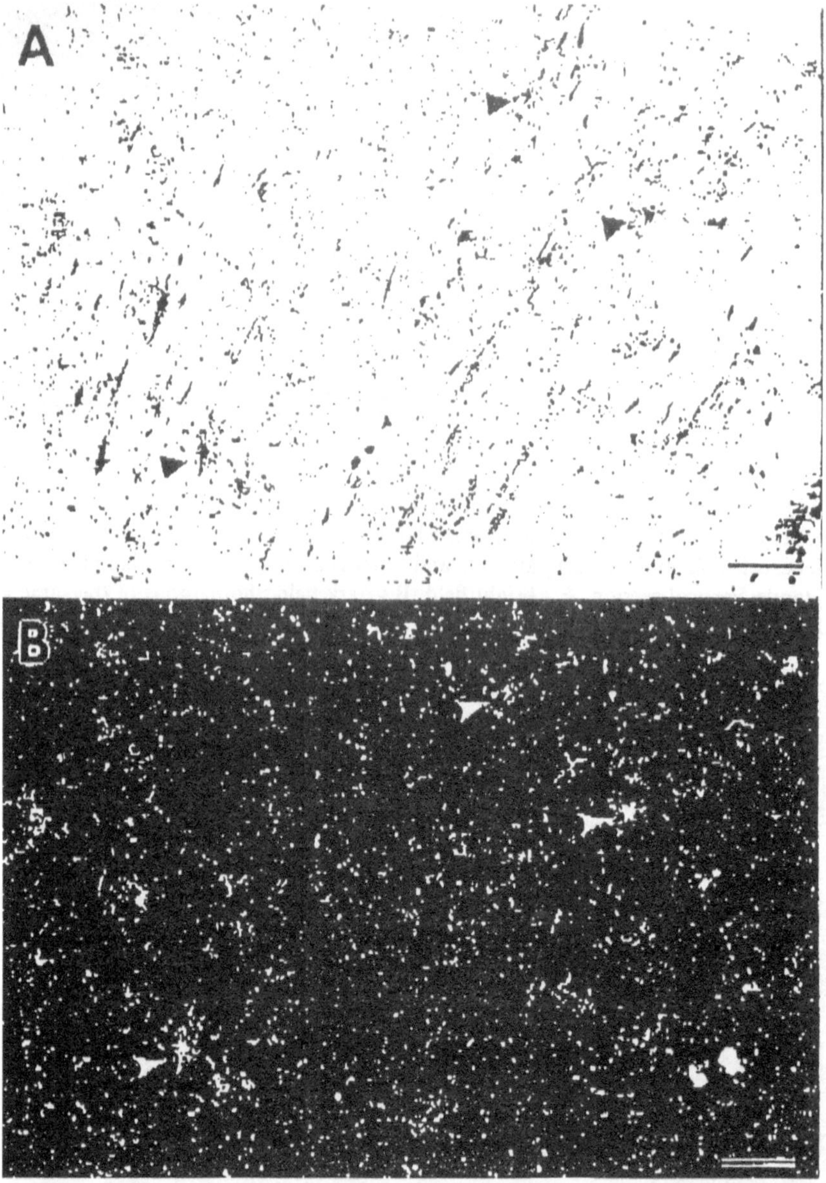

Figure 5. M3 receptor mRNA in smooth muscle cells (arrowheads) in the rat stomach. Longitudinal section. A = bright field, B = dark field photographs of the same area. Bar scales: 50 μm

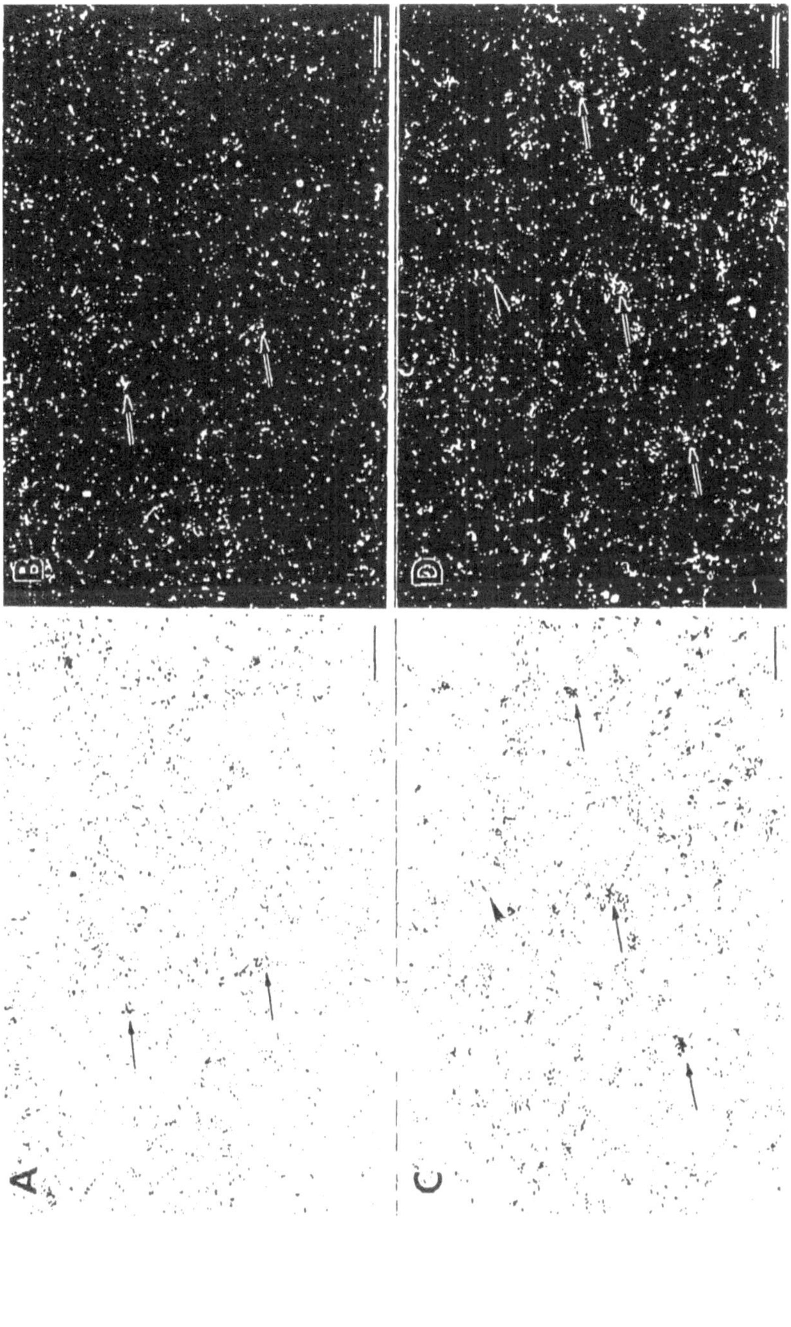

Figure 6. The density of M3 receptor mRNA signal markedly increased in immobilized rats (C,D) compared with the controls (A,B), in both epithelial (arrows) and tunica propria cells (arrowheads). Tangential sections in the middle level of the fundic glands. A and C = bright field, B and D = dark field photographs of the same areas. Bar scales: 50 μm

M1 and M3 mRNAs in tunica propria cells confirms our previous data obtained by oligonucleotide probes. Expression of muscarinic receptor mRNAs in these cells indicates the capability, while the observed elevation of M3 mRNA density in stressed rats emphasizes their role in the regulation of gastric functions.

Our data on M3-subtype mRNA in parietal cells of the rat gastric mucosa supports the findings of Pfeiffer et al. obtained by radio ligand binding assays in rats [9] and human [10], and of Kajimura et al. based on radio ligand binding and DNA blot techniques in rabbit [12]. The presence of M3 mRNA in a portion of parietal cells, obviously demonstrated by concomitant IHC and ISHH, suggests that parietal cells are not a homogeneous population. The problem of the sensitivity of the ISHH method can be one possible reason for the observed inhomogeneity. For example, the actual mRNA content of a low-activity cell might be below the detection limit, even if the mRNA is present, and only the highly active cells can be visualized. However, the question of whether this difference among the parietal cells reflects their functional status, their life cycle, or can be explained by ab ovo genetic differences, remains open for further investigations. Differential expression of M3 mRNA in parietal cells correlates with the relatively low density of muscarinic binding sites in these cells hinted at by Angus and Black [16] and Black and Shankley [7].

Demonstration of M3 mRNA in chief cells supports the finding of Culp et al. [13] but the very low level of M3 mRNA signal in mucous cells is in partial contradiction with their results. In fact, we were not able to confirm either the existence or the lack of expression of muscarinic receptor mRNAs in mucous cells. If any, there must be a very small amount compared with other labelled cells.

M1 subtype mRNA in epithelial cells, found exclusively in the prepyloric area of the stomach, might be expressed by the endocrine cells in this area. These cells cannot be easily distinguished in our hybridized sections from other epithelial cells. We could surely differentiate these cells from proton pump immunoreactive parietal cells. Considering the microscopic shape, the localization, the number of these cells, and also the cholinergic gastrin release reported by Sue et al. [14], the M1 mAChR-positive cells are certainly gastrin-producing G cells in the prepyloric area of the rat stomach. Non-parietal cells labelled for either M1 or M3 mRNAs might be, furthermore, other endocrine or paracrine cells since, for example, somatostatin-producing D cells (M1 subtype suggested) [14,15] and histamine-releasing enterochromaffin-like/mucosal mast cells (M3 subtype suggested) [7,19] are reported to respond to cholinomimetics.

In the literature, M3 and M2 mAChRs are reported in gastrointestinal smooth muscles based on pharmacological studies [21–23] and blot hybridizations [46]. We were able to detect M3 mRNA in the smooth muscle cells of the rat stomach but we failed to detect M2 receptor mRNA, although our M2 riboprobe made with a human template did label with the known distribution [46] in the control rat brain sections. This lack of detection of M2 receptor mRNA might be explained by either organ/species-specificity or very low expression of this subtype.

We were able to detect both M1 and M3 mRNAs in the enteric ganglia of the rat stomach. Presynaptic–postsynaptic differentiation is not possible at the light-microscopic level. M1-type pharmacological response of gastrointestinal smooth muscle might rather reflect to the M1 receptors in the enteric ganglia than to either prejunctional or postjunctional receptors since we did not see the M1 mRNA signal over the smooth muscle layer of the rat stomach. On the other hand, species- and/or organ-specific manifestations of receptors can be also presumed.

Further distinction of mAChR subtypes in different cell types of the stomach is in progress, combining ISHH demonstration of mRNAs and IHC detection of different cell types by specific antibodies. We hope that precise knowledge of receptors in specific cell types will lead us to a better understanding of physiological and pathological processes in the stomach, and, upon availability of highly selective compounds, opens up the possibility of more reliable therapy of gastric diseases.

ACKNOWLEDGEMENTS

The authors thank Dr Tom Bonner for the generous supply of cDNA templates, Dr Adam Smolka for the proton pump antibody and Rickardo Dreyfuss for his photographic work.

REFERENCES

1. Spiro HM. Clinical Gastroenterology, 4th edn. New York, USA: McGraw-Hill; 1993: Pt II, 141–72.
2. Taylor P. Cholinergic agonists. In: Gilman AG, Rall TW, Nies AS, Taylor P, ed. The Pharmacological Basis of Therapeutics, 8th edn. New York, USA: Pergamon Press; 1990:122–30.
3. Taylor P. Agents acting at the neuromuscular junction and autonomic ganglia. In: Gilman AG, Rall TW, Nies AS, Taylor P, eds. The Pharmacological Basis of Therapeutics, 8th edn. New York, USA: Pergamon Press; 1990:166–86.
4. Goyal RK. Identification, localization and classification of muscarinic receptor subtypes in the gut. Life Sci. 1988;43:2209–20.
5. Hulme EC, Birdsall NJ, Buckley NJ. Muscarinic receptor subtypes. Ann Rev Pharmacol Toxicol. 1990;30:633–73.
6. Ecknauer R, Thompson WJ, Johnson LR, Rosenfeld GC. Isolated parietal cells: [3H]QNB binding to putative cholinergic receptors. Am J Physiol. 1980;239:G204–9.
7. Black JW, Shankley NP. Pharmacological analysis of the muscarinic receptors involved when McN-A 343 stimulates acid secretion in the mouse isolated stomach. Br J Pharmacol. 1985;86:609–17.
8. Soll AH, Berglindh T. Physiology of isolated gastric glands and parietal cells: Receptors and effectors regulating function. In: Johnson LR, ed. Physiology of the Gastrointestinal Tract, 2nd edn. New York, USA: Raven Press; 1987;883–909.
9. Pfeiffer A, Rochlitz H, Noelke B et al. Muscarinic receptors mediating acid secretion in isolated rat gastric parietal cells are of M3 type. Gastroenterology. 1990;98:218–22.
10. Pfeiffer A, Hanack C, Kopp R et al. Human gastric mucosa express glandular M3 subtype of muscarinic receptors. Dig Dis Sci. 1990;35:1468–72.
11. Van der Zee EA, Buwalda B, Strubbe JH, Strosberg AD, Luiten PG. Immunocytochemical localization of muscarinic acetylcholine receptors in the rat endocrine pancreas. Cell Tissue Res. 1992;269:99–106.
12. Kajimura M, Reuben A, Sachs G. The muscarinic receptor gene expressed in rabbit parietal cells is the m3 subtype. Gastroenterology. 1992;103:870–5.
13. Culp DJ, Wolosin JM, Soll AH, Forte JG. Muscarinic receptors and guanylate cyclase in mammalian gastric glandular cells. Am J Physiol. 1983;245:G641–6.
14. Sue R, Toomey ML, Todisco A, Soll AH, Yamada T. Pirenzepine-sensitive muscarinic receptors regulate gastric somatostatin and gastrin. Am J Physiol. 1985;248:G184–7.
15. Yamada T, Soll AH, Park J, Elashoff J. Autonomic regulation of somatostatin release: studies with primary cultures of canine fundic mucosal cells. Am J Physiol. 1984;247:G567–73.
16. Angus JA, Black JW. The interaction of choline esters, vagal stimulation and H2-receptor blockade on acid secretion in vitro. Eur J Pharmacol. 1982;80:217–24.

17. Black JW, Leff P, Shankley NP. Further analysis of anomalous pKB values for histamine H2-receptor antagonists on the mouse isolated stomach assay. Br J Pharmacol. 1985;86:581–7.
18. Sandvik AK, Kleveland PM, Waldum HL. Muscarinic M2 stimulation releases histamine in the totally isolated, vascularly perfused rat stomach. Scand J Gastroenterol. 1988;23:1049–56.
19. Gerber JG, Payne NA. The role of gastric secretagogues in regulating gastric histamine release in vivo. Gastroenterology. 1992;102:403–8.
20. Ruoff HJ, Fladung B, Demol P, Weihrauch TR. Gastrointestinal receptors and drugs in motility disorders. Digestion. 1991;48:1–17.
21. Ladinsky H, Giraldo E, Monferini E et al. Muscarinic receptor heterogeneity in smooth muscle: binding and functional studies with AF-DX 116. Trends Pharmacol Sci. 1988;Suppl:44:44–8.
22. Hanack C, Pfeiffer A. Upper gastrointestinal porcine smooth muscle expresses M2- and M3 receptors. Digestion. 1990;45:196–201.
23. Bellido J, Fernandez JL, Gomez A, Sanchez de la Cuesta F. Otenzepad shows two populations of binding sites in human gastric smooth muscle. Can J Physiol Pharmacol. 1995;73:124–9.
24. Kilbinger H, Nafziger M. Two types of neuronal muscarine receptors modulating acetylcholine release from guinea-pig myenteric plexus. Naunyn Schmiedebergs Arch Pharmacol. 1985;328:304–9.
25. North RA, Suprenant A. Muscarinic receptors on neurones of the submucous plexus. In: Lux G, Daniel EE, eds. Muscarinic Receptor Subtypes in the GI Tract. Berlin: Springer–Verlag;1985:28–32.
26. Dammann F, Fuder H, Giachetti A, Giraldo E, Kilbinger H, Micheletti R. AF-DX 116 differentiates between prejunctional muscarinic receptors located on noradrenergic and cholinergic nerves. Naunyn Schmiedebergs Arch Pharmacol. 1989;339:268–71.
27. Soejima O, Katsuragi T, Furukawa T. Opposite modulation by muscarinic M1 and M3 receptors of acetylcholine release from guinea pig ileum as measured directly. Eur J Pharmacol. 1993;249:1–6.
28. Dietrich C, Kilbinger. Prejunctional M1 and postjunctional M3 muscarinic receptors in the circular muscle of the guinea-pig ileum. Naunyn Schmiedebergs Arch Pharmacol. 1995;351:237–43.
29. Kubo T, Fukuda K, Mikami A et al. Cloning, sequencing and expression of complementary DNA encoding the muscarinic acetylcholine receptor. Nature. 1986;323:411–16.
30. Kubo T, Maeda A, Sugimoto K et al. Primary structure of porcine cardiac muscarinic acetylcholine receptor deduced from the cDNA sequence. FEBS Lett. 1986;209:367–72
31. Bonner TI, Buckley NJ, Young AC, Brann MR. Identification of a family of muscarinic acetylcholine receptor genes [published erratum appears in Science. 1987;237(4822):237]. Science. 1987;237:527–32.
32. Peralta EG, Ashkenazi A, Winslow JW, Smith DH, Ramachandran J, Capon DJ. Distinct primary structures, ligand-binding properties and tissue-specific expression of four human muscarinic acetylcholine receptors. EMBO J. 1987;6:3923–9.
33. Bonner TI, Young AC, Brann MR, Buckley NJ. Cloning and expression of the human and rat m5 muscarinic acetylcholine receptor genes. Neuron. 1988;1:403–10.
34. Bonner TI. The molecular basis of muscarinic receptor diversity. Trends Neurol Sci. 1989;12:148–51.
35. Buckley NJ, Bonner TI, Buckley CM, Brann MR. Antagonist binding properties of five cloned muscarinic receptors expressed in CHO-K1 cells. Mol Pharmacol. 1989;35:469–76.
36. Boddeke HW, Buttini M. Pharmacological properties of cloned muscarinic receptors expressed in A9 cells; comparison with in vitro models. Eur J Pharmacol. 1991;202:151–7.
37. Miller JH, Gibson VA, McKinney M. Binding of [3H]AF-DX 384 to cloned and native muscarinic receptors. J Pharmacol Exp Ther. 1991;259:601–7.
38. Dong GZ, Kameyama K, Rinken A, Haga T. Ligand binding properties of muscarinic acetylcholine receptor subtypes (m1–m5) expressed in baculovirus-infected insect cells. J Pharmacol Exp Ther. 1995;274:378–84.
39. Ashkenazi A, Winslow JW, Peralta EF et al. An M2 muscarinic receptor subtype coupled to both adenylyl cyclase and phosphoinositide turnover. Science. 1987;238:672–5.
40. Conklin BR, Brann MR, Buckley NJ, Ma AL, Bonner TI, Axelrod J. Stimulation of arachidonic acid release and inhibition of mitogenesis by cloned genes for muscarinic receptor subtypes stably expressed in A9 L cells. Proc Natl Acad Sci USA. 1988;85:8698–702.
41. Pinkas-Kramarski R, Stein R, Zimmer Y, Sokolovsky M. Cloned rat M3 muscarinic receptors mediate phosphoinositide hydrolysis but not adenylate cyclase inhibition. FEBS Lett. 1988;239:174–8.
42. Stein R, Pinkas-Kramarski R, Sokolovsky M. Cloned M1 muscarinic receptors mediate both adenylate cyclase inhibition and phosphoinositide turnover. EMBO J. 1988;7:3031–5.
43. Jones SV, Barker JL, Buckley NJ, Bonner TI, Collins RM, Brann MR. Cloned muscarinic receptor subtypes expressed in A9 L cells differ in their coupling to electrical responses. Mol Pharmacol. 1988;34:421–6.
44. Bujo H, Nakai J, Kubo T et al. Different sensitivities to agonist of muscarinic acetylcholine receptor subtypes. FEBS Lett. 1988;240:95–100.

45. Fukuda K, Kubo T, Maeda A et al. Selective effector coupling of muscarinic acetylcholine receptor subtypes. Trends Pharmacol Sci. 1989;Suppl:4–10.
46. Maeda A, Kubo T, Mishina M, Numa S. Tissue distribution of mRNAs encoding muscarinic acetylcholine receptor subtypes. FEBS Lett. 1988;239:339–42.
47. Mezey E, Palkovits M. Localization of targets for anti-drugs in cells of the immune system [see comments]. Science. 1992;258:1662–5.
48. Mezey E, Hoffman BJ, Harta G, Palkovits M, Northup J. Potential problems in using [35S]-dATP-tailed oligonucleotides for detecting mRNAs in certain cells of the immune system. J Histochem Cytochem. 1994;42:1277–83.
49. Pare WP, Glavin GB. Restraint stress in biomedical research: a review. Neurosci Biobehav Rev. 1986;10:339–70.
50. Young S. In situ hybridization histochemical detection of neuropeptide mRNA using DNA and RNA probes. Meth Enzymol. 1989;168:702–10.
51. Bradley DJ, Towle HC, Young WS. Spatial and temporal expression of alpha- and beta-thyroid hormone receptor mRNAs, including the beta 2-subtype, in the developing mammalian nervous system. J Neurosci. 1992;12:2288–302.
52. Smolka A, Swiger KM. Site-directed antibodies as topographical probes of the gastric II,K-ATPase alpha-subunit. Biochim Biophys Acta. 1992;1108:75–85
53. Weiner DM, Levey AI, Brann MR. Expression of muscarinic acetylcholine and dopamine receptor mRNAs in rat basal ganglia. Proc Natl Acad Sci USA. 1990;87:7050–4.
54. Baumgold J, Drobnick A. An agonist that is selective for adenylate cyclase-coupled muscarinic receptors. Mol Pharmacol. 1989;36:465–70.
55. Wess J, Lambrecht G, Mutschler E, Brann MR, Dorje F. Selectivity profile of the novel muscarinic antagonist UH-AH 37 determined by the use of cloned receptors and isolated tissue preparations. Br J Pharmacol. 1991;102:246–50.
56. Wilkes JM, Kajimura M, Scott DR, Hersey SJ, Sachs G. Muscarinic responses of gastric parietal cells. J Memb Biol. 1991;122:97–110.
57. Aagaard P, McKinney M. Pharmacological characterization of the novel cholinomimetic L-689,660 at cloned and native brain muscarinic receptors. J Pharmacol Exp Ther. 1993;267:1478–83.
58. Howell RE, Laemont KD, Kovalsky MP et al. Pulmonary pharmacology of a novel, smooth muscle-selective muscarinic antagonist in vivo. J Pharmacol Exp Ther. 1994;270:546–53.
59. Doods H, Entzeroth M, Mayer N. Cardioselectivity of AQ-RA 741, a novel tricyclic antimuscarinic drug. Eur J Pharmacol. 1991;192:147–52.
60. Shannon HE, Bymaster FP, Calligaro DO et al. Xanomeline: a novel muscarinic receptor agonist with functional selectivity for M1 receptors. J Pharmacol Exp Ther. 1994;269:271–81.

Manuscript received 30 Nov. 95.
Accepted for publication 30 Nov. 95.

TS Gaginella et al. (eds.), Biochemical Pharmacology as an Approach to Gastrointestinal Disorders, 187–195

CHANGES OF SENSORY NEUROPEPTIDES IN EXPERIMENTAL GASTROINTESTINAL DISEASES

S. EVANGELISTA[1]* AND D. RENZI[2]
[1]Menarini Research, Via Sette Santi 1, 50131 Florence; [2]Gastroenterology Unit, Clinical Pathophysiology Department, University of Florence, Florence, Italy
*Correspondence

ABSTRACT

Calcitonin gene-related peptide (CGRP) is a marker of afferent fibres in the upper gastrointestinal tract, being almost completely depleted following treatment with selective neurotoxin capsaicin. Decreased levels of gastric CGRP-like immunoreactivity (li) were observed during acetic acid-, cysteamine-, concentrated ethanol- and water immersion stress-ulcers. The ulcerogens did not affect tissue content of other peptides, suggesting that reduction in gastric CGRP-li cannot be attributed only to the tissue damage and, moreover, restoration of CGRP-li was observed in animals with ulcers in healing status. These findings, together with the observation that CGRP could be released during increased acid-back diffusion, suggest the involvement of CGRP during gastric ulcer formation.

Similar results were obtained in duodenal ulcers produced by cysteamine, dulcerozine or mepirizole. Decrease in duodenal CGRP-li and substance P (SP)-li was associated with the development of gastroduodenal ulcers. In a rat model of colitis, such as that induced by trinitrobenzenesulphonic acid (TNB), decreased levels of colonic CGRP-li were observed during both acute and late phases of colitis.

These findings show that sensory neuropeptides are involved in several experimental diseases and may play a significant role in their pathogenesis.

Keywords: calcitonin gene-related peptide (CGRP), capsaicin, substance P (SP), tachykinins, ulcers

Capsaicin is the pungent ingredient in a wide variety of red peppers of the genus *Capsicum* and, chemically, it is a derivative of vanillyl amide, 8-methyl-*N*-vanillyl-6-nonenamide. Many studies have established capsaicin as an important probe to study sensory neuron mechanisms. In fact, low doses of capsaicin (in the μg/kg range) induce transient excitation of thin primary afferent neurons whilst systemic administration of high doses of the drug (in the mg/kg range) to small rodents causes long-lasting damage to these neurons [1]. The extent of injury, seen as ultrastructural changes or degeneration of unmyelinated C fibres and thinly myelinated aδ afferent fibres, depends on the dosage, route of administration and animal species [1]. Characteristically, these neurons subserve a dual afferent and local effector role. The afferent function enables information to be conveyed to the central nervous system. The local effector function arises from the release of neuropeptide transmitters from the peripheral nerve terminals of sensory endings. These peptides govern several local tissue functions, such as vasodilatation. In recent years, these latter functions have been extensively studied in the gastrointestinal tract [2].

This paper was presented at the Section of IUPHAR GI Pharmacology Symposium on 'Biochemical pharmacology as an approach to gastrointestinal disorders (basic science to clinical perspectives)', October 12–14, 1995, Pécs, Hungary.

The present article reviews the changes in neuropeptides of sensory origin caused by experimental diseases in stomach, small intestine and large intestine.

DECREASE IN CGRP-li DURING GASTRIC ULCER FORMATION

There is a wide range of experimental evidence for a protective role of capsaicin-sensitive sensory nerves in the stomach. Firstly, ablation of capsaicin-sensitive afferent neurons with high doses of capsaicin caused aggravation of experimentally induced lesion formation in the gastric mucosa produced by several stimuli [3–5]. Secondly, activation of capsaicin-sensitive fibres in the stomach enhanced the resistance of the gastric mucosa to experimentally imposed damage [3,6].

The Hungarian scientists, Szolcsanyi and Barthò, were the first, in 1981, to suggest an impaired defence mechanism in ulcers induced by pylorus ligation or acid distension in animals treated with high desensitizing doses of capsaicin [3]. They hypothesized that the basis of the mechanism leading to this aggravation was a lack of vasodilating neurotransmitters. After this fundamental observation, many studies have demonstrated the pivotal role played by CGRP, a marker of gastric sensory nerves [7], in the protective effects produced by capsaicin-sensitive afferent fibres. Capsaicin-sensitive afferent neurons in general contain a number of bioactive peptides, including CGRP, tachykinins (SP and neurokinin A (NKA)), vasoactive intestinal peptide (VIP), somatostatin, dynorphin and others [1]. Since regional and species differences might exist [8], the data reported thereafter are almost exclusively related to the rat, the species most commonly used in experimental gastrointestinal diseases. As shown in Figure 1, capsaicin pretreatment produced a selective depletion of peptides in the rat stomach. In fact, CGRP was markedly decreased after capsaicin pretreatment while galanin, neuropeptide Y (NPY), NKA and VIP were unaffected in both the secretory and non-secretory zones of the rat stomach (Figure 1). Immunohistochemical studies have shown that neonatal capsaicin pretreatment causes a depletion of fibres displaying CGRP immunoreactivity in the oesophagus and stomach of the rat [9].

Further, CGRP is considered the likely mediator of sensory neurons in the stomach. In fact, low doses of peripherally administered CGRP were effective in antagonizing certain types of experimentally induced gastric ulcers in rats [10] and the close intra-arterial infusion of the peptide, at doses without systemic hypotensive effects, produced protection against ulcers induced by ethanol, aspirin [11,12] or endothelin-1 [13]. The effect of intra-arterial CGRP, through a route which mimicks its local release in the stomach, resembles that of stimulation of afferent nerve endings by intragastric capsaicin, which likewise protects against both ethanol- and aspirin-induced lesion formation [6,14]. On the other hand, capsaicin-induced protection against ethanol lesions were dose-dependently antagonized by human (h)CGRP$_{8-37}$, the recently discovered CGRP antagonist [15], and significantly attenuated by anti-CGRP antibodies [16]. Further, worsening of the damaging effect of ethanol in the rat gastric mucosa was obtained by blocking the endogenous CGRP by active immunization [17]. These findings indicate that sensory neurons are important in maintaining the integrity of the mucosa in the face of not only injurious stimuli but also acid-pepsin digestion to

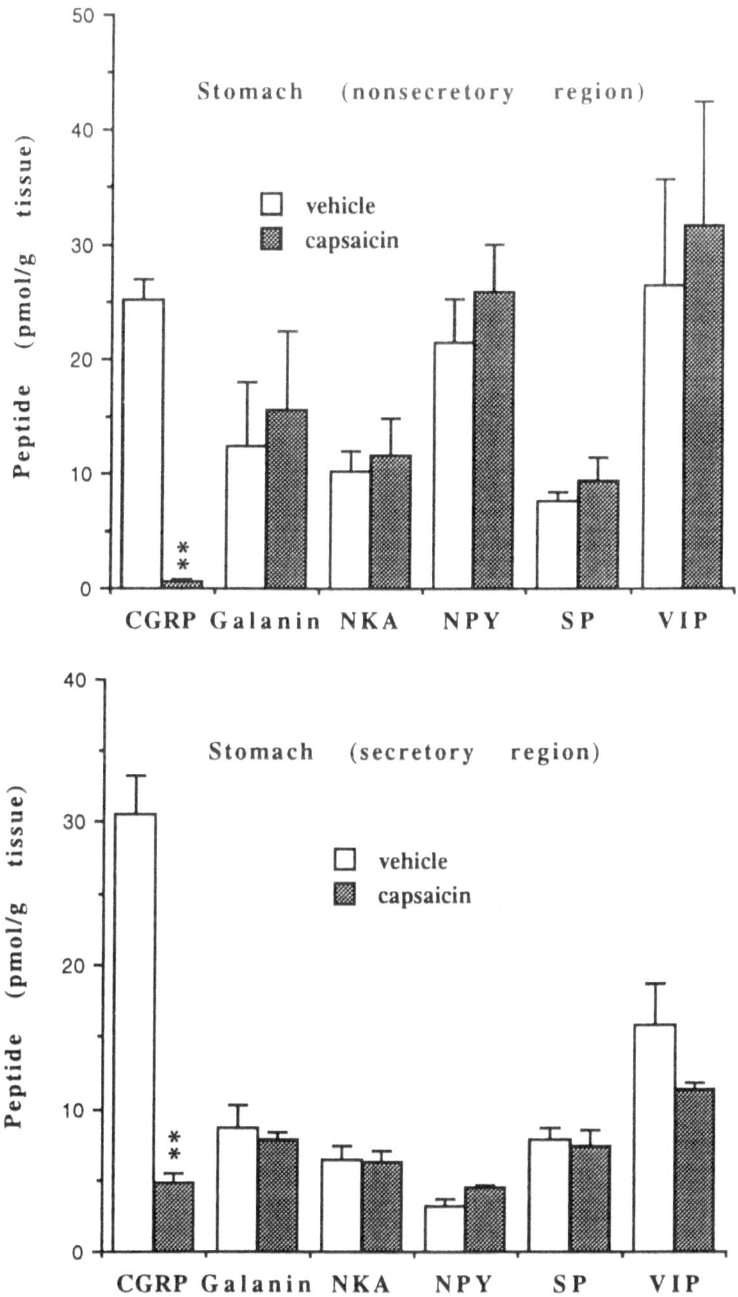

Figure 1. Effect of neonatal capsaicin pretreatment (50 mg/kg sc; solid colums) on CGRP-, galanin-, NKA-, NPY-, SP- and VIP-like immunoreactivity in the non-secretory (upper panel) and secretory (lower panel) regions of the rat stomach. Mean ± SE of 7–8 rats for each group. ** = $p < 0.01$ compared with the respective vehicle-treated group (open columns)

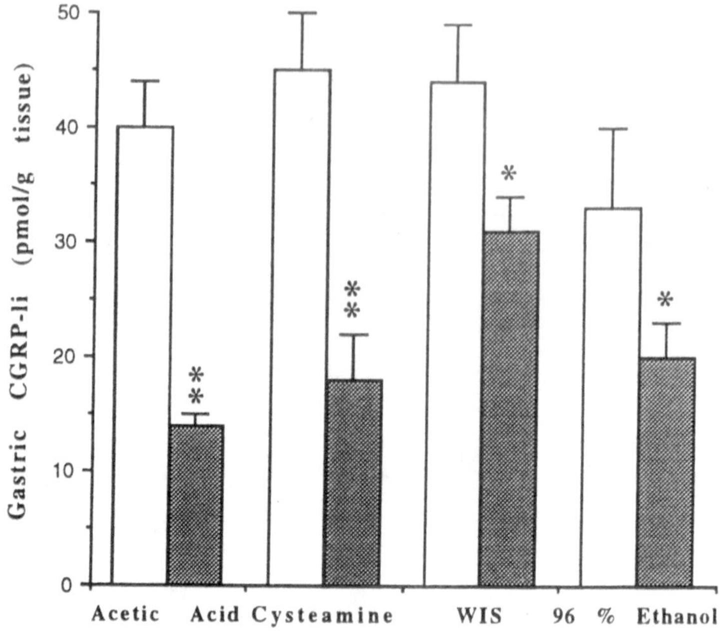

Figure 2. Effect of acetic acid (50 μl of 20% acetic acid/rat injected into the serosal region of the stomach, sacrificed 24 h later), cysteamine (900 mg/kg po, sacrificed 24 h later), water immersion stress (WIS, for 3 h) or 96% ethanol (5 ml/kg po, sacrificed 1 h later) on rat gastric CGRP-li. Open or solid columns indicate controls or treated animals, respectively. Mean ± SE of 8–12 rats for each group. * = $p < 0.05$ and ** = $p < 0.01$ compared with the respective control group

which the mucosa is exposed. In keeping with these findings, reduced tissue levels of CGRP derived from a capsaicin-sensitive pool in the rat stomach following acetic acid-, cysteamine-, concentrated ethanol- or water-immersion stress-ulcers are shown in Figure 2. The ulcerogens did not affect tissue content of other peptides [18,19] suggesting that reduction in gastric CGRP-li cannot be ascribed to generalized damage of the tissue. On the other hand, restoration of CGRP-li levels was observed in animals with ulcers that were healing [18,19]. As recently reported [18], gastric CGRP-li had already decreased 5 min after concentrated ethanol administration and returned to control values 10 days after the challenge in animals with lesions in the process of healing. Similar results were obtained in subchronic gastric ulcers induced by acetic acid injection in rats [19]. A relative decrease in gastric CGRP-li persisting up to 2 weeks after ulcer induction was observed. Lack of this potent vasodilating peptide and therefore inadequate blood supply to the ulcer bed and margins could be the cause of delayed healing observed in capsaicin-pretreated rats [19]. These findings and the observation that there is a tonic flow of CGRP, involving 80% of the peptide bulk [20], towards the peripheral endings of sensory fibres suggest that the peptide is restored in connection with the healing of ulcers after its release induced by the ulcerogen.

Taken together, these observations strongly suggest that CGRP is the likely mediator of the protective functions of sensory nerves in the stomach where it exerts a trophic effect.

DECREASE IN CGRP-li AND SP-li LEVELS IN DUODENAL ULCERS

It has been reported that, in the duodenum, the capsaicin-induced changes in vascular permeability are confined to the first centimetres caudal to the pyloric sphincter [21] and the authors of this paper have suggested that the resulting trophic effect on the duodenal mucosa might serve to counteract the irritation produced by the sudden drop in duodenal pH following gastric emptying. Recent observations indicate that acid stimulating a selective and Ca^{2+}-dependent release of sensory neuropeptides from capsaicin-sensitive primary afferents [22] can modulate acid back-diffusion [23]. Acid accumulation in the lumen and its penetration into the duodenal wall during the formation of ulcers might be the signals for these mechanisms mediated by primary afferents. Removal of these protective mechanisms by systemic capsaicin treatment leads to an increase in incidence and severity of duodenal ulcers induced by cysteamine or dulcerozine [21]. In view of the above, the observed reduction in duodenal CGRP-li following cysteamine-, dulcerozine- or mepirizole-induced ulcers [24] might originate from an intensive stimulation of the 'efferent' function of these sensory nerves. The temporal relationship of this phenomenon shows that duodenal CGRP-li decreased almost concomitantly with the formation of duodenal and gastric lesions induced by cysteamine administration [25] and there was an inverse correlation between degree of ulcers and peptide levels [24].

Unlike duodenal CGRP, which is decreased by 84% after neonatal capsaicin pretreatment [25], SP-neurons in the duodenum derive entirely from an intrinsic source [26]. In view of the above, it is noteworthy that SP-li was decreased in the presence of cysteamine ulcers [27]. On the other hand, SP has been described to be involved in neurogenic inflammation [28] and, local release of SP-li after capsaicin application in vascularly perfused rat duodenum has been reported recently [29]. Overall, extractable SP-li has been described to increase in jejunum of rats infected with *Trichinella spiralis* [30]. In spite of this and of the different mechanisms of the ulcerogenic agents used, the role of SP in small intestinal ulcers is so far unknown. Further studies are necessary to ascertain whether changes in this intrinsic neuropeptide are among the factors involved in the pathophysiology of small-intestinal ulcers rather than the results of them.

CHANGES IN NEUROPEPTIDES IN EXPERIMENTAL COLITIS

Gut calcitonin gene-related peptide (CGRP) is found in the intrinsic neurons of the myenteric and submucosal plexuses or in the extrinsic fibres arising from sensory primary neurons in dorsal root ganglia [9]. About 50% of CGRP in the rat colon is capsaicin sensitive and is characterized as α-CGRP, while the other 50% is not capsaicin sensitive and is referred to as β-CGRP [31].

Capsaicin-pretreated animals showed an increased formation of recto-colitis induced by TNB in the rat [32] or by immunocomplexes in rabbits [35] confirming the presence of afferent fibres playing a functional role at this level.

Figure 3 shows that CGRP-li is reduced in both the acute and chronic phases of TNB-induced colitis in rats. TNB colitis is known to be histologically similar to the classical inflammatory bowel diseases, namely ulcerative colitis and Crohn's disease [34]. In fact, intrarectal administration of the hapten TNB in the presence of a mucosal

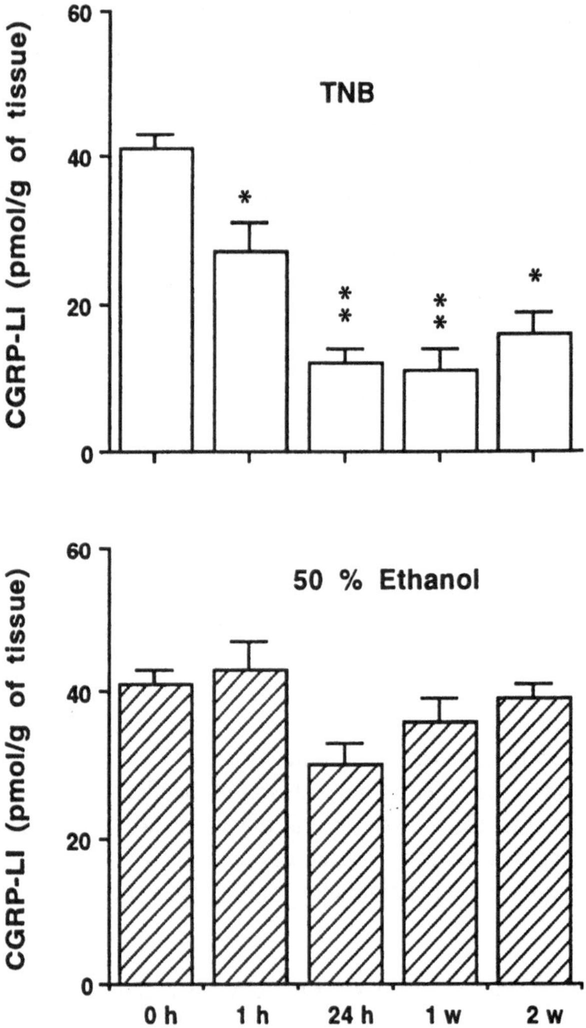

Figure 3. Time course of changes in rat recto-colon CGRP-li after intrarectal administration of trinitrobenzenesulphonic acid (TNB; upper panel) or its vehicle (50% ethanol; lower panel). Results are mean ± SE of 4–5 rats for each group * = $p < 0.05$ and ** = $p < 0.01$ compared with controls (time 0)

barrier breaker produces a colitis involving an immune-cell-mediated mechanism [34]. Ethanol, which is in itself a potent proinflammatory agent [35], did not produce any change in colonic CGRP-li (Figure 3). The decrease in CGRP was seen also in dry tissue samples, suggesting a real depletion of this peptide in spite of the tremendous increase in wet weight of the tissue [32]. The observation that tissue VIP increased after TNB suggests that CGRP depletion cannot be attributed only to tissue damage produced by the ulcerogen. Immunohistochemical studies confirmed that CGRP immunoreactivity is dramatically reduced for up to 1 week from the TNB challenge and, at 2 weeks, reinervation occurred [36].

The tissue levels of CGRP were similarly decreased using other experimental models of colitis and/or in other animal species, such as intraluminal administration of formalin and albumin immune complexes to rabbits or rats [37,38].

It has been reported that β-CGRP, which is present in the intrinsic neurons [31], might have an important role in the control of gut motility [39]. On the other hand, CGRP found in the extrinsic nerve fibres innervating the gut is involved in the regulation of intestinal blood flow [40]. At this level, the involvement of a hypothetical defensive mechanism produced by sensory fibres is supported by the observation that capsaicin desensitization worsens chronic rectocolitis induced by TNB [32] and by the findings that topical capsaicin administration [41] or exogenous CGRP [42] acutely protect against a colonic injury through the induction of mucosal colonic hyperaemia [43]. Whatever the mechanism(s), the decrease in CGRP-li in all phases of TNB colitis suggests that this peptide could be involved in inflammatory mechanism(s) leading to the ulcer.

CONCLUSION

The findings surveyed in the present article reported evidence that sensory peptides might play a role in the pathogenesis of gastrointestinal ulcers. In the stomach, it is now well established that they exert a protective role and that CGRP is the likely neurotransmitter mediator of these effects.

On the other hand, sensory neuropeptides are able to monitor noxious challenges to the tissue and dysfunction of this neural emergency system weakens resistance to the injurious stimuli and may be an aetiological factor in ulcer development in the entire gastrointestinal tract.

ACKNOWLEDGEMENTS

We would like to thank Drs C.A. Maggi and M. Tramontana (Pharmacology Dept., Menarini, Florence, Italy) and Drs A. Calabrò, C. Panerai and C. Surrenti (University of Florence) for helpful advice and suggestions. I am grateful to Mrs J. Marchant for revision of the English text.

REFERENCES

1. Holzer P. Capsaicin: cellular targets, mechanisms of action, and selectivity for thin sensory neurons. Pharmacol Rev. 1991;43:143–201.
2. Maggi CA. Capsaicin-sensitive nerves in the gastrointestinal tract. Arch Int Pharmacodyn Ther. 1990;303:157–66.
3. Szolcsanyi J, Barthò L. Impaired defense mechanism to peptic ulcer in the capsaicin desensitized rat. In: Mozsik G, Hanninen O, Javor T, eds. Gastrointestinal Defense Mechanism. Oxford and Budapest: Pergamon Press and Akademiai Kiado; 1981:39–51.
4. Evangelista S, Maggi CA, Meli A. Evidence for a role of adrenals in the capsaicin-sensitive 'gastric defence mechanism' in rats. Proc Soc Exp Biol Med. 1986;182:568–9.
5. Holzer P, Sametz W. Gastric mucosal protection against ulcerogenic factors in the rat mediated by capsaicin-sensitive afferent neurons. Gastroenterology. 1986;91:975–81.
6. Holzer P, Lippe ITh. Stimulation of afferent nerve endings by intragastric capsaicin protects against ethanol-induced damage of gastric mucosa. Neuroscience. 1988;27:981–7.
7. Green T, Dockray GJ. Characterization of the peptidergic afferent innervation of the stomach in the rat, mouse and guinea-pig. Neuroscience. 1988;25:181–93.
8. Sundler F, Ekblad E, Hakanson R. Occurrence and distribution of substance P- and CGRP-containing nerve fibers in gastric mucosa: species differences. Adv Exp Med Biol. 1991;298:29–37.
9. Sternini C, Reeve JR, Brecha N. Distribution and characterization of calcitonin gene-related peptide immunoreactivity in the digestive system of normal and capsaicin-treated rats. Gastroenterology. 1987;93:852–62.
10. Maggi CA, Evangelista S, Giuliani S, Meli A. Anti-ulcer activity of calcitonin gene-related peptide in rats. Gen Pharmacol. 1987;18:33–4.
11. Lippe ITh, Lorbach M, Holzer P. Close arterial infusion of calcitonin gene-related peptide into the rat stomach inhibits aspirin- and ethanol-induced hemorrhagic lesions. Regul Pept. 1989;26:35–46.
12. Evangelista S, Tramontana M, Maggi CA. Pharmacological evidence for the involvement of multiple calcitonin gene-related peptide (CGRP) receptors in the antisecretory and antiulcer effect of CGRP in rat stomach. Life Sci. 1992;50:PL-13–18.
13. Whittle BJR, Lopez-Belmonte J. Interactions between the vascular peptide endothelin-1 and sensory neuropeptides in gastric mucosal injury. Br J Pharmacol. 1991;102:950–4.
14. Holzer P, Pabst MA, Lippe ITh. Intragastric capsaicin protects against aspirin-induced lesion formation and bleeding in the rat gastric mucosa. Gastroenterology. 1989;96:1425–33.
15. Chiba T, Yamaguchi A, Yamatani T et al. Calcitonin gene-related peptide receptor antagonist human CGRP-(8-37). Am J Physiol. 1989;256:E331–5.
16. Lambrecht N, Burchert M, Respondek M, Muller KM, Peskar M. Role of calcitonin gene-related peptide and nitric oxide in the gastroprotective effect of capsaicin in the rat. Gastroenterology. 1993;104:1371–80.
17. Forster ER, Dockray GJ. The role of calcitonin gene-related peptide in gastric mucosal protection in the rat. Exp Physiol. 1991;76:623–6.
18. Evangelista S, Tramontana M, Panerai C, Surrenti C, Renzi D. Gastric lesions induced by concentrated ethanol are associated with a decrease in gastric calcitonin gene-related peptide-like immunoreactivity in rats. Sci J Gastroenterol. 1993;28:1112–14.
19. Tramontana M, Renzi D, Calabrò A et al. Influence of capsaicin-sensitive afferent fibers on acetic acid induced chronic gastric ulcers in rats. Sc J Gastroenterol. 1994;29:406–13.
20. Varro A, Green T, Holmes S, Dockray GJ. Calcitonin gene-related peptide in visceral afferent nerve fibres: quantification by radioimmunoassay and determination of axonal transport rates. Neuroscience. 1988;26:927–32.
21. Maggi CA, Evangelista S, Abelli L, Somma V, Meli A. Capsaicin-sensitive mechanisms and experimentally induced duodenal ulcers in rats. J Pharm Pharmacol. 1987;39:559–61.
22. Geppetti P, Tramontana M, Evangelista S et al. Differential effect of neuropeptide release of different concentrations of hydrogen ions on afferent and intrinsic neurons of the rat stomach. Gastroenterology. 1991;101:1505–11.
23. Holzer P, Livingston EH, Guth PH. Sensory neurons signal for an increase in rat gastric mucosal blood flow in the face of pending acid injury. Gastroenterology. 1991;101:416–23.
24. Evangelista S, Renzi D, Mantellini P, Surrenti C, Meli A. Duodenal ulcers are associated with a depletion of duodenal calcitonin gene-related peptide-like immunoreactivity in rats. Eur J Pharmacol. 1989;164:389–91.

25. Evangelista S, Renzi D, Tramontana M, Surrenti C, Theodorsson E, Maggi CA. Cysteamine induced-duodenal ulcers are associated with a selective depletion in gastric and duodenal calcitonin gene-related peptide-like immunoreactivity in rats. Regul Pept. 1992;39:19–28.
26. Holzer P, Gamse R, Lembeck F. Distribution of substance P in the rat gastrointestinal tract – lack of effect of capsaicin pretreatment. Eur J Pharmacol. 1980;61:303–7.
27. Evangelista S, Renzi D, Mantellini P, Surrenti C, Meli A. Duodenal SP-like immunoreactivity is decreased in experimentally induced duodenal ulcers. Neurosci Lett. 1990;112:352–5.
28. Maggi CA. Tachykinins and calcitonin gene-related peptide (CGRP) as co-transmitters released from peripheral endings of sensory nerves. Prog Neurobiol. 1995;45:1–98.
29. Fujimiya M, Kwok YN. Effect of capsaicin on release of substance P-like immunoreactivity from vascularly perfused rat duodenum. Dig Dis Sci. 1995;40:96–9.
30. Swain MG, Agro A, Blennerhassett P, Stanisz A, Collins SM. Increased levels of substance P in the myenteric plexus of trichinella-infected rats. Gastroenterology. 1992;102:1913–19.
31. Mulderry PK, Ghatei MA, Spokes RA et al. Differential expression of α-CGRP and β-CGRP by primary sensory neurons and enteric autonomic neurons of the rat. Neuroscience. 1988;25:195–205.
32. Evangelista S, Meli A. Influence of capsaicin-senstive fibers on experimentally-induced colitis in rats. J Pharm Pharmacol. 1989;41:574–5.
33. Reinshagen M, Patel A, Sottili M et al. Protective function of extrinsic sensory neurons in acute rabbit experimental colitis. Gastroenterology. 1994;106:1208–14.
34. Beck PL, Morris GP, Wase AW, Szewczuk M, Wallace JL. Immunological manipulation of disease progression in a rat model of chronic inflammatory disease of the colon. In: MacDermott RP, ed. Inflammatory Bowel Disease: Current Status and Future Approaches. Amsterdam: Elsevier Science; 1988:201–6.
35. Wallace JL, Whittle BJR, Boughton-Smith NK. Prostaglandin protection of rat colonic mucosa from damage induced by ethanol. Dig Dis Sci. 1985;30:866–76.
36. Sharkey KA. Substance P and calcitonin gene-related peptide (CGRP) in gastrointestinal inflammation. Ann NY Acad Sci (USA). 1992;664:425–42.
37. Eysselein VE, Reinshagen M, Cominelli F et al. Calcitonin gene-related peptide and substance P decrease in the rabbit colon during colitis. Gastroenterology. 1991;101:1211–19.
38. Miampamba M, Chéry-Croze S, Chayvialle JA. Spinal and intestinal levels of substance P, calcitonin gene-related peptide and vasoactive intestinal peptide following perendoscopic injection of formalin in rat colonic wall. Neuropeptides. 1992;22:73–80.
39. Mayer EA, Koelbel CBM, Snape WJ Jr, Eysselein VE, Ennes H, Kodner A. Substance P and CGRP mediate motor response of rabbit colon to capsaicin. Am J Physiol. 1990;259:G889–97.
40. Hottenstein OD, Pawlik WW, Remak G, Jacobson ED. Capsaicin-sensitive nerves modulate resting blood flow and vascular tone in rat gut. Naun Schmied Arch Pharmacol. 1992;343:179–84.
41. Goso C, Evangelista S, Tramontana M, Manzini S, Blumberg PM, Szallasi A. Topical capsaicin administration protects against trinitrobenzene sulfonic acid-induced colitis in rat. Eur J Pharmacol. 1993;249:185–90.
42. Evangelista S, Tramontana M. Involvement of calcitonin gene-related peptide in rat experimental colitis. J Physiol (Paris). 1993;87:277–80.
43. Leung FW. Role of capsaicin-sensitive afferent nerves in mucosal injury and injury-induced hyperemia in rat colon. Am J Physiol. 1992;262:G332–7.

Manuscript received 31 Oct. 95.
Accepted for publication 9 Nov. 95.

Section V

GI MUCOSAL INJURY AND PROTECTION

TS Gaginella et al. (eds.), Biochemical Pharmacology as an Approach to Gastrointestinal Disorders, 199–223

BIOCHEMICAL ENERGY BACKGROUNDS AND THEIR REGULATION IN THE GASTRIC CORPUS MUCOSA IN PATIENTS WITH DIFFERENT GASTRIC SECRETORY RESPONSES

Gy. MÓZSIK*, A. DEBRECENI, I. JURICSKAY, O. KARÁDI AND L. NAGY
First Department of Medicine, Medical University of Pécs, H-7643 Pécs, Hungary
*Correspondence

ABSTRACT

Many observations have been carried out to clarify the possible correlations between the gastric secretory responses and gastric fundic (corpus) mucosal biochemistry in animals. However, only a few studies have been performed in human beings (or patients) and even these gave contradictory results.

The aims of our observations were:

1. To evaluate the possible correlations between the gastric basal acid output (BAO) or maximal acid output (MAO) and tissue content of adenosine triphosphate (ATP), adenosine diphosphate (ADP), adenosine monophosphate (AMP), adenylate pool (ATP+ADP+AMP) and 'energy charge' [(ATP+0.5 ADP)/(ATP+ADP+AMP)] in gastric corpus mucosa of patients with 'genuine' peptic ulcer disease;

2. To identify the affinity, intrinsic activity curves and the values of pA_2, pD_2, $\alpha_{ouabain}$ and $\alpha_{pentagastrin}$ for the main hormones and drugs involved in the gastric inhibitory (ouabain) and stimulatory (pentagastrin, histamine) secretory responses.

The observations were carried out in patients with 'genuine' peptic ulcer or in their stomach (corpus) resecata obtained from surgery. The gastric basal and maximal acid output (over 1 h after 6 μg/kg sc application of pentagastrin) were measured before operation on the patients (but one week after cessation of medical treatment, except of antacids). The resecates of gastric corpus mucosa and muscular layer were obtained immediately after their resections, put into liquid nitrogen and the ATP, ADP and AMP determined from them. Adenylate pool (ATP+ADP+AMP), ratio of ATP/ADP and 'energy charge' [(ATP+0.5ADP)/(ATP+ADP+AMP)] were calculated. At the same time, the Mg^{2+}-Na^+-K^+-dependent (total), only Mg^{2+}-dependent and Na^+-K^+-dependent ATPases were prepared from the corpus mucosa and their activities expressed in μmol of P_i liberated (mg membrane protein^{-1} h^{-1}). The affinity and intrinsic activity curves for acetylcholine, pentagastrin and histamine (and pA_2 and pD_2 values) were determined on the transformations of ATP–ADP and ATP–cAMP.

It was found that:

1. A positive and close correlation exists between the:

a) BAO vs MAO ($p<0.001$, $n=41$); **b)** BAO vs. corpus mucosal (c.m.) ATP ($p<0.05$, $n=41$); **c)** MAO vs. c.m. ATP ($p<0.001$, $n=41$); **d)** BAO vs. c.m. ADP ($p<0.001$, $n=41$); **e)** MAO vs. c.m. ADP ($p<0.001$, $n=41$); **f)** BAO vs. c.m. AMP ($p<0.05$, $n=41$); **g)** MAO vs. c.m. AMP ($p<0.05$, $n=41$); **h)** BAO vs. adenylate pool ($p<0.05$, $n=41$); **i)** MAO vs. adenylate pool ($p<0.05$, $n=41$); **j)** BAO vs. adenine–adenosine ($p<0.05$, $n=41$); **k)** MAO vs. adenine–adenosine ($p<0.05$, $n=41$); **l)** BAO vs. ratio of ATP/ADP in the gastric corpus mucosa ($p<0.05$, $n=41$); **m)** MAO vs. ratio of ATP/ADP in the gastric corpus mucosa ($p<0.05$, $n=41$); **n)** c.m. ATP vs. ADP ($p<0.001$, $n=41$); **o)** c.m. ATP vs. Na^+-K^+-dependent ATPase ($p<0.001$, $n=41$); **p)** c.m. ADP vs. Na^+-K^+-dependent ATPase ($p<0.001$, $n=41$);

This paper was presented at the Section of IUPHAR GI Pharmacology Symposium on 'Biochemical pharmacology as an approach to gastrointestinal disorders (basic science to clinical perspectives)', October 12–14, 1995, Pécs, Hungary.

2. Acetylcholine stimulates, while histamine and pentagastrin inhibit, the activity of Na^+-K^+-dependent ATPase;

3. Pentagastrin and histamine stimulate the Mg^{2+}-dependent ATPase; however, Ach. had no effect on its activity;

4. The extent of ATP-cAMP transformation is stimulated by histamine and pentagastrin while it is inhibited by Ach.

It has been concluded that:

1. The gastric BAO (and MAO) secretory responses depend on the energy metabolism of the gastric corpus mucosa (ATP, ADP, AMP, adenylate pool, ratio of ATP/ADP and 'energy charge') and not only on the number of parietal cells;

2. The energy liberation from ATP (into ADP or cAMP) is regulated by acetylcholine, histamine and pentagastrin in different pathways (acetylcholine via ATP–ADP, while histamine and pentagastrin via ATP–cAMP transformation);

3. The ATP–ADP transformation is more sensitive than the ATP–cAMP pathway for energy liberation necessary for gastric H^+ secretion;

4. The gastric H^+ secretion is due to (a) ATP–ADP transformation and (b) ATP–cAMP transformation;

5. The biochemical background of energy liberation for gastric H^+ secretion – by ATP–cAMP transformation – exists only after the inhibition of ATP–ADP transformation.

Keywords: patients with 'genuine' peptic ulcer; gastric secretory responses; gastric mucosal energy metabolism; hormonal regulations; dual energy metabolism for gastric H^+ secretion

INTRODUCTION

The gastric secretory responses are consequences of an active and special metabolic process of the gastric mucosa, when the H^+, Na^+, K^+, Cl^-, Ca^{2+}, Mg^{2+} move against their chemical gradients (from the plasma into the gastric juice). The gastric H^+ is an extreme example of active transport because it is concentrated (from the plasma to gastric juice) from pH 7.4 to pH 1. No similar degree of ion transport can be found in the human body or in other living animals; however, the moving (transport) of H^+ is closely associated with Na^+, K^+, Cl^-, Ca^{2+} and Mg^{2+} [1].

The physiology, biochemistry and pathology of the transport of cations and anions across the cell membrane have been much studied in animals, however, relatively few observations have been made in patients.

The transport of Na^+ and K^+ across the cell membrane is called the 'sodium pump' in the literature. The electrophysiological background of sodium pumps has been extensively studied in the nervous system, muscle [2–5] and erythrocyte [6]. ATP–ADP transformation by Na^+-K^+-dependent ATPase, was found by Skou [6] to be the biochemical background to active transport of cations. The biochemical background and explanations of ion transport was found to be more complicated when the cAMP system was discovered and its key role in the regulation of cells was internationally accepted [7].

Gastric physiology and pathophysiology has provided a special area to study the mechanisms of ion transport across the cell membrane in the stomach during recent decades. The basic observations were usually carried out in amphibian, guinea pig or rabbit stomach [8]. Interestingly, these results obtained from animals have been applied to humans (including the discovery of H_2-antagonists, gastrin-antagonists, H^+-K^+-inhibitors) [8–11]; however, the most clinicians would like to obtain direct (or indirect) experimental data from patients too.

Many studies have been performed by our work team in human beings (patients) to clarify the basic physiological, pathophysiological and biochemical aspects of gastric secretory responses.

The aims of our observations were:

1. To study the correlation between gastric basal (BAO) and maximal (MAO) acid secretory responses in patients with 'genuine' peptic ulcer;

2. To evaluate the possible correlation between gastric acid secretory responses (BAO, MAO) and the biochemical constituents (tissue ATP, ADP, AMP, Mg^{2+}-Na^+-K^+-dependent, only Mg^{2+}-dependent and Na^+-K^+-dependent ATPases) prepared from the resecates of corpus mucosa obtained from patients (with peptic ulcers) who underwent a partial resection of the stomach;

3. To analyse the affinities and intrinsic activity curves for atropine, epinephrine, cAMP, PGE and PGE_2, pentagastrin, histamine and g-strophanthin (ouabain) on the transformations of ATP into ADP and ATP into cAMP;

4. To clarify the correlations that exist between gastric corpus mucosal levels of ATP, ADP, AMP, ratio of ATP/ADP, adenylate pool (ATP+ADP+AMP) and 'energy charge' [(ATP+0.5ADP)/(ATP+ADP+AMP)];

5. To find correlations between biochemical constituents of human gastric corpus mucosa and musculature.

MATERIALS AND METHODS

The observations were carried out in patients with 'genuine' gastric, duodenal and jejunal ulcers. The observations could be divided into two parts:

1. *In vivo studies*: The gastric BAO and MAO were determined in the patients with peptic ulcer who underwent partial gastrectomy (according to Billroth II). The gastric secretory responses were measured one week before the surgical intervention at which time the patients had received antacids only for one week. Gastric maximal acid output was provoked by sc administration of pentagastrin (6 μg/kg, Peptavlon, ICI, England). The gastric basal and maximal acid outputs were determined for one-hour periods over which the gastric juice was collected. The

quantity of gastric H^+ was measured by titration with 0.1 mol/L NaOH. The amount of 0.1 mol/L NaOH needed to reach pH 7.0 was measured (detected by a pH titrimeter, Radelkis, Budapest). The H^+ output was expressed in mmol/h (mean ± SEM) under the circumstances with (MAO) and without (BAO) a supramaximal dose of pentagastrin due to gastric acid secretory responses.

2. *In vitro studies*: Tissue specimens of human gastric corpus mucosa and musculature were obtained at the time of gastric surgery when the mucosa and musculature were separated and thereafter put into liquid nitrogen. The adenosine triphosphate (ATP), diphosphate (ADP), monophosphate (AMP) and adenine–adenosine were separated according to methods published earlier [12] from human gastric corpus mucosa and musculature. The deoxyribonucleic acid was prepared from both human gastric corpus mucosa and musculature according to the method of Schmidt and Thannhauser [13]. The tissue levels of ATP, ADP and AMP were expressed as μmol/mg DNA (mean ± SEM). The adenylate pool (ATP+ADP+AMP), ratio of ATP/ADP and 'energy charge' [(ATP+0.5ADP)/(ATP+ADP+AMP)] were calculated [5].

The Mg^{2+}-Na^+-K^+-dependent (total), Mg^{2+}-dependent and Na^+-K^+-dependent ATPases were prepared from the human gastric corpus (mucosa and musculature) according to our method published previously [1,14]. The membrane ATPase activity was measured by the liberation of inorganic phosphate (P_i) during the breakdown of ATP into ADP. The membrane ATPase activity was expressed as P_i (mg membrane protein)$^{-1}$ h^{-1} (mean ± SEM). The membrane protein content was assayed by the method of Lowry et al. [15].

The affinity and intrinsic activity curves for atropine, epinephrine, cAMP, PGE_2 and PGI_2, histamine, pentagastrin and g-strophanthin (ouabain) were identified according to the method of Csáky [16]. The values of pA_2, pD_2 and intrinsic activity ($\alpha_{ouabain} = 1.00$) were also determined for these drugs.

Statistical analysis

The results were expressed as mean ± SEM. The values of pA_2, pD_2 and intrinsic activities ($\alpha_{atropine}$ is 1.00 for the drugs inhibiting the extent of ATP–ADP transformation, while $\alpha_{pentagastrin}$ is 1.00 for stimulating the extent of ATP–cAMP transformation) were calculated from the dose–response curves. The correlation, equation of regression line, correlation and *p* values were calculated and expressed by the method of Fisher [described in Reference 17].

RESULTS

Correlation between the gastric BAO and MAO in patients with 'genuine' (gastric, duodenal and jejunal) ulcer diseases

The gastric secretory responses were expressed as mmol/h (mean ± SEM; $n = 41$):

BAO = 2.40 ± 0.34
MAO = 14.75 ± 1.04

The regression equation is $y = 2.5x + 8.2$; $r = 0.80$; $p < 0.001$.

Gastric BAO and gastric corpus mucosal biochemistry in patients

The results were (Figures 1–7):

a) BAO (2.68 ± 0.33 mmol/h) vs. gastric mucosal ATP (476.1 ± 47 μmol/mg DNA); $y = 1739x - 0.456$; $n = 41$; $r = 0.31$; $p < 0.05$;

b) BAO (2.68 ± 0.33 mmol/h) vs. gastric mucosal ADP (291.5 ± 63 μmol/mg DNA); $y = 46x + 166$; $n = 41$; $r = 0.24$; p-value not significant (NS);

c) BAO (2.68 ± 0.33 mmol/h) vs. ratio of ATP/ADP in gastric mucosal (1.63 ± 0.35); $y = 0.16x + 0.65$; $n = 41$; $r = 0.56$; $p < 0.001$;

d) BAO (2.68 ± 0.33 mmol/h) vs. gastric mucosal AMP (4994 ± 2435 μmol/mg DNA); $y = 2375x - 1.38$; $n = 41$; $r = 0.32$; $p < 0.05$;

e) BAO (2.68 ± 0.33 mmol/h) vs. gastric mucosal adenylate pool (5762 ± 2558 μmol/mg DNA); $y = 2564x - 1.115$; $n = 41$; $r = 0.33$; $p < 0.05$;

f) BAO (2.68 ± 0.33 mmol/h) vs. 'energy charge' in the corpus mucosa (0.41 ± 0.03); $y = 0.03x + 0.49$; $n = 41$; $r = -0.38$; $p < 0.05$;

g) BAO (2.68 ± 0.33 mmol/h) vs. gastric mucosal adenine–adenosine (5222 ± 1499 μmol/mg DNA); $y = 165x + 687$; $n = 41$; $r = 0.36$; $p < 0.05$.

The gastric MAO and gastric corpus mucosal biochemistry in patients

The results were (Figures 8–14):

a) MAO (14.75 ± 1.04 mmol/h) vs. gastric mucosal ATP (476.1 ± 47 μmol/mg DNA); $y = 61x - 0.42$; $n = 41$; $r = 0.43$; $p < 0.05$;

b) MAO (14.75 ± 1.04 mmol/h) vs. gastric mucosal ADP (291.5 ± 63 μmol/mg DNA); $y = 27x - 103$; $n = 41$; $r = 0.44$; $p < 0.05$;

c) MAO (14.75 ± 1.04 mmol/h) vs. ratio of ATP/ADP in gastric mucosa (1.63 ± 0.35); $y = 0.04x + 0.42$; $n = 41$; $r = 0.45$; $p < 0.05$;

d) MAO (14.75 ± 1.04 mmol/h) vs. gastric mucosal AMP (4995 ± 2435 μmol/mg DNA); $y = 849x - 7.5$; $n = 41$; $r = 0.36$; p-value NS;

e) MAO (14.75 ± 1.04 mmol/h) vs. gastric mucosal adenylate pool (5762 ± 2558 μmol/mg DNA); $y = 937x - 8.06$; $n = 41$; $r = 0.38$; $p < 0.05$;

f) MAO (14.75 ± 1.04 mmol.h) vs. 'energy charge' in the corpus mucosa (0.41 ± 0.03); $y = 0.009x + 0.43$; $n = 41$; $r = 0.04$; p-value NS;

g) MAO (14.75 ± 1.04 mmol/h) vs. gastric mucosal adenine–adenosine (5222 ± 1499 μmol/mg DNA); $y = 637x + 357$; $n = 41$; $r = 0.44$; $p < 0.05$.

The gastric BAO, MAO and gastric corpus musculature energy metabolism in patients

The ATP, ADP, AMP and adenine–adenosine were measured directly and the ratio of ATP/ADP, adenylate pool and energy charge were calculated from the above parameters in the gastric corpus musculature in patients.

The correlation between each of biochemical parameters and gastric BAO or MAO values were studied; however, no significant correlation could be proved ($n = 21$) (Figures 1–14).

Affinity and intrinsic activity curves for acetylcholine, histamine and pentagastrin on the membrane ATPases and adenylate cyclase prepared from the human gastric mucosa

The atropine, epinephrine, cAMP, PGI_2, PGE_2, pentagastrin, histamine and ouabain inhibit the Na^+-K^+-dependent ATPases prepared from human gastric corpus mucosa. The actions of these compounds offered a new speculative (or causal) approach to possible correlations between the transformation of ATP–ADP (by membrane ATPase) and ATP–cAMP (by adenylate cyclase).

The analysis of the actions of acetylcholine, histamine and pentagastrin was chosen for further analysis on adenylate pool. Surprisingly, we found that the values of pD_2 and pA_2 for these compounds are higher for transformation of ATP–cAMP than for transformation of ATP–ADP (Table 1).

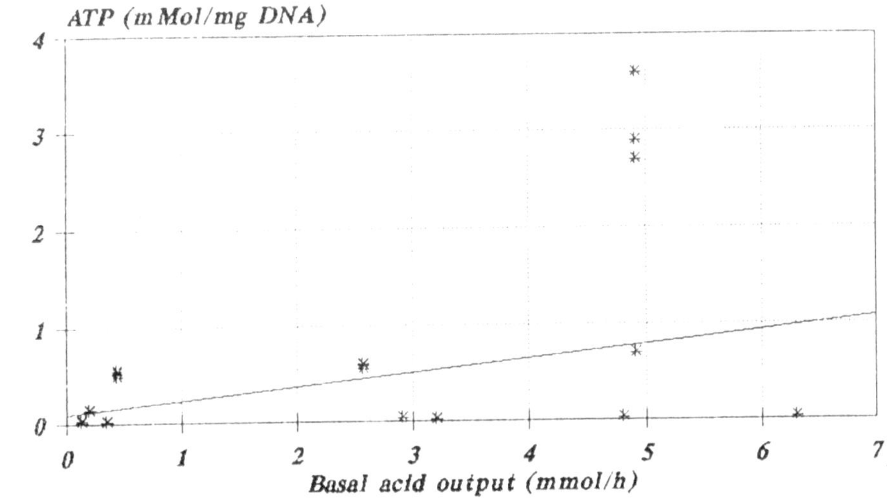

N=41; r=0.31; p<0.05
Y=1739*X-0.456

BAO (Mean ± S.E.M) = 2.68 ± 0.33

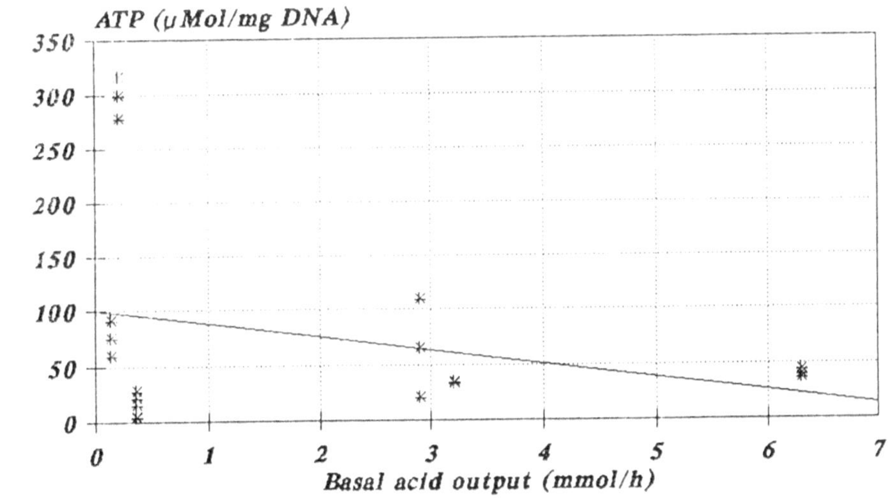

N=21; r=-0.31; N.S.
Y=-13*X+102

Figure 1. Correlation between the corpus mucosal (above) and musculature (below) ATP vs. BAO in patients

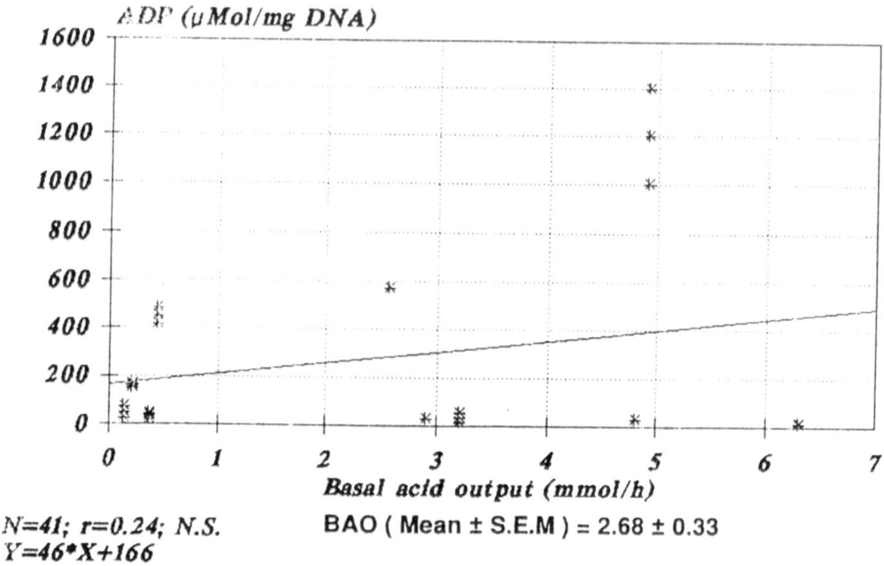

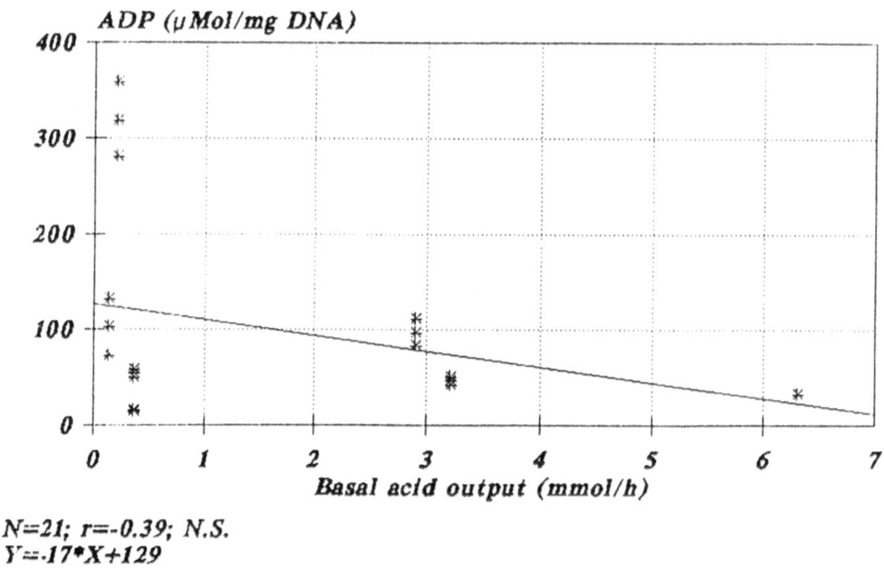

Figure 2. Correlation between the corpus mucosal (above) and musculature (below) ADP vs. BAO in patients

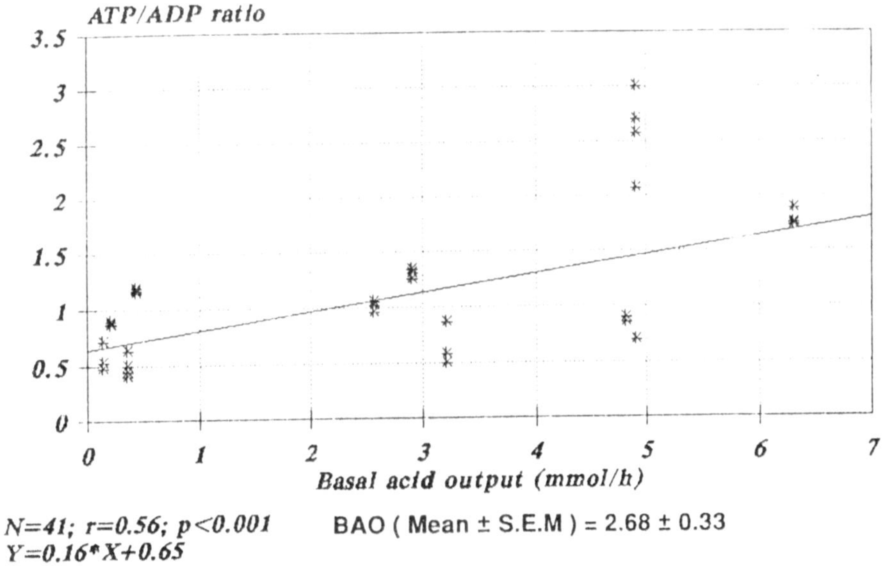

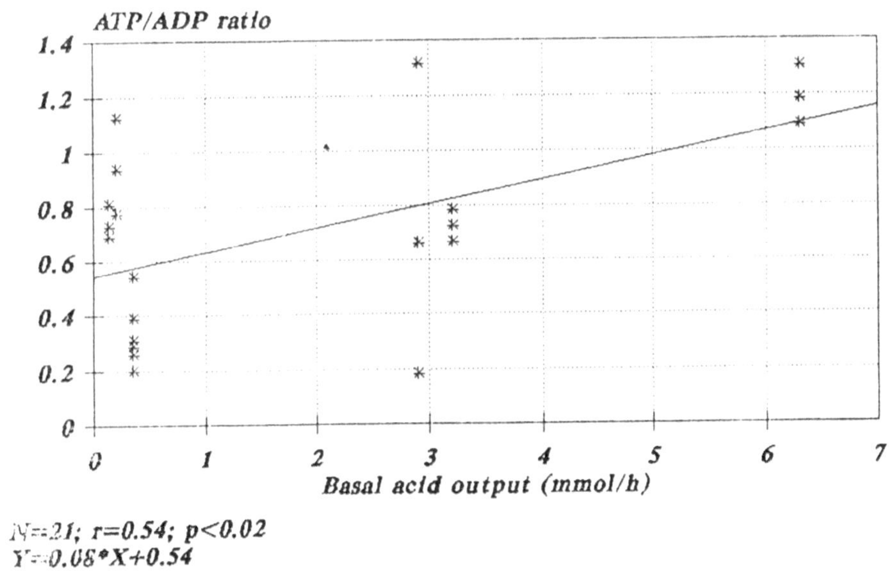

Figure 3. Correlation between the corpus mucosal (above) and musculature (below) ratio of ATP/ADP vs. BAO in patients

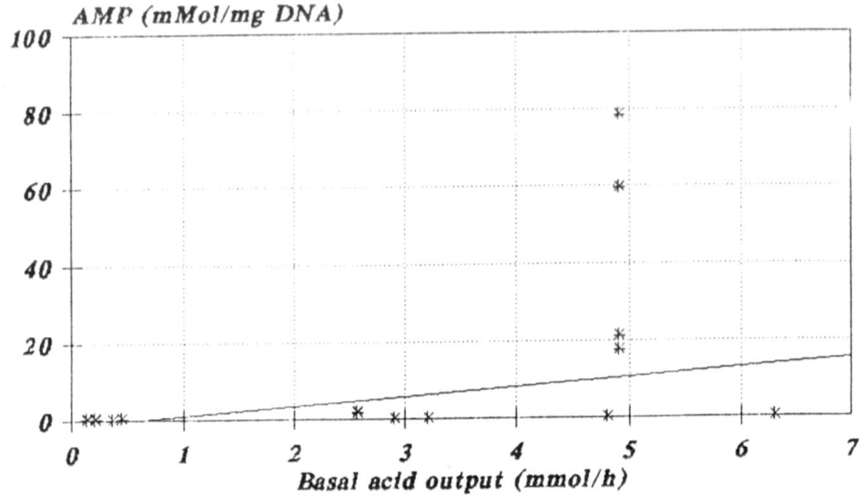

N=41; r=0.32; p<0.05
*Y=2375*X-1.380*

BAO (Mean ± S.E.M) = 2.68 ± 0.33

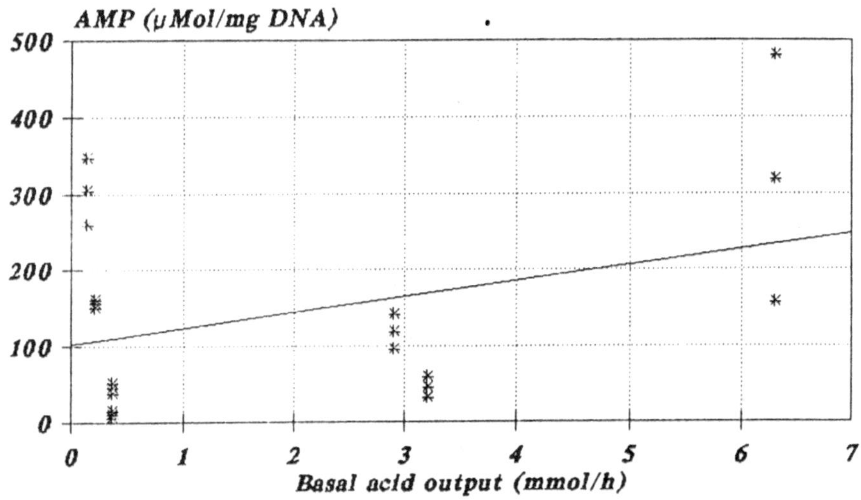

N=21; r=0.34; N.S.
*Y=19*X+104*

Figure 4. Correlation between the corpus mucosal (above) and musculature (below) AMP vs. BAO in patients

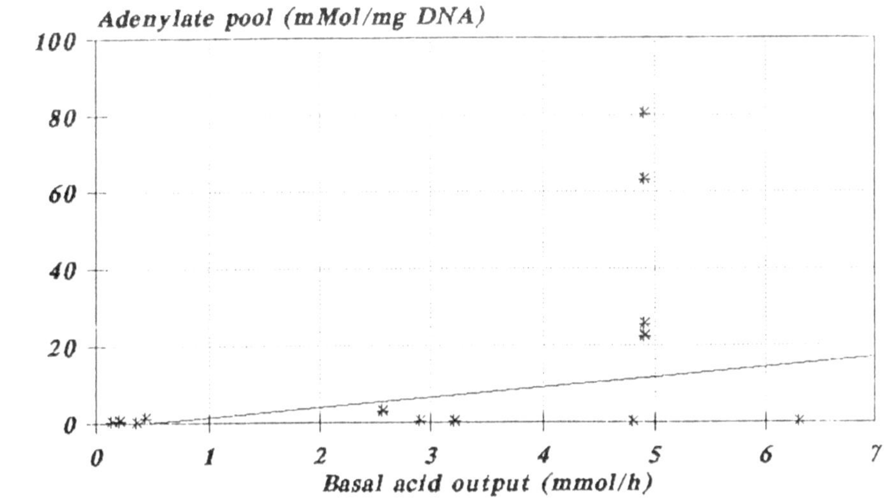

N=41; r=0.33; p<0.05 BAO (Mean ± S.E.M) = 2.68 ± 0.33
*Y=2564*X-1.115*

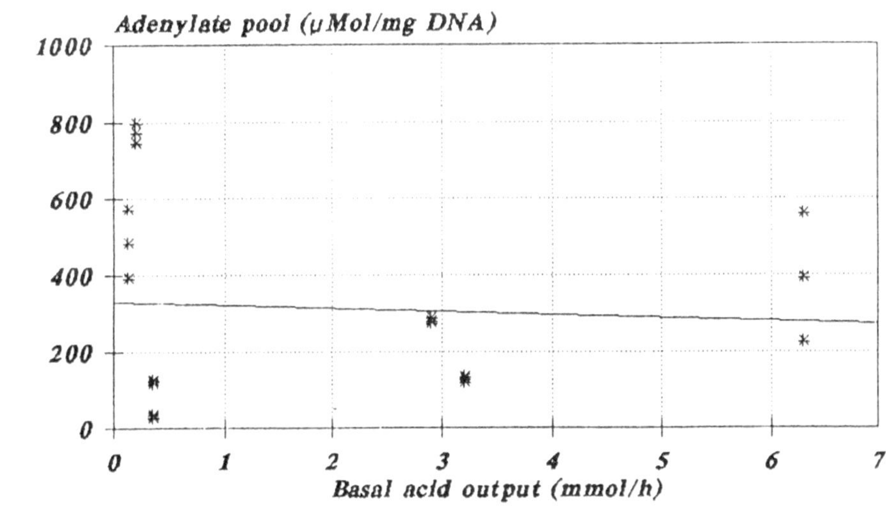

N=21; r=-0.09; N.S.
*Y=-11*X+334*

Figure 5. Correlation between the corpus mucosal (above) and musculature (below) adenylate pool vs. BAO in patients

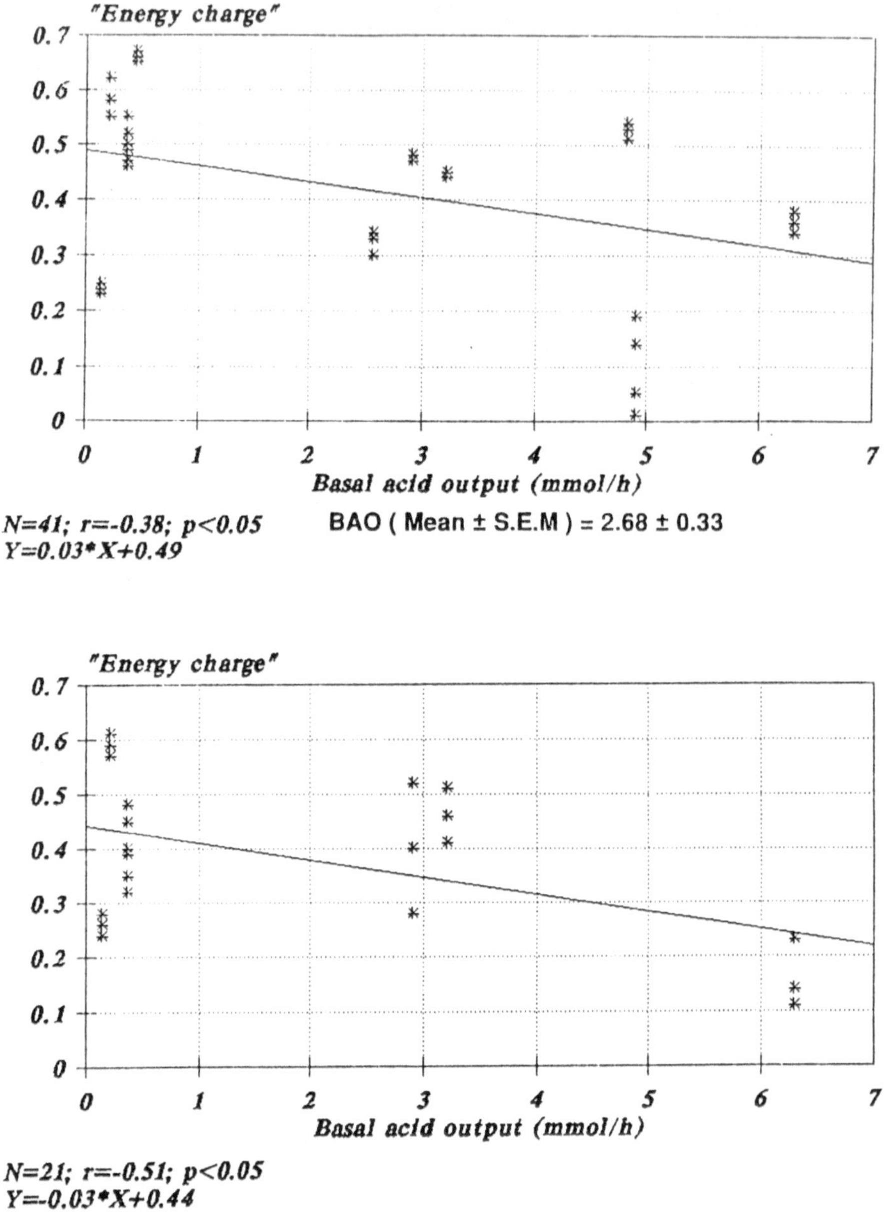

Figure 6. Correlation between the corpus mucosal (above) and musculature (below) 'energy charge' vs. BAO in patients

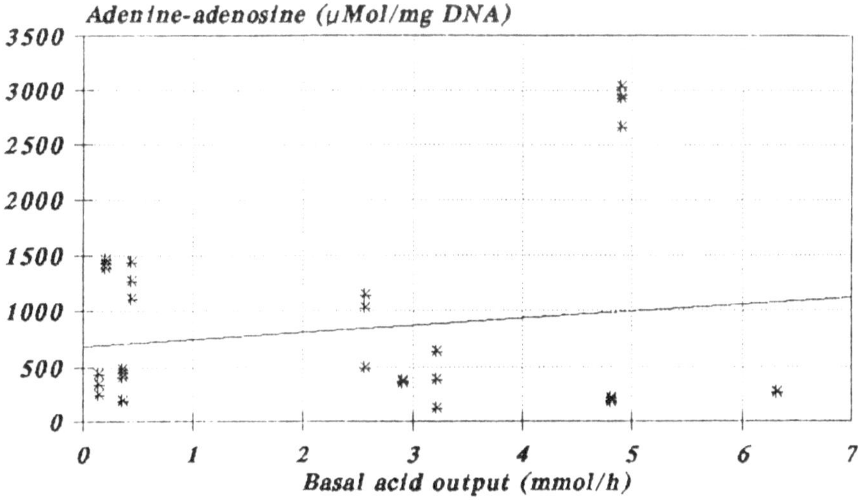

N=41; r=0.36; p<0.05 BAO (Mean ± S.E.M) = 2.68 ± 0.33
*Y=165*X+687*

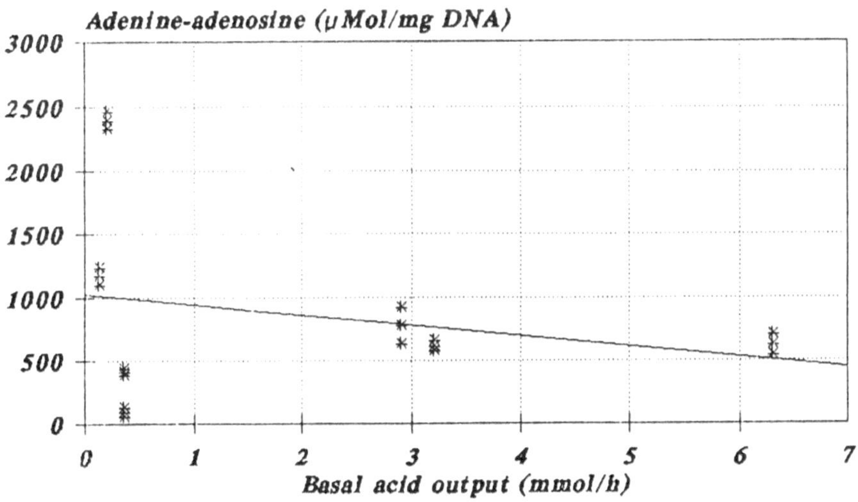

N=21; r=-0.28; N.S.
*Y=-90*X+1036*

Figure 7. Correlation between the corpus mucosal (above) and musculature (below) adenine–adenosine vs. BAO in patients

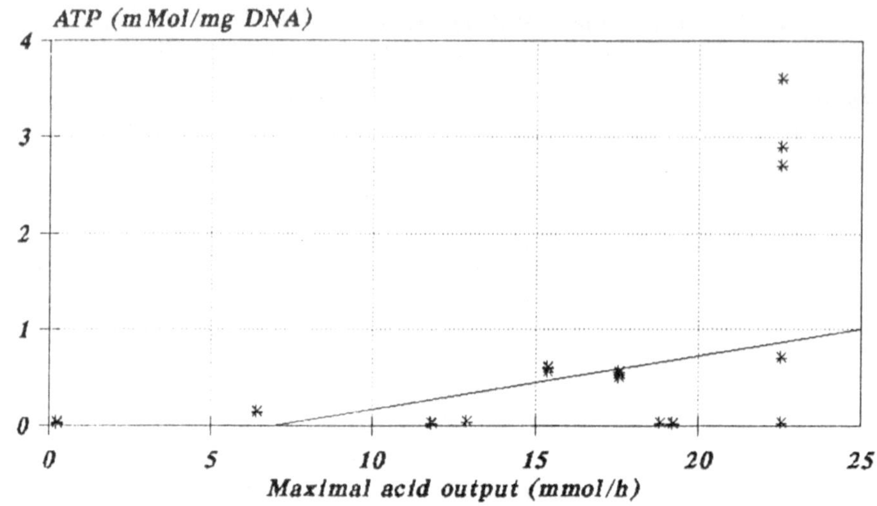

N=41; r=0.43; p<0.05 MAO (Mean ± S.E.M) = 14.75 ± 1.04
*Y=61*X-0.42*

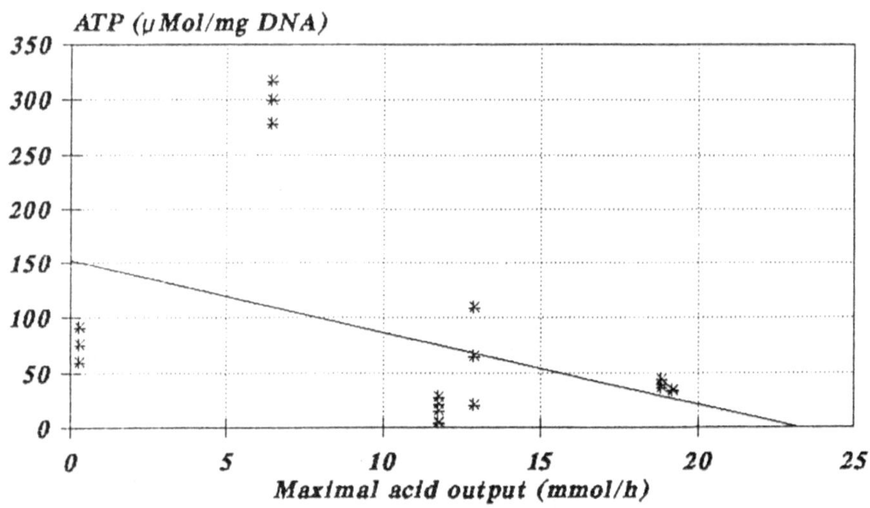

N=21; r=-0.38; N.S.
*Y=-6.6*X+147*

Figure 8. Correlation between the corpus mucosal (above) and musculature (below) ATP vs. MAO in patients

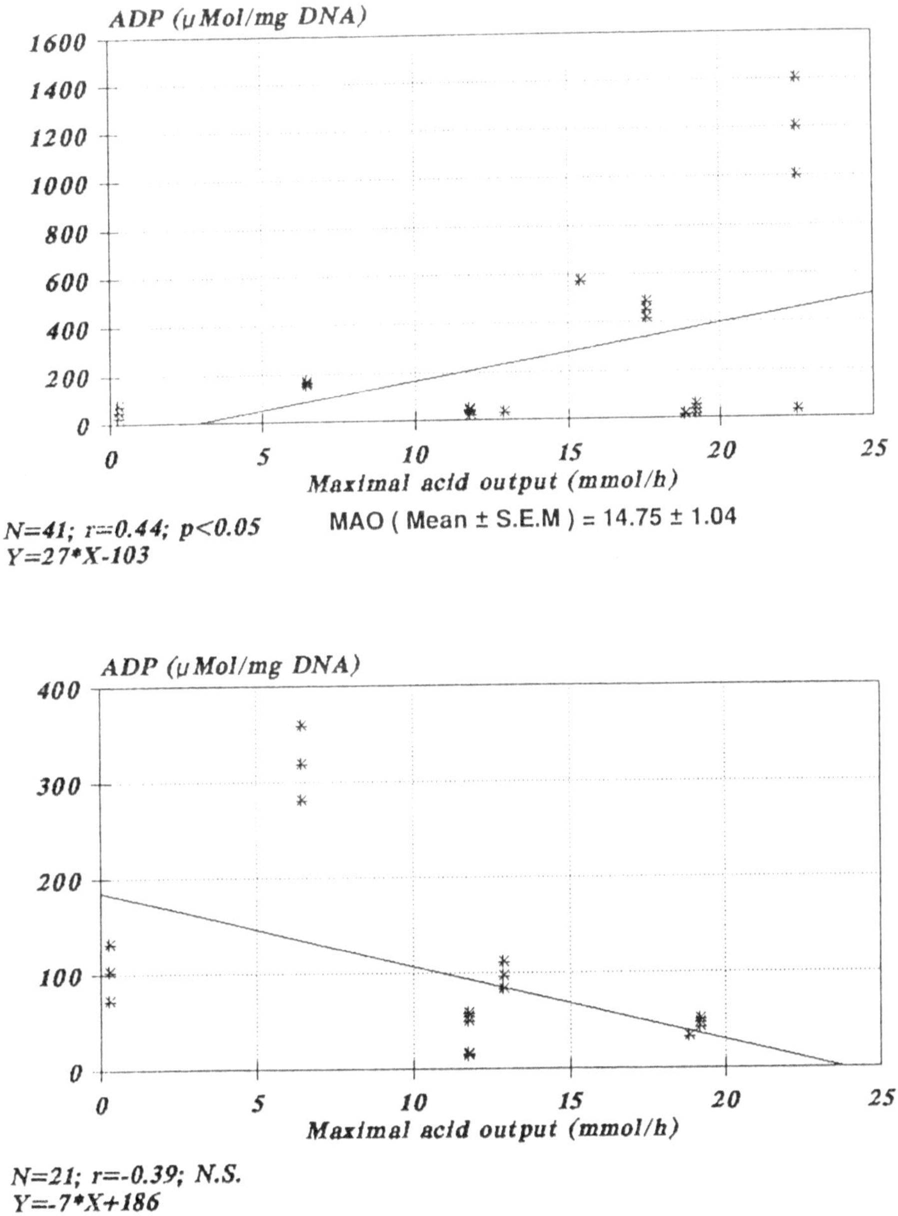

Figure 9. Correlation between the corpus mucosal (above) and musculature (below) ADP vs. MAO in patients

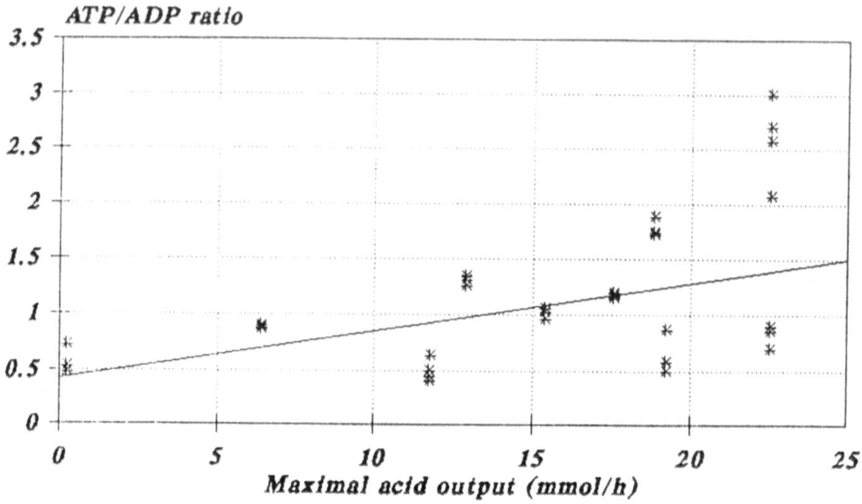

N=41; r=0.45; p<0.05
Y=0.04•X+0.42

MAO (Mean ± S.E.M) = 14.75 ± 1.04

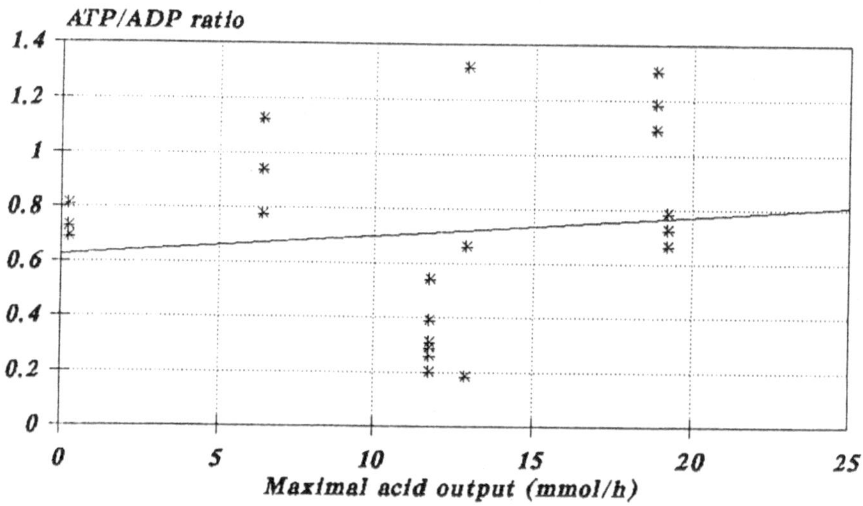

N=21; r=0.13; N.S.
Y=0.007•X+0.63

Figure 10. Correlation between the corpus mucosal (above) and musculature (below) ratio of ATP/ADP vs. MAO in patients

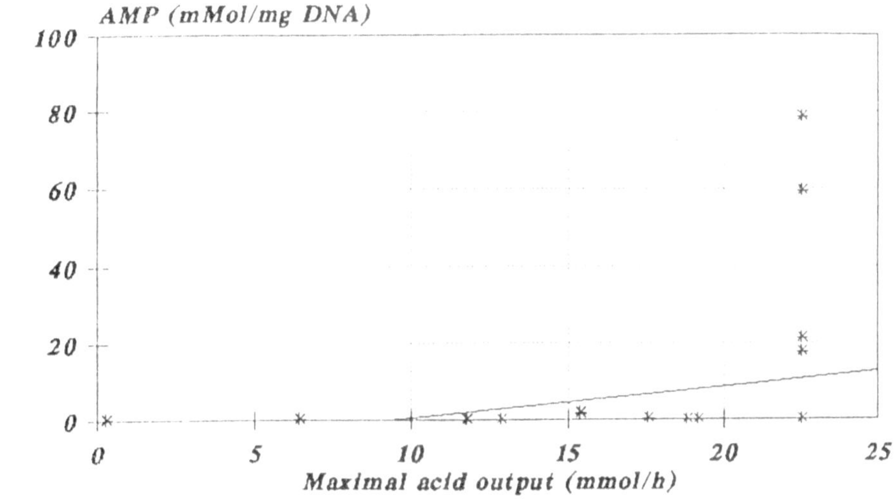

N=41; r=0.36; N.S.
Y=849*X-7.5

MAO (Mean ± S.E.M) = 14.75 ± 1.04

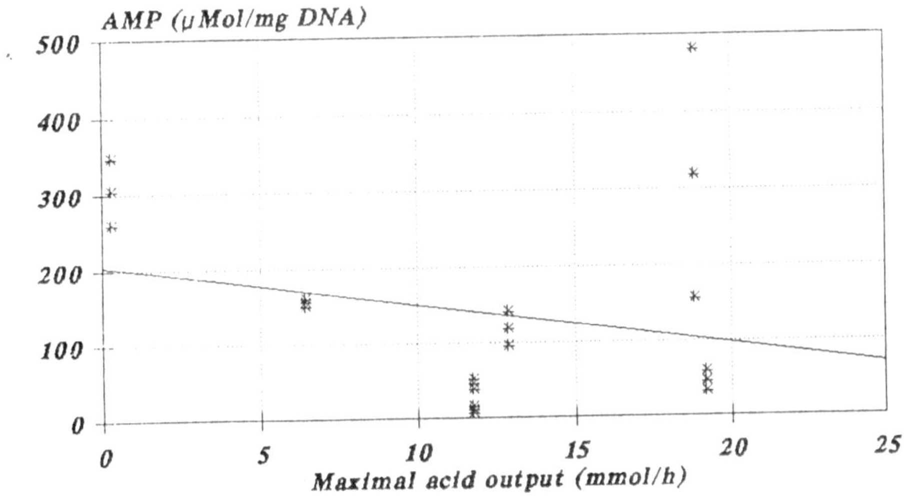

N=21; r=-0.66; p<0.05
Y=-15*X+197

Figure 11. Correlation between the corpus mucosal (above) and musculature (below) AMP vs. MAO in patients

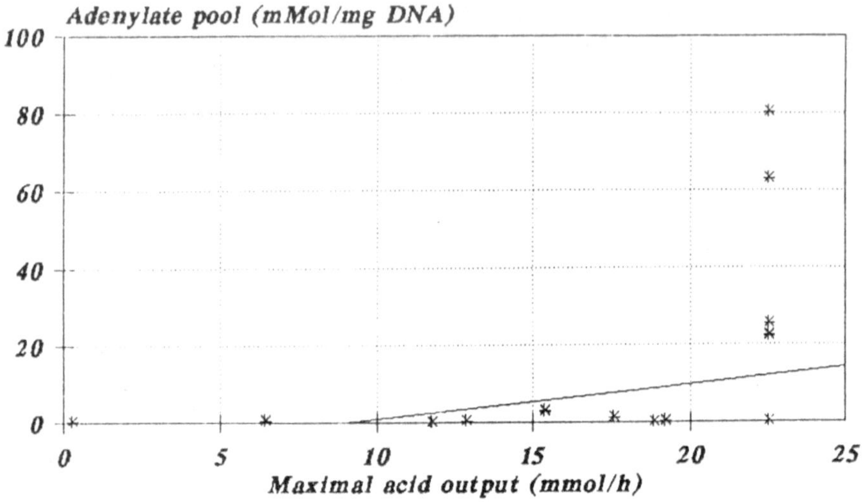

N=41; r=0.38; p<0.05
Y=937*X-8.06

MAO (Mean ± S.E.M) = 14.75 ± 1.04

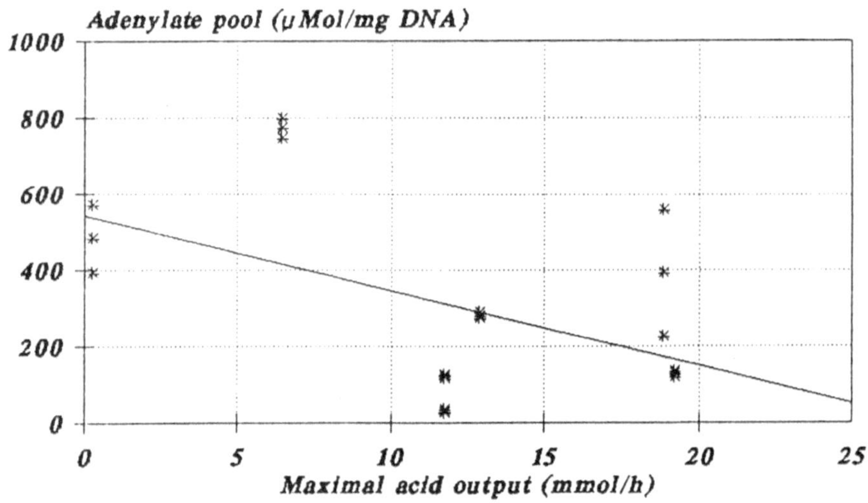

N=21; r=-0.641 p<0.02
Y=-29*X+586

Figure 12. Correlation between the corpus mucosal (above) and musculature (below) adenylate pool vs. MAO in patients

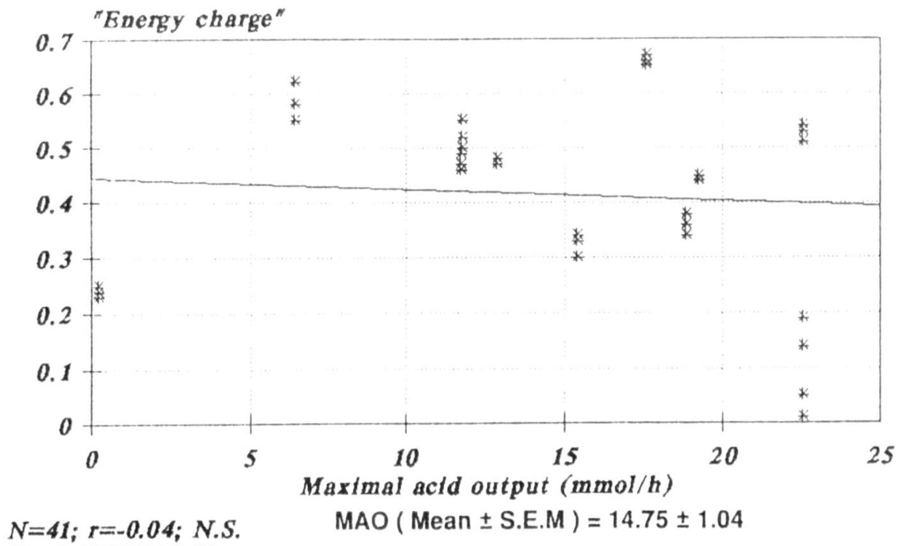

N=41; r=-0.04; N.S.
Y=-0.009*X+0.43

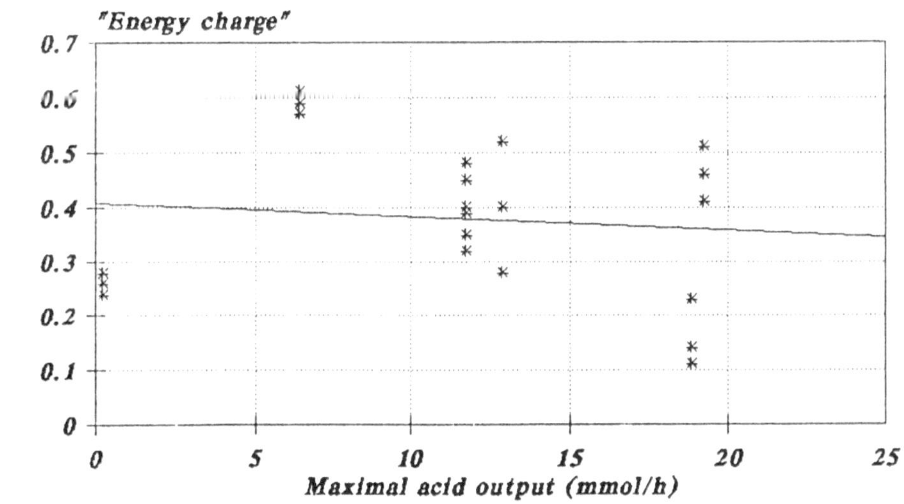

N=21; r=0.29; N.S.
Y=-0.007*X+0.41

Figure 13. Correlation between the corpus mucosal (above) and musculature (below) 'energy charge' vs. MAO in patients

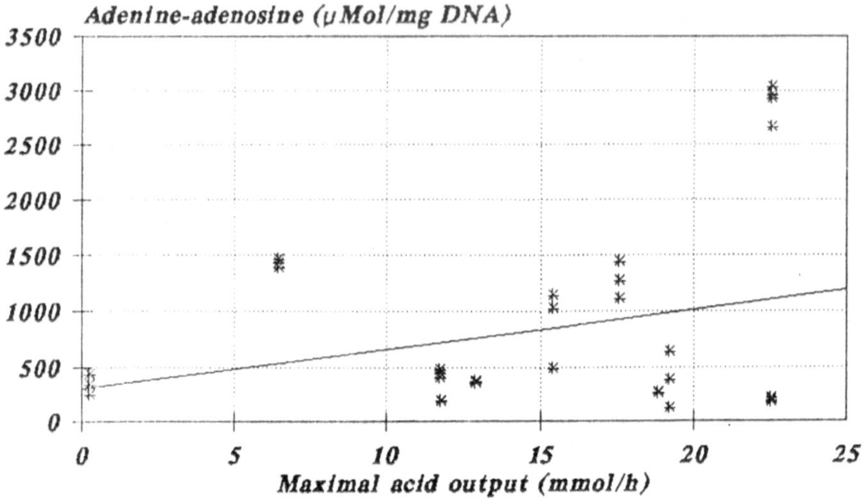

N=41; r=0.44; p<0.05
*Y=637*X+357*

MAO (Mean ± S.E.M) = 14.75 ± 1.04

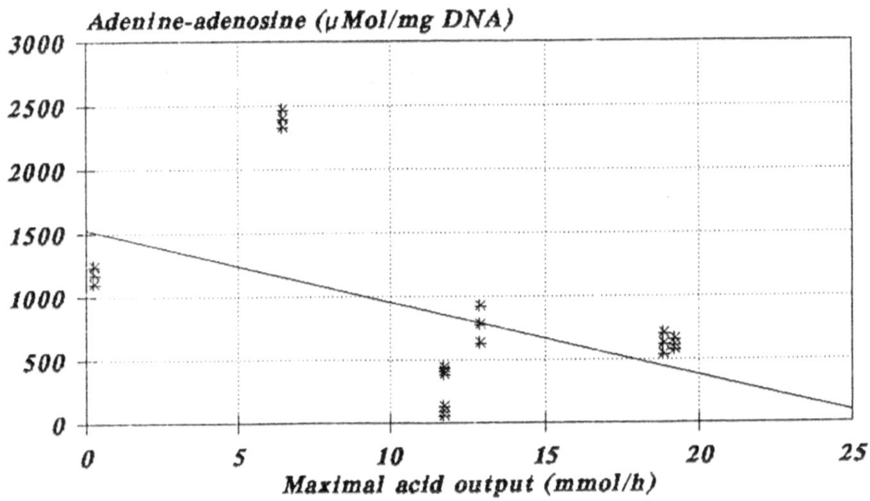

N=21; r=-0.48; p<0.05
*Y=-62*X+1489*

Figure 14. Correlation between the corpus mucosal (above) and musculature (below) adenine–adenosine vs. MAO in patients

TABLE 1
Actions of acetylcholine, histamine and pentagastrin in human beings

			Intrinsic activities	
Mediators	Actions	Affinity values (pD_2)	α	pA_2
ATP–membrane ATPase–ADP				
Acetylcholine	Stimulation	5.50	1.00_{Ach}	5.50
Histamine	Inhibition	9.70	$1.00_{Ouabain}$	9.70
Pentagastrin	Inhibition	10.55	$0.87_{Ouabain}$	10.55
ATP–adenylate cyclase–cAMP				
Acetylcholine	Inhibition	5.30	$-0.70_{Pentagastrin}$	5.30
Histamine	Stimulation	9.30	$1.00_{Pentagastrin}$	9.30
Pentagastrin	Stimulation	9.40	1.00	9.40

DISCUSSION

The biochemical background of gastric H^+ secretion is closely associated with changes of cations and anions in the gastric juice of patients. Positive and significant correlation exists between total chloride vs. H^+ ($r=0.46$; $n=32$; $p<0.01$); Ca^{2+} vs. H^+ ($r=0.498$; $n=31$; $p<0.01$); total chloride vs. Na^+ ($r=0.40$; $n=32$; $p<0.05$); neutral chloride (total chloride – chloride related to gastric H^+) vs. Na^+ ($r=0.74$; $n=32$; $p<0.001$); meanwhile a negative and mathematically significant correlation exists between Na^+ vs. H^+ ($r=-0.41$; $n=32$; $p<0.02$); and neutral chloride vs. H^+ ($r=-0.50$; $n=32$; $p<0.01$) [20].

Details of the biochemical backgrounds were studied mainly between 1970 and 1980 in animal experiments; however, only a few observations were made in human beings.

The existence of Na^+-K^+-dependent and Mg^{2+}-dependent ATPase [14] and adenylate cyclase [18] in the human gastric mucosa was proved by us.

Later on, a positive and significant correlation was proved between gastric BAO and Na^+-K^+-dependent ATPase activity [19]; a biochemical and energy background existed between gastric corpus vs. antral, antral vs. duodenal mucosa [12] in patients.

A causal and mathematically positive correlation was proved between the gastric BAO, corpus mucosal ATP, ADP and Na^+-K^+-dependent ATPase [20]. Some similar observations were obtained between the gastric MAO and gastric corpus mucosal biochemical parameters [21,22]. However, the other biochemical parameters – such as AMP, adenylate pool, ratio of ATP and 'energy charge' – were not measured. On the other hand, these studies were carried out in patients with gastric BAO and MAO responses, who underwent gastric surgery for various reasons (resection of stomach, perforation, polyps).

The regulatory mechanisms of tissue energy content in the human gastric corpus mucosa are not clearly understood; the details are extremely complicated. It has been shown that the ATP–ADP transformation occurs under cholinergic influence [20,26,27], while it is inhibited by histamine and pentagastrin [23].

In the present work, the study of biochemistry of gastric corpus mucosa was carried out in patients with 'genuine' peptic ulcer who underwent surgical resection of stomach or small intestine.

Energy release is necessary for the active transport of anions and cations and the energy comes from the tissue ATP (in which the energy is stored) by membrane-located ATPase [2–4] and adenylate cyclase [7] in the presence of Mg^{2+}. The ATP is a common substrate for both membrane ATPase (ATP–ADP transformation) and adenylate pool (ATP–cAMP transformation) [21,22,24].

In our present study, the complex adenosine metabolism was studied simultaneously in patients' gastric corpus mucosa and musculature. This type of biochemical evaluation is needed to understand tissue biochemistry in a complex way.

The calculation ratio of ATD/ADP is widely accepted as a fundamental method to the biochemical background to transport processes (under various circumstances in animals and humans).

The calculation of 'energy charge' [(ATP+0.5ADP)/(ATP+ADP+AMP)] was introduced by Atkinson [5]. According to this formula, the value of 'energy charge' is one when the adenosine compounds are in phosphorylated form, while its value theoretically (practically) is 0 when adenosine compounds are in dephosphorylated form.

The presented results clearly indicate that the gastric secretory responses (BAO, MAO) correlated with not only membrane-bound ATP-dependent energy systems, but with the whole metabolism of adenosine compounds. Interestingly, the 'energy charge' is the same in the corpus mucosa of patients with different gastric acid secretory responses (BAO, MAO).

Earlier, it was proved that the gastric secretory responses and the number of parietal cells correlate well [25]. The levels of ATP, ADP, AMP, adenylate pool and 'energy charge' were expressed in relation to 1.0 mg DNA, representing the same proportion of cells to parietal cells, and their biochemical make-up changes significantly in the corpus mucosa of patients with different secretory responses.

The results of affinity, intrinsic activity curves, pA_2, pD_2 and $\alpha_{ouabain}$ (for drugs inhibiting the ATP–ADP transformation) and $\alpha_{pentagastrin}$ (for drugs stimulating the ATP–cAMP transformation) for acetylcholine, pentagastrin and histamine indicate clearly that energy metabolism (in the human gastric fundic mucosa) can be separated biochemically into two parts due to gastric acid secretion: the ATP–ADP transformation gives the biochemical background for BAO, while the ATP–cAMP transformation supplies the energy liberation for MAO (Figure 15).

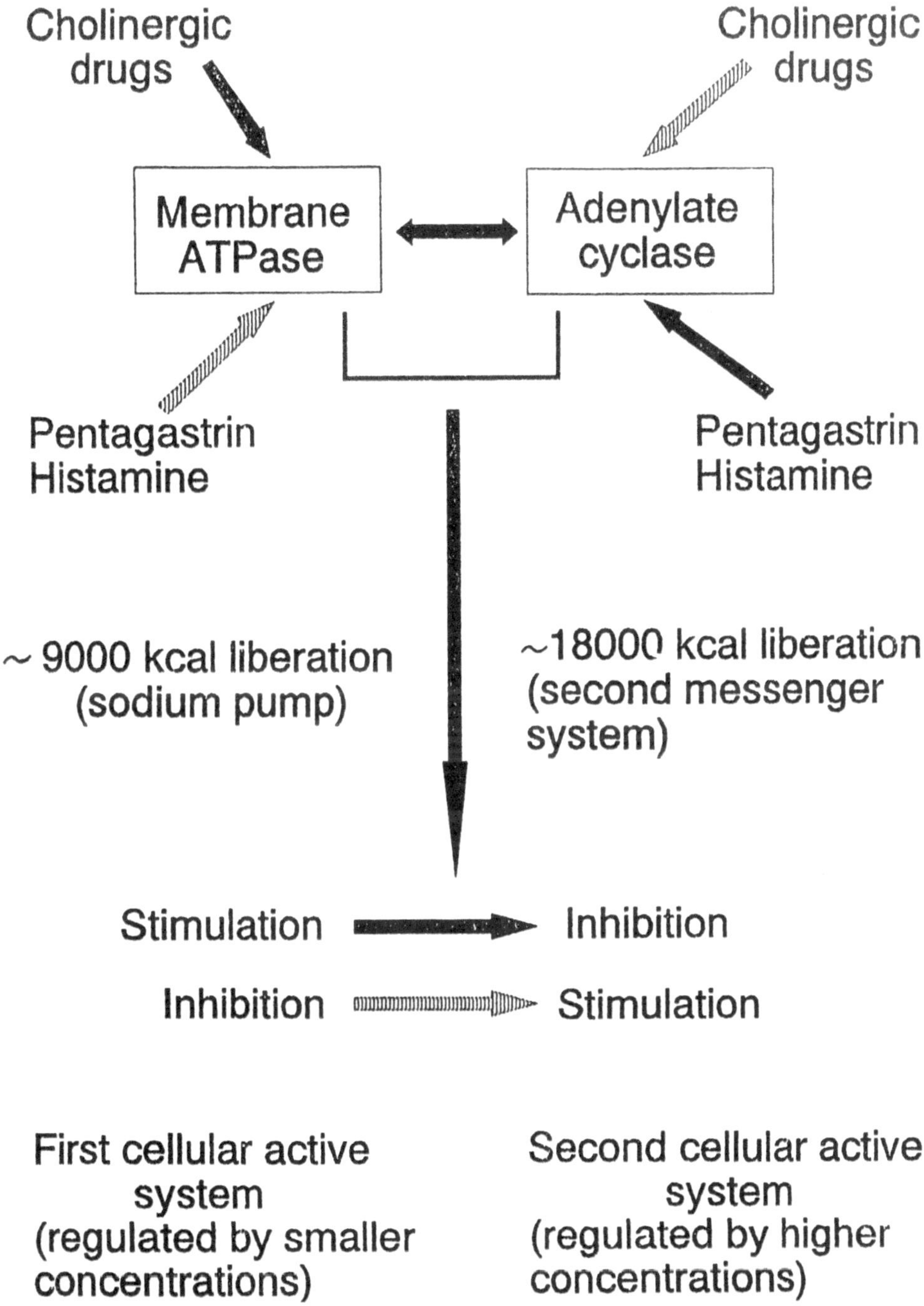

Figure 15. Schematic diagram of the relationships between ATP–membrane ATPase–ADP and ATP–adenylate cyclase–cAMP ATP-splitting enzymes

ACKNOWLEDGEMENTS

The authors wish to express their thanks to Mrs Margaret Jermás, Rosalie Nagy, Drs Beáta Bódis, Csaba Kövesdy and János Kutas for their excellent technical assistance.

REFERENCES

1. Mózsik Gy, Nagy L, Kutas F, Tárnok F. Interaction of cholinergic function with Mg-Na-K-dependent ATPase system of cells in the human fundic gastric mucosa. Scand J Gastroenterol. 1974;9:741–5.
2. Albers RW. Biochemical aspects of active transport. Ann Rev Biochem. 1967;36:727–56.
3. Schwartz A, Lindenmayer GE, Allen CJ. Sodium–potassium–adenosine triphosphatase: Pharmacological, physiological and biochemical aspects. Pharmacol Rev. 1975;27:3–134.
4. Askari A. Properties and functions of Na-K-activated adenosine-triphosphatase. Ann NY Acad Sci. 1974;242:1–741.
5. Atkinson DE. The energy charge of the adenylate pool as a regulatory parameter. Interaction with feedback modifiers. Biochemistry. 1968;7:4030–4.
6. Skou JC. Enzymatical basis for active transport of Na and K across the cell membrane. Physiol Rev. 1965;45:596–617.
7. Robinson GA, Butcher RW, Sutherland EW. Cyclic AMP. New York: Academic Press; 1971.
8. Sachs G. The gastric H-K-ATPase. In: Johnson LR, ed. Physiology of the Gastrointestinal Tract. Third Edn. New York: Raven Press; 1994;1119–38.
9. Soll AH, Berglindh T. Receptors that regulate gastric acid-secretory function. In: Johnson LR, ed. Physiology of the Gastrointestinal Tract. Third Edn. New York: Raven Press; 1994:1138–69.
10. Hakanson R, Chen D, Sundler F. The ECL cells. In: Johnson LR, ed. Physiology of the Gastrointestinal Tract. Third Edn. New York: Raven Press; 1994:1171–84.
11. Lloyd KCK, Debas HT. Peripheral regulation of gastric acid secretion. In: Johnson LR, ed. Physiology of the Gastrointestinal Tract. Third Edn. New York: Raven Press; 1994:1185–226.
12. Mózsik Gy, Vizi F, Kutas J. A cellular-biochemical evaluation of gastric body mucosa and muscular layer in patients with different basal acid outputs. Scand J Gastroenterol. 1976;11:205–11.
13. Schmidt G, Thannhauser SJ. Method for determination of deoxyribonucleic acid, ribonucleic acid and phosphoproteins in animal tissues. J Biol Chem. 1945;161:83–9.
14. Mózsik Gy, Øye I. The preparation of Na-K-dependent ATPase from human gastric mucosa. Biochem Biophys Acta. 1969;183:640–1.
15. Lowry OH, Rosenbrough NJ, Farr AR, Randal RJ. Protein measurements with Folin phenol reagent. J Biol Chem. 1951;193:265–75.
16. Csáky TZ. Introduction to General Pharmacology. New York: Appleton–Century–Crofts Educational Division, Meredith Corporation; 1969:17–34.
17. Kleinbaum D, Kupper L. The correlation coefficient and its relationship to straight-line regression analysis. In: Kleinbaum D, Kupper L, eds. Applied Regression Analysis. Boston, Duxbury Press; 1986:78–81.
18. Mózsik Gy, Morón F, Jávor T. Examination of adenyl cyclase system prepared from human gastric mucosa. In: Riis P, Anthonisen P, Baden H, eds. Advance Abstracts, 4th World Congress of Gastroenterology, Copenhagen. The Danish Gastroenterological Association; 1978:381.
19. Mózsik Gy, Nagy L, Tárnok F, Vizi F, Kutas J. H^+ secretion and Na-K-dependent ATPase system in the human gastric mucosa. Experientia (Basel), 1970;30:1024–5.
20. Mózsik Gy, Kutas J, Nagy L, Tárnok F, Vizi F. Interrelationships between the cholinergic influences, gastric mucosa Na-K-dependent ATPase, ATP, ADP, ions of gastric juice and basal secretion in patients. Acta Physiol Scand. 1978;Suppl:199–208.
21. Mózsik Gy, Nagy L, Tárnok F, Vizi F. The energy systems of gastric tissues, their neural, hormonal and pharmacological regulations in order to gastric H^+ secretion and ulcerogenesis. (A review of animal experiments and clinical biochemical studies). Acta Med Acad Sci Hung. 1979;36:1–29.
22. Mózsik Gy, Nagy L, Tárnok F. Feed-back mechanism system between the ATP–adenylate cyclase–cAMP system and ATP-Na^+-K^+-dependent ATP-ase–ADP in the rat and human gastric fundic mucosa in relation to gastric acid secretion. In: Gáti T, Szollár LG, Ungváry Gy, eds. Advances in Physiological Sciences, Vol.12. Nutrition, Digestion, Metabolism. Oxford: Pergamon Press/Budapest: Akadémiai Kiadó; 1981:157–73.

23. Mózsik Gy, Nagy L, Tárnok F, Kutas F. Effects of histamine on transport Na-K-dependent ATP-ase system (EC 3613) prepared from human gastric mucosa. Pharmacology. 1974;12:193–200.
24. Mózsik Gy. Some feedback mechanisms by drugs in the interrelationship between the active transport system and adenyl cyclase system localized in the cell membrane. Eur J Pharmacol. 1970;7:319–27.
25. Saub LS, Myren J, eds. The Physiology of Gastric Secretion. Oslo: Universitets Forlaget/Baltimore: Williams–Wilkins Company; 1968.
26. Mózsik Gy. Direct inhibitory effects of adenosine monophosphates on Na-K-dependent ATP-ase prepared from human gastric mucosa. Eur J Pharmacol. 1970;9:207–10.
27. Mózsik Gy, Vizi F, Nagy L, Beró T, Tárnok F, Kutas J. Na-K-dependent ATPase system and the gastric H^+ secretion by the human gastric mucosa. In: Mózsik Gy, Jávor T, eds. Progress in Peptic Ulcer. Budapest: Publishing House of the Hungarian Academy of Sciences; 1976.

Manuscript received 26 Nov. 95.
Accepted for publication 29 Dec. 95.

TS Gaginella et al. (eds.), Biochemical Pharmacology as an Approach to Gastrointestinal Disorders, 225–237

OXIDATIVE STRESS AND ITS PREVENTION IN TOXIC LIVER LESIONS. AN OVERVIEW

J. FEHÉR*, A. BLÁZOVICS AND G. LENGYEL
2nd Department of Medicine, Semmelweis University, Budapest, Hungary
*Correspondence

ABSTRACT

The yearly intake of alcoholic beverages in the population of Hungary is very high. It is about 12 L/y per capita. The mortality rate from micronodular liver cirrhosis is 43/100 000 each year; the cumulative survival over 5 years is 50% of the total number of patients, including those treated and untreated. The mechanism by which the alcohol produces a toxic effect on the liver is oxidative stress. The different diseases are: fatty liver, alcoholic hepatitis and liver cirrhosis. Much evidence is presented that nutritional antioxidants, e.g. vitamin E and certain drugs, namely flavonoids from *Silibum marianum*, exert a protective effect on several immune dysfunctions. The toxic reactions of the liver can be investigated by different methods. In clinical and experimental studies, silymarin and silibinin exerted favourable effects on acute and chronic hepatitis, liver cirrhosis and toxic hepatic injury. Our studies show that, in hyperlipidaemic rats and in patients with chronic alcoholic liver disease, the extra-hepatically detectable oxidative stress state is favourably influenced by silymarin treatment. Therapy should achieve decreased lipid peroxidation and improve the antioxidant protection of patients.

Keywords: oxidative stress, liver disease, alcoholism, silibinin

INTRODUCTION

In recent years, there has been growing interest concerning the role of free oxygen radicals in several physiological and pathological processes. Free radicals may play a role in the pathomechanism of fatty liver, alcoholic liver cirrhosis and in metabolic alterations [1–7].

Medical plants and their curative effects have been known for hundreds of years, but the mechanisms of their medical actions are not very well established even nowadays. Aromatic and medical plants have many free radical scavenger molecules, some of them are excellent antioxidants and have anti-inflammatory effect in wonderful variations [6–10].

Among the active compounds of medical plants, free radical scavengers are the flavonoids, flavolignanes, polyphenols, catechines, non-steroidal sesquiterpenes and so on [3–5,11,12].

Since flavonoid-type compounds exert cytoprotection, we examined whether silibinin and its isomers are able to decrease the damaging effect of free-radical reactions and lipid peroxidation in experimental hyperlipidaemia and in alcoholic liver disease.

This paper was presented at the Section of IUPHAR GI Pharmacology Symposium on 'Biochemical pharmacology as an approach to gastrointestinal disorders (basic science to clinical perspectives)', October 12–14, 1995, Pécs, Hungary.

Silibinin is a well-known free-radical scavenger and antioxidant. This drug is widely used in the therapy of liver diseases of different aetiologies.

The aim of this study was to prove the exact effect of silibinin with in-vitro physicochemical and biochemical methods, as well as with in-vivo experimental and clinicopharmacological studies.

IN-VITRO PHYSICOCHEMICAL STUDIES

Azide radicals produce tryptophan radicals via oxidation and subsequent deprotonation of the amino acid. Tryptophan radicals decayed by second-order kinetics, with $2k = 6 \times 10^8\ dm^{-3}\ mol^{-1}\ s^{-1}$, in good agreement with earlier data [13]. In the presence of silibinin, the decay observed at the absorption maximum, 510 nm, turns into pseudo-first order in silibinin concentration ($k = 1 \times 10^7\ dm^{-3}\ mol^{-1}\ s^{-1}$) and is accompanied by the build-up of the oxidized silibinin radical, $\lambda_{max} = 390$ nm. This is illustrated by the oscilloscope traces shown in Figure 1 [13].

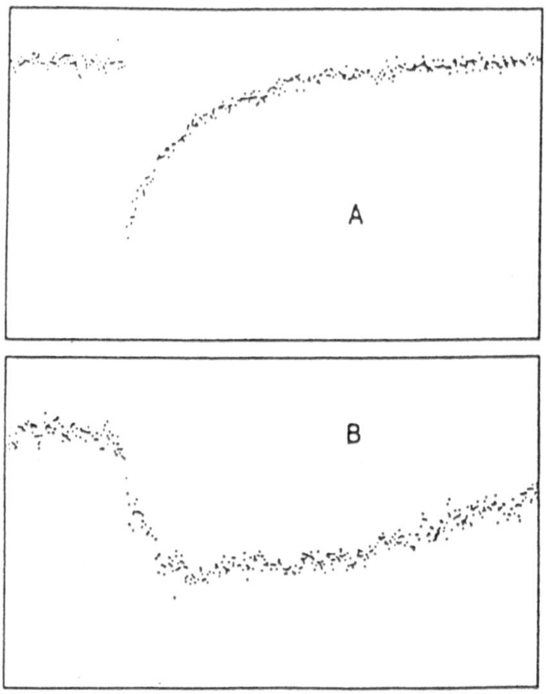

Figure 1. Oscilloscope traces of transients produced by an 80-ns pulse of 8 Gy dose in a solution containing 0.1 mol/L NaN_3, 4 mmol/L tryptophan, 0.4 mmol/L silibinin saturated with N_2O at pH 7.4. Full scale represents 2 ms; **A** 510 nm (λ_{max} of tryptophan radical); **B** 390 nm (λ_{max} of silibinin radical)

IN-VITRO CLINICAL STUDIES

Free radical formation was detected by the chemiluminometric method with a CLD-1 Medicor–Medilab luminometer. Luminescent light was measured with a sensitive photomultiplier. The electrical signals of the multiplier are processed by means of an MMT microprocessor system. In the $H_2O_2/{}^{\cdot}OH$-luminol system, we demonstrated a dose-dependent effect of silibinin on oxygen free radicals (Figure 2).

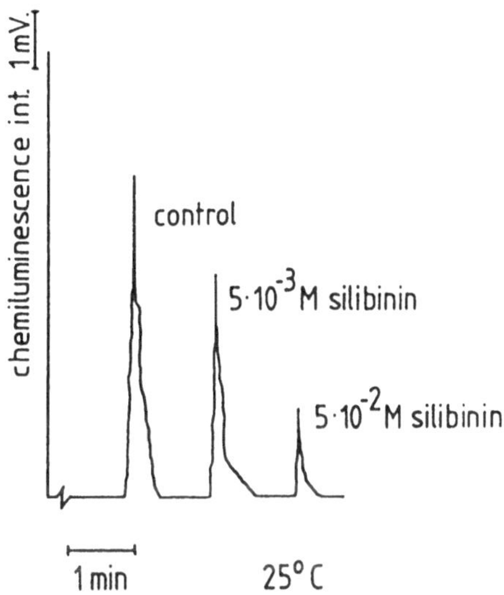

Figure 2. H_2O_2 scavenging activity of silibinin

BIOCHEMICAL EXPERIMENTS

Wistar rats weighing 150–200 g were fed a fat-rich diet (2% cholesterol, 0.5% cholic acid and 20% sunflower oil added to the normal LATI chow). Sunflower oil had the worst parameters (Table 1) in view of the content of diene conjugates and intensity of chemiluminescence. This is why sunflower oil was chosen for feeding.

In a 'short-term' experiment rats were treated with 15 mg (kg body weight)$^{-1}$ day^{-1} silibinin which was given intraperitoneally for 5 days from the 4th day to decapitation. After the 5 days treatment followed by decapitation, their livers were removed in ice-cold potassium chloride isotonic solution and microsomal fractions were prepared by ultracentrifugation. The microsomal pellet was irradiated with Co^{60} isotope (γ).

The malondialdehyde content, and activities of NADPH cytochrome c, NADH b_5 reductases and *N*-demethylase were measured by standard methods. Statistical analysis

TABLE 1
Changes in diene conjugation and in chemiluminescence intensity of commercial quality edible oil

Samples ($n = 5$)	Diene conjugates (ABS. 233 nm) (in 100 µl sample)	Chemiluminescence intensity (mV × 180 s)
Sunflower oil	8.74	200.62×10^3
Soya oil	4.44	8.80×10^3
Corn oil	2.50	5.12×10^3

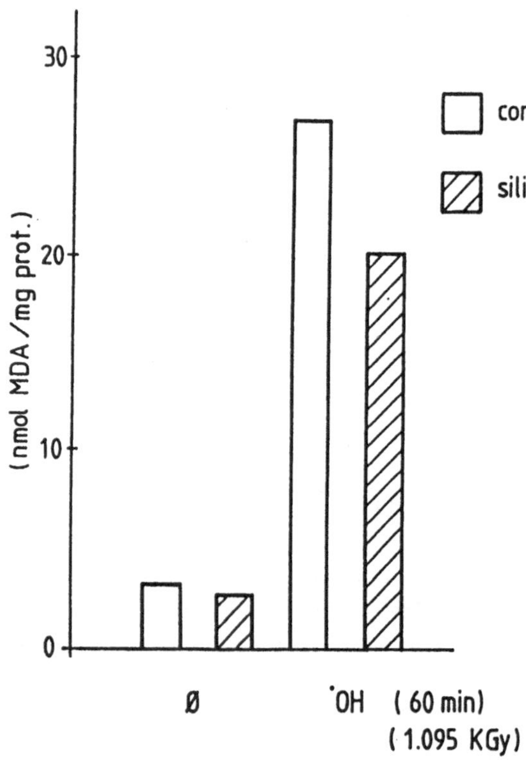

Figure 3. In-vitro effect of silibinin treatment on the lipid peroxidation of rat liver microsomes in an in-vitro ^{60}Co (γ) irradiated system

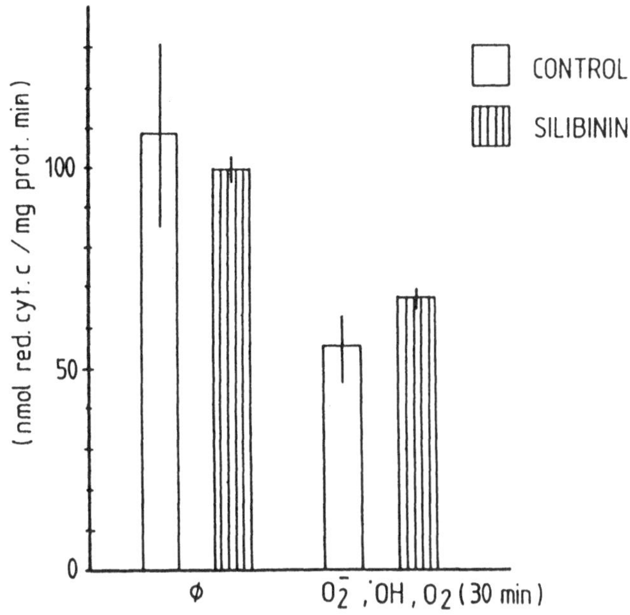

Figure 4. Effect of in-vivo silibinin treatment on the activity of NADPH cytochrome c reductase in an in-vitro ^{60}Co (γ) irradiated system

was performed with the Student's *t*-test. Confidence limits were added at $p < 95\%$.

At a silibinin concentration of 10^{-5} mol/L in vitro, MDA content was lowest in comparison with the untreated sample. On the figures, each point represents five experiments in duplicate (Figure 3). NADPH cytochrome c reductase was sensitive to lipid peroxidation, and the enzyme integrity could be protected by silibinin (Figure 4).

In-vivo antioxidant treatment produced a protective effect on the activity of NADH b_5 reductase (Figure 5) and of *N*-demethylase (Figure 6). The activity was higher than that of irradiated controls, showing the improved results of treatment.

Free radicals generate chain reactions, causing damage to membranes and leading to the production of lipid peroxides with the destruction of membrane-bound enzymes, such as NADPH cytochrome c reductase, NADH b_5 reductase, cytochrome P_{450} and cytochrome b_5 and *N*-demethylase. The silibinin treatment non-significantly increased: the rate of NADPH cytochrome c (Figure 7) and NADH b_5 reductases (Figure 8), *N*-demethylase activity (Figure 9), cytochrome b_5 content (Figure 10) and, considerably, the P_{450} concentrations (Figure 11) when the rats were fed on a fat-rich diet.

These data demonstrate that silibinin has a membrane-protecting effect and is able to increase the natural scavenger capacity [3].

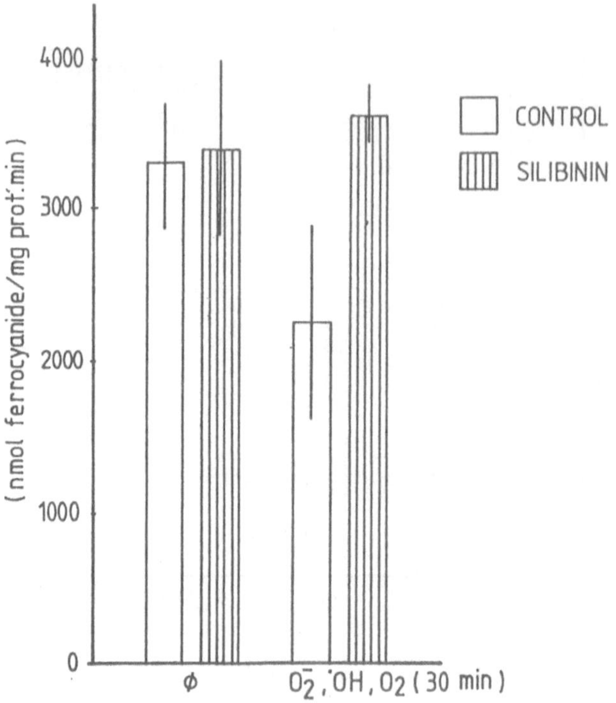

Figure 5. Effect of in-vivo silibinin treatment on the activity of NADH ferricyanide reductase in an in-vitro ^{60}Co (γ) irradiated system

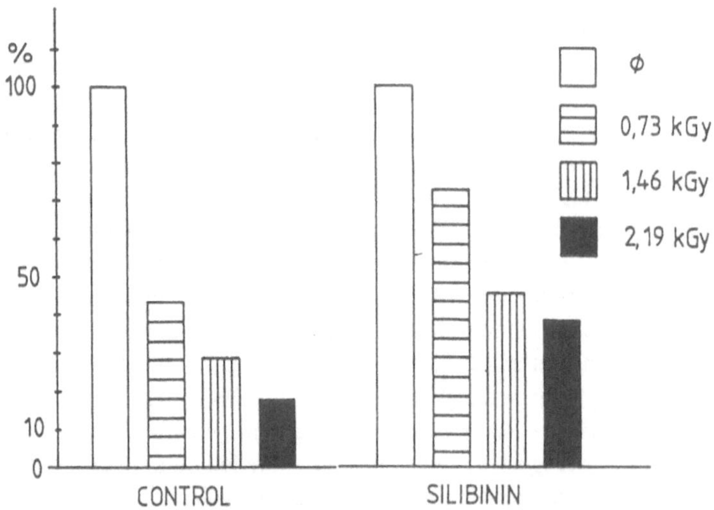

Figure 6. Effect of in-vivo antioxidant treatment on the activity of *N*-demethylase in an in-vitro ^{60}Co (γ) irradiated system

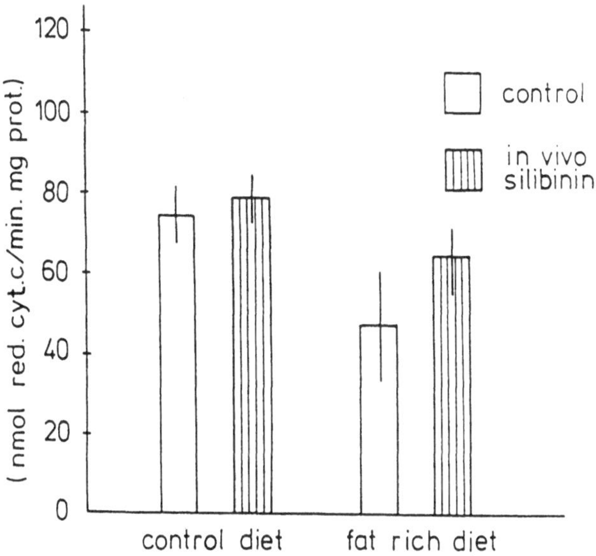

Figure 7. Effect of silibinin treatment on the activity of NADPH cytochrome c reductase

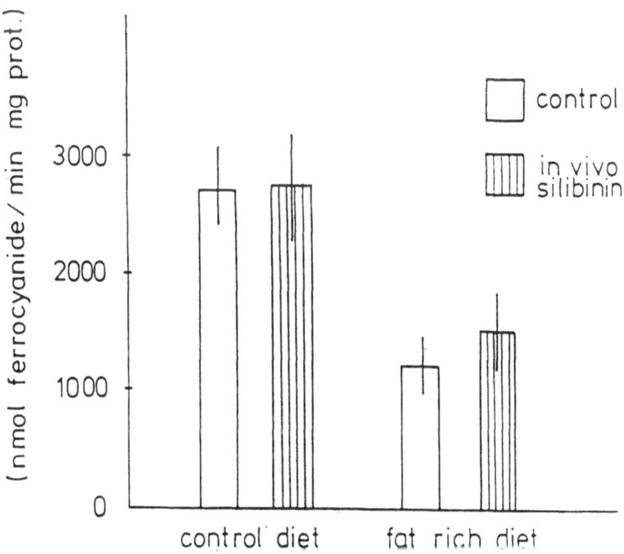

Figure 8. Effect of silibinin treatment on the activity of NADH ferricyanide reductase

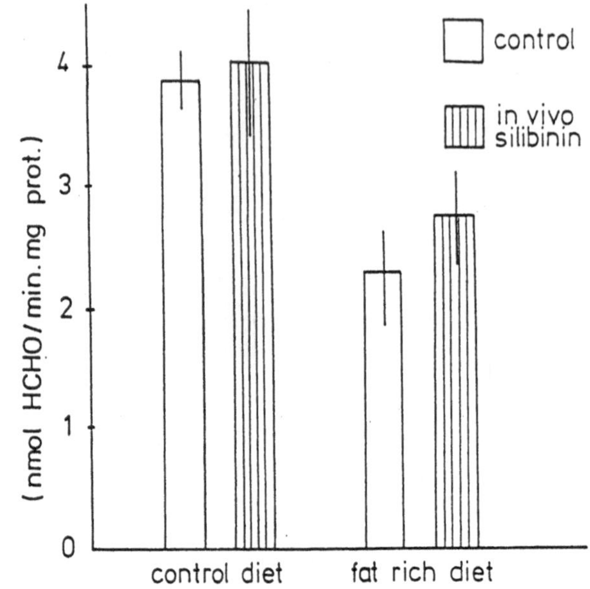

Figure 9. Effect of silibinin treatment on the activity of *N*-demethylase

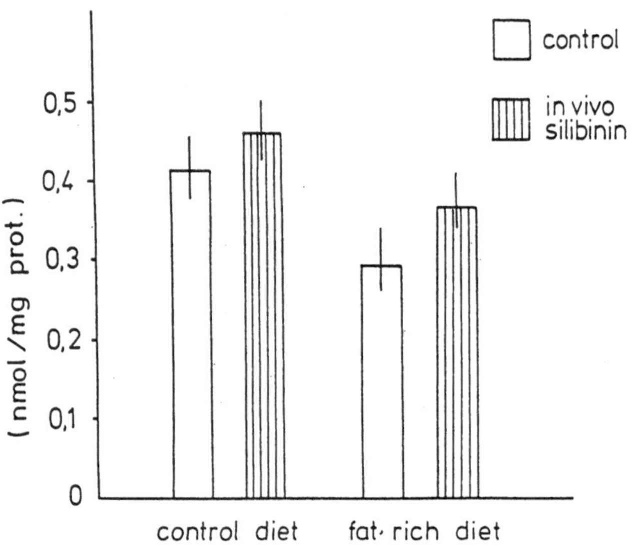

Figure 10. Effect of silibinin on the cytochrome b_5 content

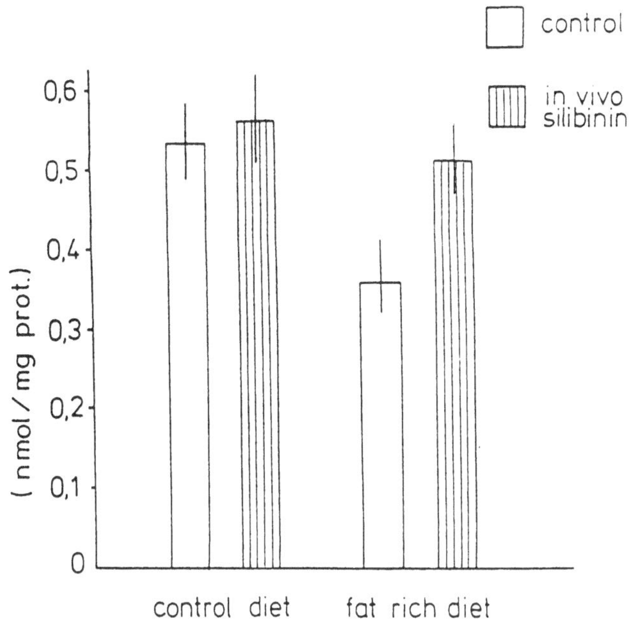

Figure 11. Effect of silibinin on the cytochrome P_{450} content

HUMAN CLINICOPHARMACOLOGICAL STUDIES

The yearly intake of alcoholic beverages in the population of Hungary is very high. It is about 12 L/y per capita. The mortality rate of micronodular liver cirrhosis is 43/100 000. The increase in alcohol consumption in Hungary is demonstrated in Figure 12.

Because of the high mortality rate in alcoholic liver cirrhosis, we examined the protective effect of silymarin in patients with alcoholic liver disease.

The efficacy of silymarin (Legalon) was investigated in a double-blind study, in patients with chronic alcoholic liver disease. Thirty-six patients with chronic alcoholic liver disease participated in this study: 27 men, 9 women (average age 46 ± 7 years). Daily alcohol consumption exceeded 60 g in men and 30 g in women. Period of chronic alcohol consumption was 8 ± 4 years. The patients were vascularly compensated, symptoms of encephalopathy were not observed, malnutrition did not occur and there was no other associated disease. The virus and immunological (antinuclear antibody, anti-smooth muscle antibody) markers were negative. Silymarin–placebo randomization was done by the pharmaceutical company (MADAUS, Cologne); the placebo contained the vehicle of silymarin in the same form. The treatment lasted for 6 months [3–5].

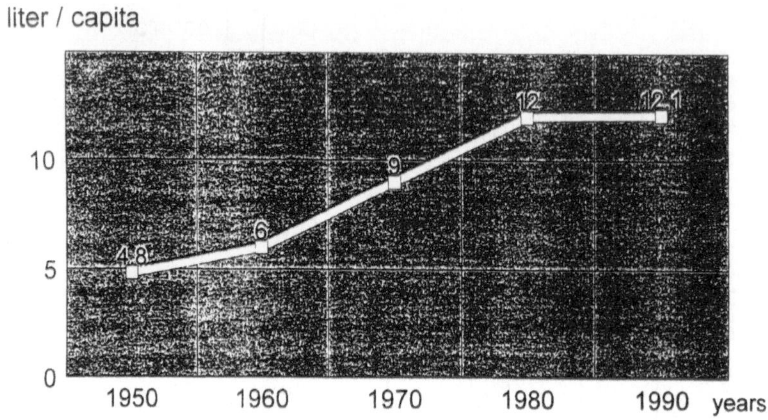

Figure 12. Alcohol consumption in Hungary

TABLE 2
Liver function after six months' therapy with silymarin

Group	SeBi (μmol/L) (2–26)	AST (U/L) (1–20)	ALT (U/L) (1–30)	GGT (U/L) (1–25)	AP (U/L) (70–170)
Silymarin					
I: 0 months	38.4±11.7	37.3±7.5	33.9±8.2	263.7±49.5	152.3±26.6
II: 3 months	17.2±3.7	21.4±4.8	20.1±4.4	79.1±18.9	151.1±21.4
III: 6 months	19.4±3.9	22.8±5.1	21.7±5.3	111.2±21.3	143.6±17.3
Placebo					
IV: 0 months	37.8±10.2	38.5±9.6	32.7±7.4	224.9±42.3	143.1±24.2
V: 3 months	30.4±8.3	35.6±8.1	28.7±6.3	156.5±34.9	135.3±17.7
VI: 6 months	32.5±7.6	31.3±4.5	27.4±5.6	170.4±37.1	163.9±18.6
Significance					
I vs IV	NS	NS	NS	NS	NS
I vs II	$p<0.01$	$p<0.02$	$p<0.05$	$p<0.001$	NS
I vs III	$p<0.02$	$p<0.02$	$p<0.05$	$p<0.01$	NS
IV vs V	NS	NS	NS	$p<0.05$	NS
IV vs VI	NS	NS	NS	$p<0.05$	NS
II vs V	$p<0.05$	$p<0.02$	NS	$p<0.02$	NS
III vs VI	$p<0.05$	$p<0.05$	NS	$p<0.02$	NS

TABLE 3
Effect of silymarin treatment on lipid peroxidation and antioxidant system in chronic alcoholic liver diseases, in a six-month double-blind investigation (average ± SEM)

Group (n)	MDA (nmol/ml)	Serum GPX (U/g plasma protein)	Free SH (μmol/ml)	Erythrocyte SOD (U/ml)	Lymphocyte SOD (U/ml)
Silymarin					
I: 0 months	15.1 ± 2.5	0.65 ± 0.28	0.44 ± 0.20	72.9 ± 14.5	32.6 ± 10.3
II: 6 months	10.2 ± 1.0	0.94 ± 0.25	0.63 ± 0.17	130.8 ± 19.6	74.9 ± 19.3
Placebo					
III: 0 months	14.7 ± 2.3	0.67 ± 0.21	0.45 ± 0.12	76.5 ± 20.1	29.4 ± 14.2
VI: 6 months	15.9 ± 2.1	0.54 ± 0.26	0.43 ± 0.15	85.7 ± 21.7	27.7 ± 16.1
Significance					
I vs II	$p<0.02$	$p<0.05$	$p<0.05$	$p<0.001$	$p<0.01$
II vs IV	$p<0.02$	$p<0.02$	$p<0.05$	$p<0.01$	$p<0.01$

The code was disclosed by the factory after the end of treatment. Seventeen (15 men and 2 women, average age 38 ± 7 years) took 3 × 140 mg silymarin per day (3 × 1 Legalon capsule) and 19 patients (12 men and 7 women, average age 44 ± 6 years) took 3 × 1 capsules of placebo. For statistical analysis, the two-sample Student's t-test was used.

The liver function test showed a significant improvement in the therapy group (Table 2). The level of malondialdehyde (MDA), a marker of serum lipid peroxidation (LPO) decreased significantly during the silymarin treatment ($p<0.02$). There was a significant difference between the values for the two groups following treatment ($p<0.02$; Table 3).

Following silymarin administration, serum glutathione peroxidase (GPX) activity significantly increased ($p<0.05$) and the values between placebo and therapy groups following treatment were significantly different ($p<0.02$; Table 3). Silymarin treatment significantly enhanced the SH group level ($p<0.05$). The values of the two groups following treatment were also significant ($p<0.05$).

During silymarin treatment the superoxide dismutase (SOD) activity of erythrocytes and lymphocytes significantly increased regarding both types of cells (erythrocyte SOD: $p<0.001$, lymphocyte SOD: $p<0.01$). The values for the two groups following treatment were significantly different (erythrocyte SOD: $p<0.01$, lymphocyte SOD: $p<0.01$; Table 3). During the 6-month administration of placebo, considerable changes in SOD expression of lymphocytes were not observed.

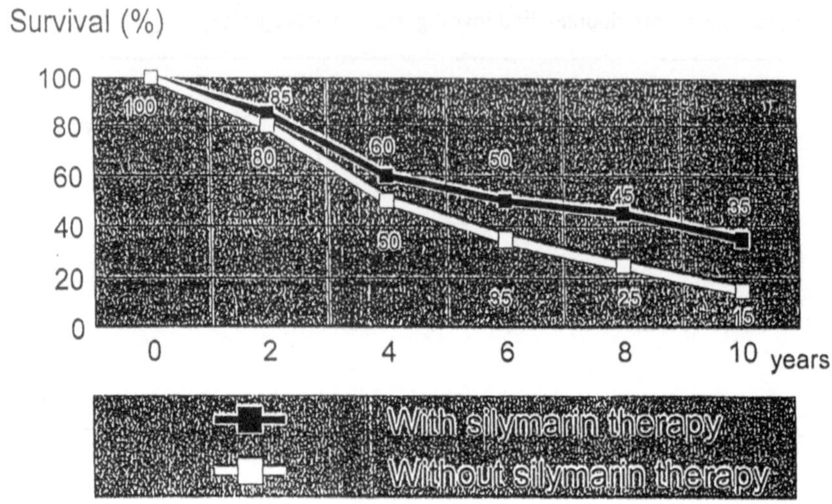

Figure 13. Ten-year follow-up of patients with alcoholic liver cirrhosis

Furthermore, we have found, in follow-up observations, that the silymarin treatment reduced the mortality rate and diminished hepatic collagen deposition. Figure 13 shows the ten-year follow-up of patients with alcoholic liver cirrhosis. The survival rate after 10 years is 0.15 without treatment and 0.35 with silymarin therapy.

CONCLUSION

These studies show that experimentally induced toxic liver lesions and the extrahepatically detectable oxidative stress state – its typical biochemical parameters – in patients with chronic alcoholic liver disease were favourably influenced by silibinin or silymarin treatment.

Applied therapy decreased lipid peroxidation and improved the patients' antioxidant protection. Following the six-month treatment, all these favourable effects resulted in the setting or significant improvement of liver function values of patients, proving the liver protective effect of the silymarin.

Follow-up observation of patients with alcoholic liver disease showed that long-term silymarin treatment could increase the survival time of patients.

On the basis of these results, we can recommend free radical scavenger therapy in alcohol-induced liver injury, with, of course, alcohol abstinence.

REFERENCES

1. Bus JS, Gibson JEL. Mechanisms of superoxide radical mediated toxicity. J Toxicol Clin Toxicol. 1982–3;19:689.
2. Csomós G, Fehér J. Free Radicals and the Liver. Berlin, Heidelberg, New York, London, Paris, Tokyo, Hong Kong, Barcelona, Budapest: Springer Verlag; 1992.
3. Fehér J, Blázovics A, Matkovics B, Mézes M. Role of Free Radicals in Biological Systems. Budapest: Akadémiai Kiadó; 1993.
4. Fehér J, Csomós G, Vereckei A. Free-Radical Reactions in Medicine. Berlin, Heidelberg, New York, London, Paris, Tokyo, Hong Kong, Barcelona, Budapest: Springer Verlag; 1987.
5. Fehér J, Vereckei A, Lengyel G. Role of free-radical reactions in liver diseases. Acta Phys Hung. 1992;80:351–61.
6. Ryle PR. Free-radicals, lipid peroxidation and ethanol hepatotoxicity. Lancet. 1984;2:461–8.
7. Stage TE, Mischke BS, Cox GW, Daniels KA. The role of free-radical inhibitors on acetaldehyde induced increases in lipid peroxidation. Fed Proc. 1983;47:513–18.
8. Garcia-Bunuel L. Lipid peroxidation in alcoholic myopathy and cardiomyopathy. Med Hypotheses. 1984;13:217–20.
9. Heikkila RE, Cohen G. 6-Hydroxydopamine: evidence for superoxide radical as an oxidative intermediate. Science. 1973;181:456–9.
10. Pár A, Jávor T. Alternatives in hepatoprotection: cytoprotection-influences on monoxidase system-free radical scavengers. Acta Physiol Hung. 1984;64:409–18.
11. Shaw S, Jayatilleke E, Ross WA, Gordon EF, Lieber CS. Ethanol-induced lipid peroxidation potentiation by long-term alcohol feeding and attenuation by methionine. J Lab Clin Med. 1981;98:417–20.
12. Shaw S, Rubin KP, Lieber CS. Depressed hepatic glutathione and increased diene conjugates in alcoholic liver disease. Evidence of lipid peroxidation. Dig Dis Sci. 1983;28:585–9.
13. György I, Blázovics A, Fehér J, Földiák G. Reactions of inorganic free radicals with liver protecting drugs. Radiat Phys Chem. 1990;36:165–7.

Manuscript received 25 Nov. 95.
Accepted for publication 29 Nov. 95.

TS Gaginella et al. (eds.), Biochemical Pharmacology as an Approach to Gastrointestinal Disorders, 239–247

THE EFFECT OF DRUGS ON LIVER FUNCTION AND BILIARY SECRETION

F. LIRUSSI[1] AND L. OKOLICSANYI[2]
[1]Institute of Internal Medicine, University of Padova, Padova; [2]Chair of Gastroenterology, University of Parma, Parma, Italy

ABSTRACT

A number of different agents are used for the quantitative assessment of deranged hepatic function which includes abnormalities of:

1. Various metabolic processes,

2. Hepatic flow, and

3. Biliary secretion.

In the last 10–15 years, we have gained considerable experience in assessing liver function in relation to the stage and/or the progression of chronic liver disease (CLD) by means of antipyrine clearance, the galactose elimination capacity and, more recently, the cytochrome P_{450}-mediated formation of monoethylglycinexylidide (MEGX) following lidocaine administration. The changes in the metabolism of these agents provide a useful tool to monitor the influence of other drugs (for example, silymarin, ursodeoxycholic acid and interferon) on CLD of different aetiology. Moreover, evaluation of drug metabolizing activity is also used to optimize the timing of liver transplantation and to quantify the functioning liver mass in potential liver donors. As regards biliary secretion, it is well known that a number of drugs may influence biliary flow, biliary lipid output and biliary bile acid composition. For example, ursodeoxycholic acid reduces biliary cholesterol secretion and is used as a litholytic agent for cholesterol gallstones. However, it is also beneficial in chronic cholestatic and non-cholestatic liver disease because of its choleretic, membrane-stabilizing and immunomodulatory effects. Conversely, silymarin, which is currently used in the management of acute poisoning as well as of CLD, may be regarded as a potential litholytic agent since it reduces biliary cholesterol concentration and secretion. In conclusion, the study of the pharmacokinetics of different drugs may provide useful information to the clinicians about the stage and the progression of CLD. On the other hand, it seems important to evaluate the influence on biliary secretion of cytoprotective agents commonly used in the treatment of CLD with or without cholestatic features.

Keywords: quantitative liver function tests, interferon treatment, hepatitic C virus, biliary secretion

INTRODUCTION

The liver plays a key role in the metabolism of lipophilic substances which are converted into polar metabolites. These are excreted into bile and eliminated from the body. Usually the metabolites produced by this process are less active and less toxic than their parent compounds and the process is termed *detoxification*. Sometimes, however, reactive metabolites are formed and the process is called *toxification*.

This paper was presented at the Section of IUPHAR GI Pharmacology Symposium on 'Biochemical pharmacology as an approach to gastrointestinal disorders (basic science to clinical perspectives)', October 12–14, 1995, Pécs, Hungary.

A number of different enzymes, including cytochrome P_{450}, oxidases, reductases, hydrolases and transferases, are involved in these reactions. Genetic polymorphism creates subpopulations of patients with either decreased, absent or increased activities of certain enzymes. Besides, environmental factors, such as the intake of other drugs, diet, alcohol, and cigarette smoking, may induce or inhibit the drug-metabolizing activity and cause intra-individual variations. Drug toxicity develops as a result of an imbalance between detoxification and toxification, with an excess of the latter.

Given this background, we will first focus our attention on a particular aspect of drug metabolism, that is the use of some drugs in the assessment of liver (dys)function and of the influence of different cytoprotective/therapeutic agents in chronic liver disease (CLD). Second, we will look at the effect of a few compounds on biliary secretion. The two topics may appear unrelated but a link between them may be found, for example, in the role of bile acids in bile formation as well as in their use in the evaluation of biliary secretion in chronic cholestatic disorders [1].

QUANTITATIVE LIVER FUNCTION TESTS

It is well known that, whatever the cause of CLD (viral, drug- or alcohol-induced or autoimmune), the period of compensated liver disease lasts much longer than the period of decompensation which ultimately leads to a stage which is incompatible with life. From this point of view, we definitely need some biochemical tests which are reproducible, not or little invasive (unlike liver biopsy) and which are able to assess reliably the functional capacity and integrity of the liver. Besides, they must provide information about the stage of CLD, the rate of progression of CLD and the prognosis of CLD. These tests are called quantitative or 'dynamic' liver function tests (LFTs) to distinguish them from the 'static' conventional LFTs (serum bilirubin, transaminase, etc.). Quantitative LFTs are usually divided into:

1. Those evaluating metabolic homeostasis,

2. Those estimating detoxification reactions, and

3. Those assessing biliary secretion.

Table 1 shows the most commonly used substrates together with the main functions studied and their location within the hepatocyte. The galactose tolerance test reflects the capacity of hepatocytes to phosphorylate carbohydrates by galactokinase, whereas the functional capacity for urea synthesis can be estimated by infusion of amino acids.

Drug-metabolizing activity (DMA) can be estimated by the administration of drugs metabolized by the hepatic cytochrome P_{450} isoenzyme system. Examples of detoxification reactions include the aminopyrine breath test, antipyrine and caffeine clearances, and the conversion of lidocaine to monoethylglycinexylidide (MEGX-test). Apart from the estimation of serum bilirubin as a classical excretory test, a more up-to-date approach to evaluate the secretory function of the liver is based on the iv

TABLE 1
Quantitative liver function tests

Location	Substrate	Function
Cytosol	Galactose	Phosphorylation
	Amino acids	Urea synthesis
Microsomes (cytochrome P_{450})	Aminopyrine	*N*-Demethylation
	Caffeine	*N*-Demethylation
	Lidocaine	*N*-De-ethylation
	Antipyrine	Hydroxylation Demethylation
Hepatocellular membranes	^{75}SeHCAT	Bile acid uptake/ excretion

injection of a γ-labelled bile acid analogue – ^{75}Selena–homocholic acid–taurine (^{75}SeHCAT). This bile acid analogue behaves like the naturally occurring taurocholate with regard to the enterohepatic circulation of bile acids [2] and is specifically taken up and excreted by the liver [3], thus providing information on these two important steps of bile secretion. Jazrawi and co-workers have recently employed the hepatic scintigraphy with ^{75}SeHCAT to study the kinetics of hepatic bile acid handling in cholestatic liver diseases. They found that hepatic excretion, but not hepatic uptake, of the bile acid analogue was deranged during cholestasis, thus confirming that bile acid retention is a feature of cholestasis in man [1]. They also used this test to evaluate the effect of ursodeoxycholic acid (UDCA) treatment in patients with primary biliary cirrhosis [1].

INFLUENCE OF DRUGS ON LIVER FUNCTION

We have prospectively evaluated the cytoprotective effect of UDCA and of an antioxidant agent, silymarin, (given alone or in combination) on conventional LFTs and on liver function in patients with compensated active cirrhosis of the liver [4]. At the end of the two-year treatment period, we observed a 31–43% decrease in the serum markers of liver cell necrosis as well as the maintenance of the functioning liver mass as assessed by the GEC test and of the detoxification function as estimated by APCL.

These results confirm those reported by Lotterer et al. [5] and Leuschner et al. [6] who showed no significant changes in GEC, indocyanine green or aminopyrine breath tests during treatment of primary biliary cirrhosis with UDCA. Further support for the safety of UDCA in advanced non-cholestatic CLD comes from a retrospective study in which we looked at the long-term (4 years) effect of UDCA treatment in patients with compensated cirrhosis of different aetiologies. The response to UDCA was greater in patients with alcoholic or cryptogenic cirrhosis than in those with hepatitis-C-related cirrhosis. However, GEC values remained, on average, stable over the four-year follow-up study, irrespective of the aetiology, and only diminished in the patients experiencing one or more episodes of ascites [7].

By contrast, a number of reports suggest that interferon (IFN) depresses DMA, at least after short-term administration of the drug [8–11]. Such an effect has been shown to occur after a single dose, ranging from 4.5 to 18.0 MU of recombinant leukocyte IFN-α in patients with chronic active hepatitis B and healthy controls [8,9], as well as following administration of lymphoblastoid IFN-α for 4 weeks at a dose of 6 MU/day, or after iv injection of IFN-β (3–9 MU/day) for 8 weeks [10,11]. The mechanism(s) by which IFN depresses hepatic DMA is still unclear, although it might be mediated by several cytokines [11]. However, all the studies mentioned above suggest that the depressant effect of IFN on DMA might be a property which is inseparable from its antiviral or antitumour activity.

These reports prompted us to set up a clinical study with the aims of verifying whether standard treatment with IFN actually impairs the DMA and whether there is any correlation between the dose of, and response to, IFN and the degree of DMA inhibition. These questions appear to be of particular clinical relevance since nowadays IFN is increasingly associated with other drugs, both in hepatological and oncological patients to enhance the response rate. Hence, depression of hepatic mixed function oxidases by IFN might result in potentially toxic drug interactions.

Instead of evaluating antipyrine or theophylline clearances following IFN administration [8,11], we studied the kinetics of MEGX formation from lidocaine (1 mg/kg body weight as an iv bolus injection). The reaction is catalysed by the cytochrome P_{450} system in the microsomes (Table 1) and represents, therefore, a quantitative estimation of hepatic DMA. Besides, as lidocaine undergoes first-pass clearance, MEGX formation may be partly affected by changes in splanchnic haemodynamics.

The test was first validated by Oellerich and colleagues in Hannover in 1987 [12]. They employed this dynamic test to evaluate liver function in healthy volunteers, liver donors and patients with liver cirrhosis. Subsequently, MEGX formation was specifically used by these authors as a measure of pre-transplant liver function in order to estimate the probability of survival in graft recipients [13]. They found that a cut-off value of 90 ng/ml of MEGX determined 15 min after lidocaine injection could reliably predict short-term survival in transplanted patients [13]. Besides, the test is easy to perform and MEGX concentrations can be rapidly determined in the laboratory using a fluorescence polarization immunoassay [12].

We used the 45-min MEGX concentration as a measure of liver function since, in previous kinetics studies, it was shown that the 45-min and the 60-min samples had the best sensitivity, specificity, diagnostic accuracy and predictive values [14]. We also performed the GEC test in order to gain information about the functioning liver mass, using a low-extraction rate compound.

CHRONIC HEPATITIS C, INTERFERON AND LIVER FUNCTION

Twenty-one patients with HCV-related CLD were selected for the trial. All had a biopsy-proven diagnosis of chronic active hepatitis ($n = 13$) or cirrhosis ($n = 8$). HCV genotypes were also determined and were classified according to Okamoto et al. [15]. Patients received recombinant IFN-α 2b at a dose of 6 MU three times a week (tiw) for 4 months, followed by 3 MU tiw for 8 months in cases with response to treatment. Patients were usually asked to stop treatment if no decrease in serum transaminase was observed by month four. Conventional markers of liver function were determined monthly, whereas MEGX formation and GEC were measured at month 0, 4 and 12 and, in 8 patients, also 6 months after IFN withdrawal. Complete or partial response was seen in 10 patients; 8 patients were considered non-responders, whereas the remaining three withdrew from treatment for severe side-effects. As expected, response was associated with less-advanced CLD and a lower percentage of type II HCV (the type more resistant to IFN therapy) in comparison with the non-responder group [16].

In responders, the 45-min MEGX values at entry were 63 ± 6 ng/ml (mean $\pm$ SEM) and did not vary significantly at months 4 and 12 during treatment (68 ± 7 ng/ml and 65 ± 8 ng/ml, respectively) or 6 months after IFN withdrawal (70 ± 7 ng/ml). In the non-responders, MEGX values increased by 21% at month 4, although not significantly so. Pre-treatment GEC values were similar in responders and non-responders (2.3 ± 0.2 mmol/min and 1.9 ± 0.2 mmol/min, respectively) and remained stable throughout the treatment period as well as after IFN withdrawal in both groups. Thus, long-term therapy (6–12 months) with IFN-α given at a standard dose of 3–6 MU three times a week, does not seem to impair the detoxification function and the functioning liver mass as assessed by MEGX formation and GEC test, respectively. These results do not support previous reports in which different IFN treatment schedules were used (higher doses of IFN given for shorter periods).

If confirmed in larger study groups, these results would encourage the association of IFN with other drugs, such as antioxidants (*N*-acetyl-cysteine, glutathione, silibinin), antivirals (ribavirin) or UDCA in HCV-related CLD, and/or would not contraindicate the concomitant intake of other agents which may represent life-long therapy for individual patients, such as theophylline.

BILIARY SECRETION: A REAPPRAISAL

Moving now to the influence of drugs on biliary secretion, we extensively reviewed this topic ten years ago [17]. Since then, a lot of progress has been made in the understanding of the bile secretory process mainly at intracellular level, including the role of hormonal regulation and of bile ductular cells [18–20]. However, a fundamental concept remains: hepatocytes behave as epithelial cells and possess various secondary and tertiary active transport systems located either on the basolateral or the canalicular membrane. These transporters are specific for certain anions or cations and show coordination between sinusoidal uptake and canalicular secretion for a number of compounds, including bile acids, lipids, protein and various anions and cations which are found in bile.

Of paramount importance in drug metabolism is the Na^+–K^+-ATPase system which is located on the basolateral membrane of hepatocytes. Drugs and hormones decreasing or increasing the bile-acid-independent fraction of bile flow usually decrease or increase the activity of this pump. Na^+–K^+-ATPase is also essential for sodium-dependent uptake of bile acids, which are the most potent agents which increase bile flow. Hepatocyte uptake of sodium taurocholate is inhibited by a number of compounds such as progesterone, bumetamide, furosemide, verapamil, phalloidin and also cyclosporin A.

Bile acids are transported within the hepatocytes by three different mechanisms:

1. By means of cytosolic binding proteins (Y′, glutathione-*S*-transferase and fatty acid binding protein), which represent the major mechanism for transcytotic bile acid movement;

2. Through the vesicular pathway, which is estimated to account for less than 10% of total bile flow under basal conditions and is inhibited by colchicine, which blocks the polymerization of tubulin to form microtubules;

3. By means of a rapid vesicular transport which is not blocked by colchicine and is likely to involve intracellular organelles, such as the Golgi apparatus and the endoplasmic reticulum.

At least three transport systems have been so far identified at canalicular levels:

1. A bile acid transport system;

2. A separate multiple organic anion transporter, and

3. A transporter for organic cations.

The latter seems to be responsible for canalicular secretion of a number of drugs, including daunomycin, vinblastine, vincristine and adriamicin [21].

The integrity of the tight junctions joining adjacent hepatocytes is essential for the maintenance of the osmotic gradient between blood and bile which is necessary for bile secretion. In certain experimental conditions, phalloidin and oestradiol make this barrier 'leaky' and cause cholestasis [22,23].

The role of intracellular messengers, such as cAMP, protein kinase C and cytosolic Ca^{2+} or various hormones, on bile formation and secretion has also been characterized in the last few years [18,24].

Similarly, recent studies have investigated some of the mechanisms involved in ductular secretion (and their hormonal regulation) which seems to account for 40% of basal bile flow, at least in man. Hepatocellular bile is extensively modified while flowing through the biliary system by secretion and/or reabsorption of water, electrolytes, including HCO_3^- and Cl^-, and other solutes [25]. Also, bile duct epithelium is involved in the so-called cholehepatic shunting where dihydroxy bile acids, such as ursodeoxycholic acid, are passively reabsorbed in the unconjugated form at ductular level, then are conjugated with glycine and taurine and subsequently excreted from the basolateral membrane to the periductular plexus. By this mechanism, a bicarbonate-rich hypercholeresis is produced. It is still controversial whether the increase in bile flow and biliary bicarbonate secretion originates from the hepatocytes or the ductular cells. Experimental studies in isolated rat hepatocyte couplets would favour this second hypothesis [26–28].

EFFECTS OF DRUGS ON BILIARY SECRETION

UDCA-induced hypercholeresis is not the only effect exerted by this bile acid. UDCA improves liver function and survival in patients with primary biliary cirrhosis [29] and other cholestatic disorders [30]. A possible explanation for the improvement of cholestasis is the enrichment of bile with more hydrophilic (and therefore less toxic) bile acids [31]. This has been shown also in the rat model with ethinyl oestradiol-induced intrahepatic cholestasis [32].

We too have observed amelioration of conventional LFTs during treatment with UDCA in patients with non-cholestatic CLD (chronic active hepatitis plus cirrhosis) of different aetiology [4]. Although we did not measure the changes in the pattern of biliary bile acids, the 30-fold increase of UDCA in the serum of treated patients suggests that the spill-over of this agent from the enterohepatic circulation into the blood could mirror the enrichment of bile with less detergent bile acids. In addition to these properties, UDCA also inhibits the intestinal absorption of other bile acids [33] and possesses immunomodulatory effects which are likely to contribute to the beneficial effect in patients with cholestatic disorders of autoimmune origin [34].

Thus, UDCA represents an interesting example in clinical pharmacology of a drug which was originally contraindicated in CLD and was used as a litholytic agent for cholesterol stones and which, by contrast, has been increasingly used in chronic cholestatic and non-cholestatic liver disease [17] since the first report by Leuschner et al. (1985) on its beneficial effect in chronic hepatitis [35].

An opposite story applies to silymarin, a drug which was originally used in acute poisoning of the liver due to the stimulation of protein synthesis and to its membrane-stabilizing effects and subsequently employed also in CLD of various aetiologies because of its free-radical scavenger properties. In 1989, Ferenci and his group [36] clearly showed that survival was significantly better in the patients treated with silymarin than in those receiving placebo, and this was especially true in those with alcoholic cirrhosis.

We were interested to see whether silibinin, which is the main component of silymarin, could influence biliary lipid composition and, if that was the case, by which mechanism(s). We investigated this both in the rat and in gallstone and cholecystectomized patients. Rats treated with silibinin for 7 days at a dose of 100 mg/kg body weight showed a significant decrease in biliary cholesterol concentration and secretion and also in biliary phospholipid secretion but no changes in bile acid secretion or bile flow [37]. The decrease in hepatic cholesterol output was confirmed in the clinical studies following oral administration of silymarin at a daily dose of 420 mg for four weeks [37]. As regards the possible mechanisms explaining the reduction of biliary cholesterol secretion, we found a dose-dependent inhibition of the activity of hydroxy-methyl-glutaryl Co-A reductase, suggesting a reduction of cholesterol neosynthesis in the liver [37].

CONCLUSIONS

Thus, its seems advisable to consider and/or set up experimental studies to investigate possible effects on bile flow and composition of drugs which are mainly eliminated by the biliary route. Although some of them may adversely affect bile flow and/or biliary lipid secretion (fibrates, somatostatin, ocreotide, ceftriaxone) or even gallbladder contraction (for example nifedipine), others might be given in combination in order to potentiate their favourable influence on bile flow and composition and decrease drug-related side-effects.

REFERENCES

1. Jazrawi RP, de Caesteker JS, Goggin P et al. Kinetics of hepatic handling of cholestatic liver disease: effect of ursodeoxycholic acid. Gastroenterology. 1994;5:373–81.
2. Jazrawi BP, Ferraris R, Bridges C et al. Kinetics of the synthetic bile acid ^{75}SeHCAT in man: comparison with 14C taurocholate. Gastroenterology. 1988;95:164–9.
3. Galatola G, Jazrawi RP, Bridges C et al. Direct measurement of first-pass ileal clearance of a bile acid in humans. Gastroenterology. 1991;100:1100–5.
4. Lirussi F, Nassuato G, Orlando R et al. Treatment of active cirrhosis with ursodeoxycholic acid and a free radical scavenger: a two year prospective study. Med Sci Res. 1995;23:31–3.
5. Lotterer E, Stiehl A, Raedsch R et al. Ursodeoxycholic acid in primary biliary cirrhosis: no evidence for toxicity in the stages I to III. J Hepatol. 1990;10:284–90.
6. Leuschner U, Fischer H, Kurtz W et al. Ursodeoxycholic acid in primary biliary cirrhosis: results of a controlled double-blind trial. Gastroenterology. 1989;97:1268–74.
7. Lirussi F, Bortolato L, Beccarello A, Okolicsanyi L, Crepaldi G. Long-term treatment with ursodeoxy-cholic acid (UDCA) of active cirrhosis. Efficacy and evaluation of liver function (LF). Hepato-Gastroenterology. 1993;III(Suppl 1):75.
8. Williams SJ, Farrel GC. Inhibition of antipyrine metabolism by interferon. Br J Clin Pharmacol. 1986;22:610–12.
9. Williams SJ, Baird-Lambert JA, Farrel GC. Inhibition of theophylline metabolism by interferon. Lancet. 1987;2:939–41.
10. Okuno H, Kitao Y, Takasu M et al. Depression of drug metabolizing activity in the human liver by interferon-α. Eur J Clin Pharmacol. 1990;39:365–7.
11. Okuno H, Takasu M, Kano H, Seki T, Shiozaki Y, Inoue K. Depression of drug-metabolizing activity in the human liver by interferon-β. Hepatology. 1993;17:65–9.
12. Oellerich M, Raude E, Burdelski M et al. Monoethylglycinexylidide formation kinetics: A novel approach to assessment of liver function. J Clin Chem Clin Biochem. 1987;25:845–53.
13. Oellerich M, Ringe B, Gubernatis G et al. Lignocaine metabolite formation as a measure of pre-transplant liver function. Lancet. 1989;1:640–2.
14. Fabris L, Iemmolo RM, Viaggi S et al. Ability of monoethylglycinexylidide (MEGX) formation test in discriminating severity of liver cirrhosis. J Hepatol. 1994;21(Suppl 1):S158.
15. Okamoto H, Sugiyama Y, Okada S et al. Typing hepatitis C virus by polymerase chain reaction with type-specific primers: Application to clinical surveys and tracing infectious sources. J Gen Vir. 1992;73:673–9.

16. Lirussi F, Crovatto M, Santini G et al. Interferon (IFN), chronic hepatitis C and HCV genotypes. Any influence on liver function? Proceedings of the X International Congress of Liver Diseases: Acute and Chronic Liver Diseases: Molecular Biology and Clinics, Oct 19–21, Basel; 1995:119.
17. Okolicsanyi L, Lirussi F, Strazzabosco M et al. The effect of drugs on bile flow and composition. An overview. Drugs. 1986;31:430–48.
18. Nathanson MH, Boyer JL. Mechanisms and regulation of bile secretion. Hepatology. 1991;14:551–66.
19. Suchy FJ. Hepatocellular transport of bile acids. Semin Liver Dis. 1993;13:235–47.
20. Radominska A, Treat S, Little J. Bile acid metabolism and the pathophysiology of cholestasis. Semin Liver Dis. 1993;13:219–34.
21. Kamimoto Y, Gatmaitan Z, Hsu J, Arias IM. The function of Gp170, the multidrug resistance gene product, in rat liver canalicular membrane vesicles. J Biol Chem. 1989;264:11693–8.
22. Elias E, Hruban Z, Wade JB, Boyer JL. Phalloidin-induced cholestasis: a microfilament-mediated change in junctional complex permeability. Proc Natl Acad Sci USA. 1980;77:2229–33.
23. Boyer JL. Tight junction in normal and cholestatic liver: does the paracellular pathway have functional significance? Hepatology. 1983;3:614–7.
24. Beuers U, Nathanson MH, Boyer JL. Effects of tauroursodeoxycholic acid on cytosolic Ca^{2+} signals in isolated rat hepatocytes. Gastroenterology. 1993;104:604–12.
25. Strazzabosco M, Okolicsanyi L, Boyer JL. Acid/base transport systems in isolated bile duct epithelial cells. In: Gentilini P, Dianzani MU, eds. Experimental and Clinical Hepatology. Amsterdam: Elsevier; 1991:133–41.
26. Gautam A, Ng OC, Boyer JL. Isolated rat hepatocyte couplets in short-term culture: structural characteristics and plasma membrane reorganization. Hepatology. 1987;7:216–23.
27. Gautam A, Ng OC, Strazzabosco M, Boyer JL. Quantitative assessment of canalicular bile formation in isolated rat hepatocyte couplets using microscopic optical planimetry. J Clin Invest. 1989;83:565–73.
28. Strazzabosco M, Sakisaka S, Hayakawa T, Boyer JL. Effect of UDCA on intracellular and biliary pH in isolated rat hepatocyte couplets and perfused livers. Am J Physiol. 1991;260:G58–69.
29. Poupon RE, Poupon R, Balkau B and the UDCA–PBC Study Group. Ursodiol for the long-term treatment of primary biliary cirrhosis. N Engl J Med. 1994;330:1342–7.
30. Reichen J. Pharmacologic treatment of cholestasis. Semin Liver Dis. 1993;13:302–15.
31. Lirussi F, Okolicsanyi L. Cytoprotection with ursodeoxycholic acid: effect in chronic non-cholestatic and chronic cholestatic liver disease. Ital J Gastroenterol. 1992;24:31–5.
32. Jacquemin E, Dumont M, Mallet A, Erlinger S. Ursodeoxycholic acid improves ethinyl estradiol-induced cholestasis in the rat. Eur J Clin Invest. 1993;23:794–802.
33. Stiehl A, Raedsch R, Rudolph G. Acute effects of ursodeoxycholic and chenodeoxycholic acid on the small intestinal absorption of bile acids. Gastroenterology. 1990;98:424–8.
34. Poupon RE, Balkau B, Eschwège E, Poupon R and the UDCA–PBC Study Group. A multicenter, controlled trial of ursodiol for the treatment of primary biliary cirrhosis. N Engl J Med. 1991;324:1548–54.
35. Leuschner U, Leuschner M, Sieratzki J, Kurtz W, Hubner K. Gallstone dissolution with ursodeoxycholic acid in patients with chronic active hepatitis and two years follow-up. Dig Dis Sci. 1985;30:642–9.
36. Ferenci P, Dragosics B, Dittrich H et al. Randomized controlled trial of silymarin treatment in patients with cirrhosis of the liver. J Hepatol. 1989;9:105–13.
37. Nassuato G, Iemmolo RM, Strazzabosco M et al. Effect of silibinin on biliary lipid composition. Experimental and clinical study. J Hepatol. 1991;12:290–5.

Manuscript received 21 Nov. 95.
Accepted for publication 25 Nov. 95.

TS Gaginella et al. (eds.), Biochemical Pharmacology as an Approach to Gastrointestinal Disorders, 249–259

ALTERATION OF MICROVASCULAR REGENERATION AND PERMEABILITY DURING ACETIC ACID-INDUCED GASTRIC ULCER HEALING: EFFECT OF BASIC FIBROBLAST GROWTH FACTOR

M. NAKAMURA[1], Y. AKIBA[1], H. ISHII[1] AND M. KITAJIMA[2]
[1]Department of Internal Medicine, [2]Department of Surgery, School of Medicine, Keio University, Tokyo 160, Japan

ABSTRACT

The microvascular network of the gastrointestinal tract is characterized by the rich distribution of the perivascular autonomic nerves.

During the process of acetic acid-induced gastric ulcer healing, an increase in vascular permeability has been shown in the regenerated vessels by the intra-aortic infusion of horseradish peroxidase. During the healing process, the immunoreactivities of basic fibroblast growth factor and platelet-derived growth factor were increased in the granulation tissues. The administration of CS23, acid-stable human recombinant basic fibroblast growth factor, decreased the increase in vascular permeability and accelerated the regeneration of a microvascular network from the point of localization of the E-selectin and CD36 immunoreactivity.

In conclusion, bFGF was shown to stimulate microvascular regeneration as well as autonomic reinnervation in the healing process of acetic acid-induced gastric ulcers.

Keywords: gastric microcirculation, acetic acid-induced gastric ulcer, microvascular permeability, basic fibroblast growth factor, platelet-derived growth factor

INTRODUCTION

The microvascular network of the gastrointestinal tract, especially of the stomach, is characterized by the rich distribution of perivascular autonomic nerves [1]. On the other hand, few microvessels regenerated after ulcer formation were found to be accompanied by autonomic reinnervation. Our recent histochemical studies on the effect of basic fibroblast growth factor (bFGF) have demonstrated an accelerated regeneration of perivascular autonomic nerves in granulation tissues after acetic acid-induced gastric ulcer formation [2]. However, the interaction of autonomic nervous and microcirculatory regeneration remains to be determined.

In the present study, the histochemical characteristics of regenerated microvessels after acetic acid-induced gastric ulcer formation were studied using Wistar strain male rats. In addition, alteration of the distribution of bFGF and platelet-derived growth factor (PDGF) immunoreactivities and the effect of human recombinant bFGF on the regeneration of the microvessels were discussed.

This paper was presented at the Section of IUPHAR GI Pharmacology Symposium on 'Biochemical pharmacology as an approach to gastrointestinal disorders (basic science to clinical perspectives)', October 12–14, 1995, Pécs, Hungary.

MATERIALS AND METHODS

Wistar strain male rats, weighing 200–250 g, were used in the following experiments. Rats were divided into the following five groups: control, three and seven days after acetic acid alone, and three days and seven days after acetic acid plus CS23 (acid-stable recombinant human bFGF, Takeda Chemical Industries Ltd., Osaka, Japan) [3]. Ulcers were induced by the application of 100% acetic acid to the anterior serosal surface of the rat stomach at the border of the fundic and antral region for 30 s three or seven days prior to the experiments. Uniform gastric ulcers with a diameter of 5 mm developed three days after treatment. In the CS23-treated groups, CS23 was dissolved in 0.01 mol/L phosphate-buffered saline (pH 7.4) with 5.0% fetal calf serum; 0.5 ml of an aqueous solution of CS23 (1 μg/100 g body weight) was given via oral gastric intubation every 12 h after the formation of the gastric ulcers until just before fixation.

Histochemical procedures to observe the microvascular network, autonomic nerves and permeability

The chronological changes in the microvascular architecture were observed by the intra-aortic infusion of horseradish peroxidase (HRP; Sigma type II; 20 mg/100 g body weight, Sigma Chemical Company, St. Louis, MO., USA), followed by the reaction with diaminobenzidine [4,5].

For immunohistochemical observation of CD36, Factor VIII, E-selectin and laminin, the stomach tissues were fixed with Zamboni's fixative, followed by treatment with phosphate-buffered saline (PBS) with graded concentration of sucrose. The cryostat sections were made and indirect immunoperoxidase staining was performed using monocloncal antibody against CD36, Factor VIII, E-selectin or laminin (Cambridge Research Biochemicals, Cheshire, UK).

To observe the localization of unmyelinated nerve fibres in the gastric mucosa, small tissue blocks were fixed with a mixed solution of 4% formaldehyde and 1% glutaraldehyde in 0.06 mol/L phosphate buffer (pH 7.4) for 6 h at 4°C, followed by postfixation with 1% osmic acid for 2 h. After dehydration in a graded ethanol series, all the tissue blocks were embedded in Epon. The ultrathin sections were made using LKB ultramicrotome, stained with lead citrate and uranyl acetate and observed with a Hitachi H-300 electron microscope [1].

Histochemical procedures to observe the localization of bFGF and PDGF immunoreactivity

For immunohistochemical observation of bFGF and PDGF, the stomach tissues were fixed as mentioned above and the cryostat sections were made and indirect immuno-peroxidase staining was performed using monoclonal antibody against bFGF (MAb 3H3, Wako Pure Chemicals Industries, Osaka, Japan) and against PDGF-AA and BB (Chemicon International Inc., Temecula, CA, USA).

To verify the intensity of the immunoreactivity, images were digitized using an image processing and analysis software Ultimage (Graftek, France) [6]. The images were managed in the computer as 512 × 512-pixel matrices with 256 grey levels. Three hundred images were transferred for analysis of grains. The area having silver grains was calculated using grey-level threshold. Student's *t*-test was used in this study.

Radioautographic procedures to observe the localization of [^{125}I]PDGF–BB-binding sites

The effector sites of PDGF–BB were studied by the radioautography of soluble compounds using [^{125}I]PDGF–BB. The binding sites of PDGF–BB were studied by the intra-aortic infusion of [^{125}I]PDGF–BB, followed by freeze-drying, fixation of osmium gas, direct Epon embedding, semithin sectioning with ethylene glycol, and application of radioautographic emulsion film by the wire-loop method. After 30–60 days exposure, the sections were developed, fixed and observed by light and electron microscopy [7,8]. The specificity of the binding sites was assessed by the addition of cold PDGF to the infusion solution.

RESULTS

Microvascular structure revealed by the histochemical method

The microvascular structure in gastric mucosa is composed of the true capillary network and the collecting venules that drain the blood flow from the capillaries in the tip portion of the gastric mucosa into the submucosal venules. The microvessels in the mucosal and submucosal layer were clearly visualized by the immunohistochemical method using anti-Factor VIII or CD36 monoclonal antibodies (Figure 1). The anti-Factor VIII immunoreactivity was rather stronger in the venules than in the arterioles and capillaries.

CD36 immunoreactivity also had a similar distribution in the rat stomach. Unmyelinated nerve fibres were seen adjacent to the microvessels by the electron microscopic observation of the gastric mucosa. Most of the synaptic vesicles of these nerves were small, agranular and characteristic of cholinergic nerves.

Alterations in microvascular permeability and related immunoreactivities during healing of acetic acid-induced gastric ulcers

During the healing process of acetic acid-induced gastric ulcers, an increase in vascular permeability is seen in the regenerated vessels by the intra-aortic infusion of horseradish peroxidase (HRP; Sigma type II), while CS23 treatment decreases the alteration in vascular permeability [2]. Laminin and E-selectin immunoreactivities increased surrounding the regenerated microvessels in acetic acid-treated gastric mucosa (Figure 2).

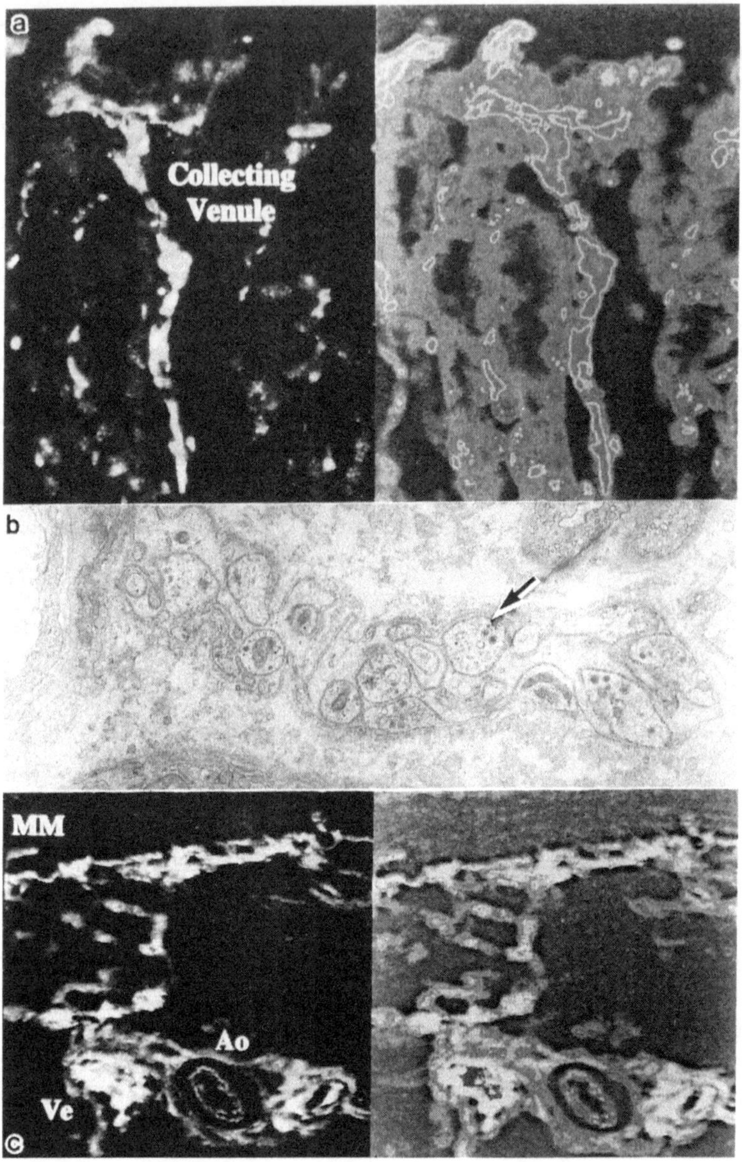

Figure 1. Immunohistochemical observation of anti-Factor VIII immunoreactivity and electron microscopic observation in the control rat stomach. **a**: In the mucosal layer, immunoreactivity is seen on the collecting venules as well as the surrounding true capillaries. ×640. **b**: By electron microscopic observation, unmyelinated nerve fibres (arrow) are seen adjacent to the microvessels in control rat gastric mucosa. ×6400. **c**: In the submucosal layer, immunoreactivity is clearly seen on the endothelial cells of the venules (Ve) and hardly found on the arterioles (Ao). ×360. Left half: Original pictures. Right half: Pictures processed for enhancement of FITC-fluorescence

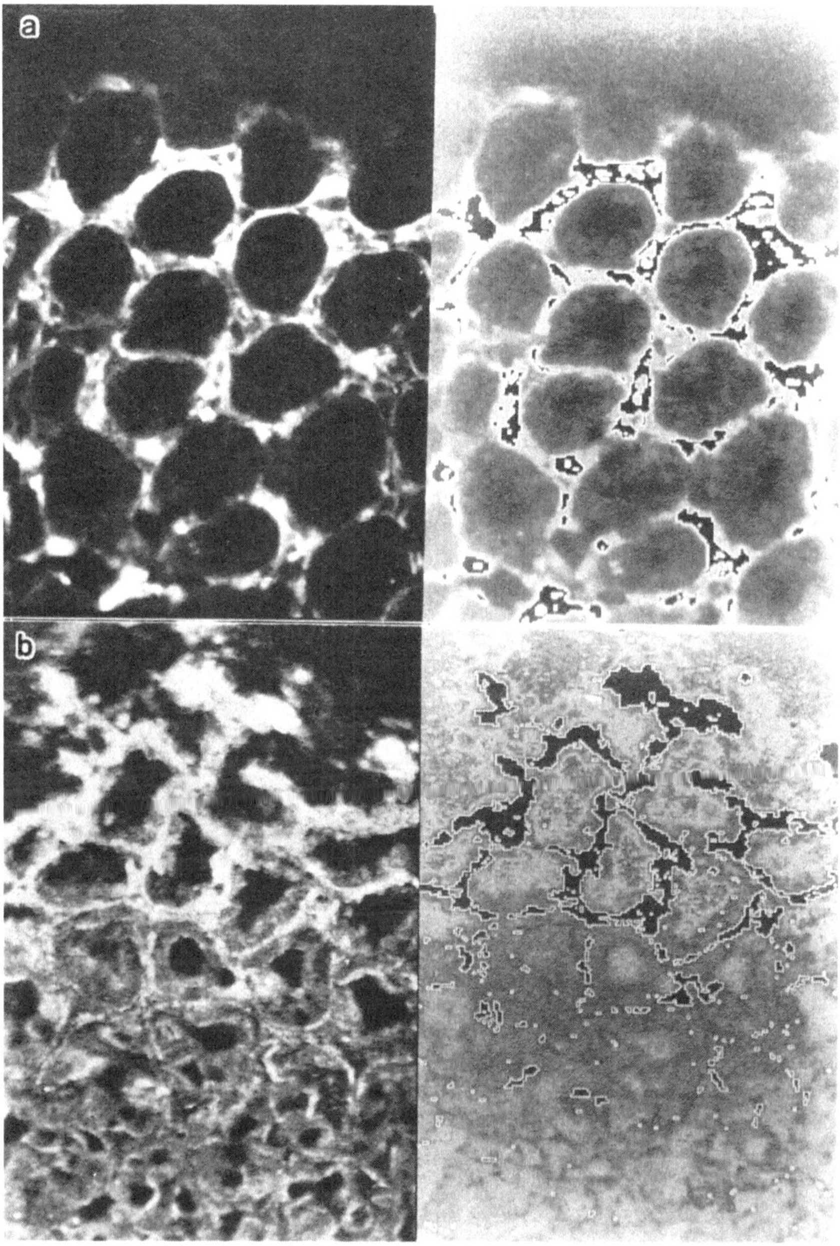

Figure 2. Immunohistochemical observation of antilaminin immunoreactivity in control and acetic acid-treated rat gastric mucosa. **a**: In the control mucosal layer, immunoreactivity is found surrounding the true capillaries and basement membrane of the epithelial cells. The immunoreactivity is very strong near the tip portion of the gastric mucosa. ×640. **b**: In the acetic acid-treated gastric mucosa three days after the acetic acid treatment, a marked increase in immunoreactivity is detected in the erosive region. ×640

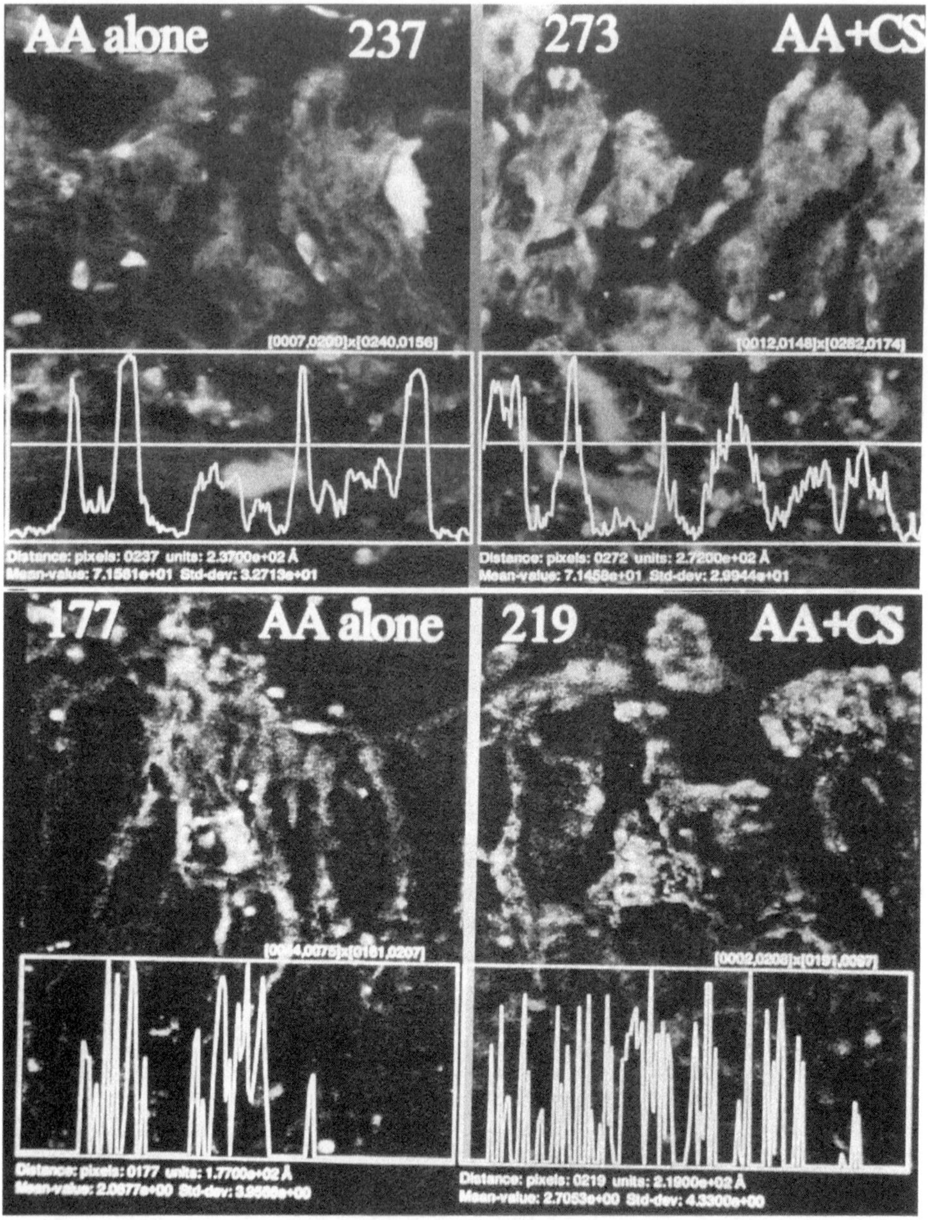

Figure 3. Comparison of the immunoreactivity of CD36 and E-selectin in gastric mucosa treated with acetic acid alone and acetic acid plus CS23. **a**: The relative amplitude of the CD36 immunoreactivity in the gastric mucosa treated with acetic acid alone is 237 ± 32.7 units, while, in rats treated with acetic acid plus CS23, the strength of the fluorescence is 273 ± 25.4 units ($p = 0.088$). $\times 240$. **b**: The amplitude of E-selectin immunoreactivity in the gastric mucosa treated with acetic acid alone is 177 ± 39.6 units, and that in the gastric mucosa treated with acetic acid plus CS23 is 219 ± 30.1 units ($p = 0.096$). $\times 240$

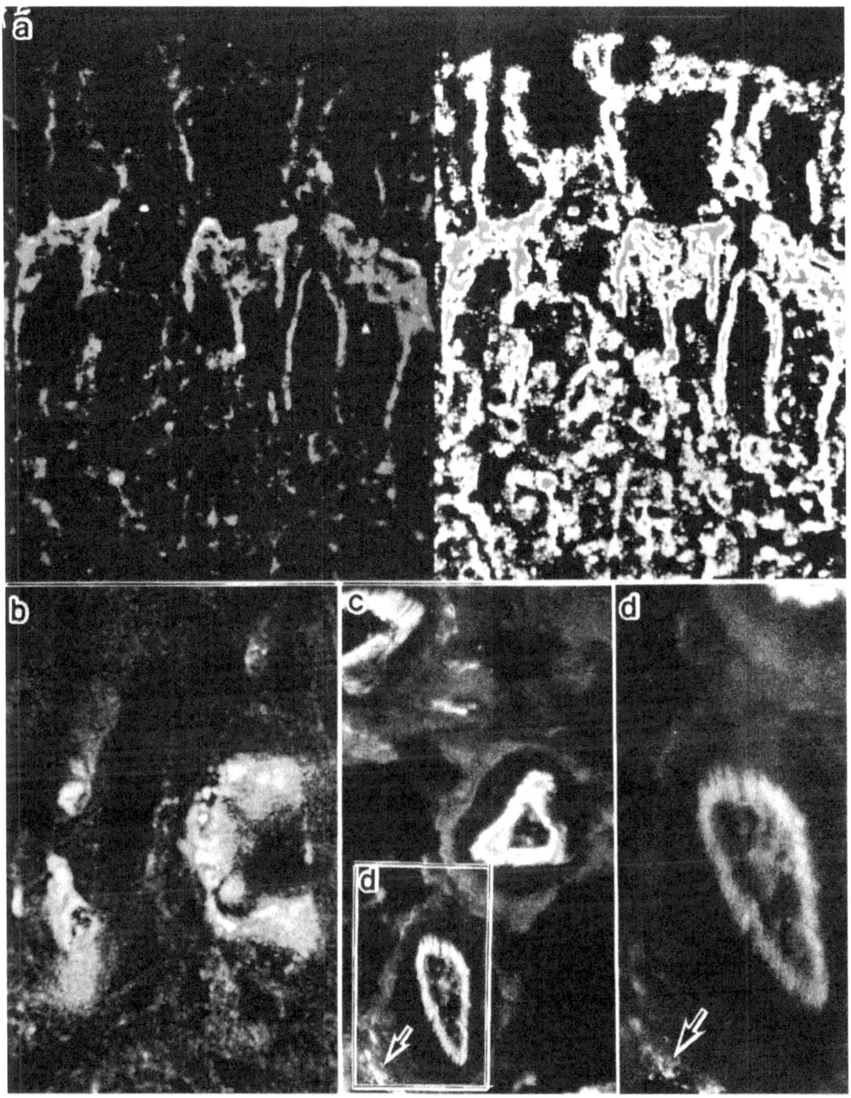

Figure 4. Immunohistochemical observation of bFGF immunoreactivity in the control rat stomach. **a**: In the mucosal layer, bFGF immunoreactivity is seen exclusively in the true capillary network. ×480. **b**: In the proper muscular layer, immunoreactivity is seen in the myenteric plexus. ×320. **c,d**: In the submucosal layer, immunoreactivity is found in the endothelial cells of the venules and in the perivascular nerve plexuses (arrows). c: ×320, d: ×640

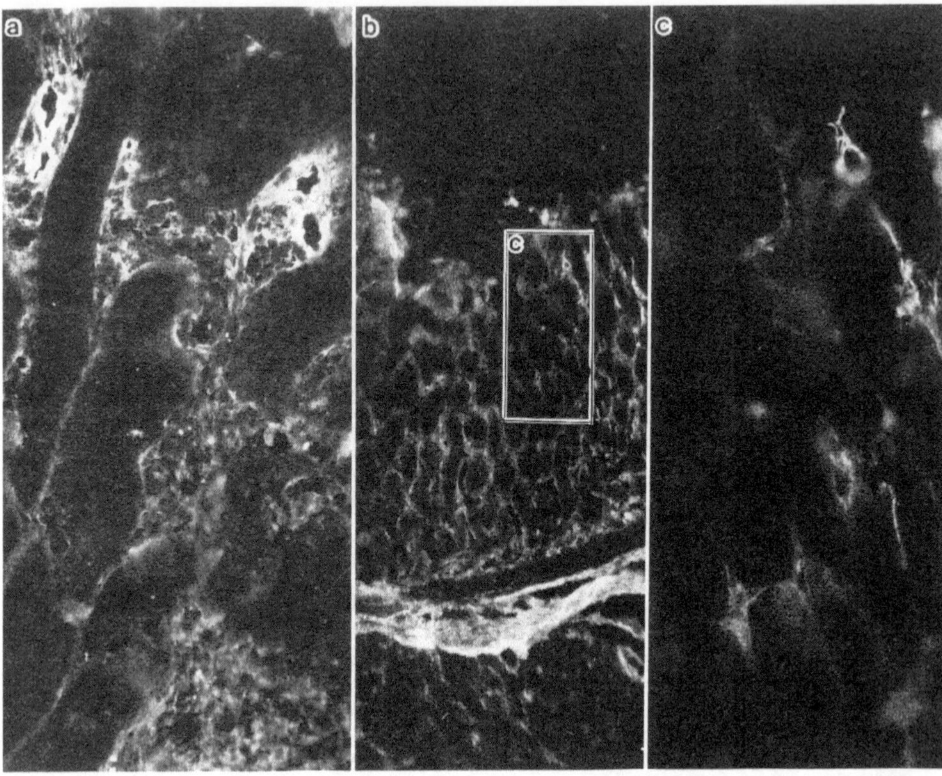

Figure 5. Immunohistochemical observation of bFGF immunoreactivity in the rat gastric mucosa treated with acetic acid. **a**: Three days after acetic acid treatment, immunoreactivity is detected in the endothelial cells of the regenerated gastric mucosa as well as in the interstitial cells of the granulation tissues. ×260. **b,c**: Seven days after acetic acid treatment, immunoreactivity is mostly seen on the endothelial cells of the capillary network. b: ×200, c: ×600

By repeated treatment with CS23, increased immunoreactivities of CD36, E-selectin (Figure 3) and laminin were observed three and seven days after the acetic acid treatment, compared with the group treated with acetic acid alone.

Localization of bFGF and PDGF immunoreactivity and effector sites of PDGF–BB in the gastric mucosa

The bFGF immunoreactivity in control rats was mostly seen in the microvascular network as well as in the autonomic nerves, including myenteric plexuses (Figure 4). After acetic acid treatment, immunoreactivity of bFGF was seen not only in the endothelial cells of the microcirculatory system but also in the interstitial cells in the granulation tissues, composed of macrophages and monocytes (Figure 5).

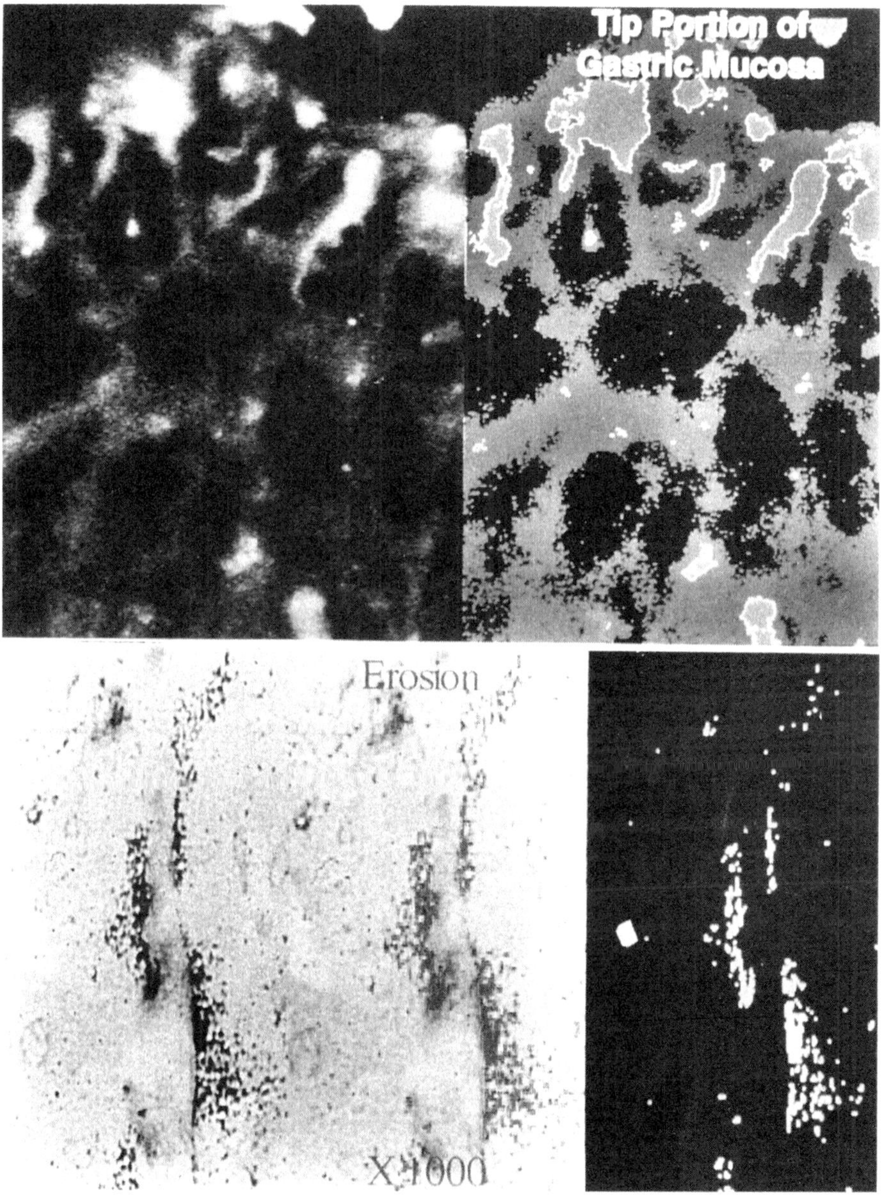

Figure 6. Immunohistochemical and radioautographic observation of PDGF–BB immunoreactivity and [^{125}I]PDGF-BB binding sites in the rat stomach three days after the acetic acid treatment. **a**: PDGF–BB immunoreactivity is strongly detected in the tip portion of the gastric mucosa. × 320. **b**: [^{125}I]PDGF–BB binding sites are accumulated on the interstitial cells just under the erosive lesion, probably corresponding to the fibroblasts. × 320. Left: original picture; Middle: enhanced by image processor; Right: silver grains are selected by image processing

PDGF–AA and PDGF-BB immunoreactivity in control rats was also seen in the microvascular system and in the autonomic nerves. In the acetic acid-treated gastric mucosa, the immunoreactivity was seen in the tip portion of the gastric mucosa, coinciding with the localization of platelet aggregation in the collecting venules and true capillaries (Figure 6). [^{125}I]PDGF-BB binding sites were seen on the fibroblasts and undifferentiated mesenchymal cells, both in the control and acetic acid-treated rats by the radioautography of soluble compounds.

DISCUSSION

Revascularization during epithelial repair is thought to be composed of various kinds of cells, including endothelial cells, smooth muscle cells, fibroblasts and other undifferentiated mesenchymal cells. Cytokines and growth factors are possible mediators between these cells but the relative significance of these factors varies from tissue to tissue. The present study shows that bFGF and PDGF immunoreactivities are richly distributed both in the endothelial cells and the enteric nerves in control rats. External addition of rhbFGF increased the immunoreactivity of E-selectin [9] and CD36, two of the markers of endothelial cells, during the healing of acetic acid-induced gastric ulcers. These results show that bFGF plays an important role in the healing process of the gastric ulcer.

PDGF is another candidate for an important role in gastric ulcer healing because this growth factor is localized adjacent to the ulcerative lesion, especially in the congested microvessels, as shown in this study.

Vascular permeability is a very useful marker to clarify the maturation of the microvascular network. In the present study, HRP intra-aortic infusion was used and this method has already been proved to be a very useful tool to investigate the alteration in permeability at a very early stage [5].

CONCLUSIONS

Cell adhesion molecules, cytokines and extracellular matrices have been shown to play some roles in the healing process of acetic acid-induced gastric ulcer.

bFGF was shown to have normalizing effects on microvascular permeability, as well as accelerating microvascular regeneration and autonomic reinnervation.

REFERENCES

1. Nakamura M, Watanabe N, Tsukada N et al. Demonstration of the adrenergic nerves in the rat gastric mucosa – a histofluorescence and electron microscopic study in comparison with the distribution of the cholinergic nerves. Okajimas Folia Anat Jpn. 1982;59:65–86.
2. Nakamura M, Oda M, Inoue J et al. Effect of basic fibroblast growth factor on reinnervation of gastric microvessels: possible relevance to ulcer recurrrence. Dig Dis Sci. 1995;40:1451–8.

3. Seno K, Sasada R, Iwane M et al. Stabilizing basic fibroblast growth factor using protein engineering. Biochem Biophys Res Commun. 1988;151:701–8.
4. Graham RC, Karnovsky MJ. The early stages of absorption of injected horseradish peroxidase in the proximal tubules of mouse kidney: ultrastructural cytochemistry by a new technique. J Histochem Cytochem. 1966;14:291–302.
5. Kitajima M, Nakamura M, Tsuchiya M. Effect of basic fibroblast growth factor on microvascular regeneration from gastric ulcerative lesion – increased binding sites of bFGF after CS23 treatment. Microvasc Res. 1995;50:133–8.
6. Nakamura M, Oda M, Inoue J et al. Binding sites for calcitonin gene-related peptide in regenerating gastric mucosa. J Clin Gastroenterol. 1993;17(Suppl. 1):S46–S52.
7. Nagata T, Nawa T, Yokota S. A new technique for electron microscopic dry-mounting radioautography of soluble compounds. Histochemie. 1969;18:241–9.
8. Nakamura M, Oda M, Kaneko K et al. Autoradiographic demonstration of gastrin-releasing peptide-binding sites in the rat gastric mucosa. Gastroenterology. 1988;94:968–76.
9. Nguyen M, Strubel NA, Bishoff J. A role for sialyl Lewis-X/A glycoconjugates in capillary morphogenesis. Nature. 1993;365:267–9

Manuscript received 14 Oct. 95.
Accepted for publication 25 Nov. 95.

TS Gaginella et al. (eds.), Biochemical Pharmacology as an Approach to Gastrointestinal Disorders, 261–268

MODULATION OF GASTRIC WOUND REPAIR BY HEPATOCYTE GROWTH FACTOR AND BASIC FIBROBLAST GROWTH FACTOR

S. WATANABE*, M. HIROSE, X.-E. WANG, H. OIDE, T. KITAMURA, H. MIWA, T. MURAI, O. KOBAYASHI, K. OTAKA, A. MIYAZAKI AND N. SATO
Department of Gastroenterology, Juntendo University School of Medicine, 2-1-1 Hongo Bunkyo-ku, Tokyo 113, Japan
*Correspondence

ABSTRACT

The process of wound repair and the role of growth factors were investigated using primary cultured rabbit gastric mucosal cells. A confluent monolayer gastric epithelial cell sheet or fibroblasts was wounded to make a cell-free area of constant size. The changes in the cell-free area were analysed quantitatively by image analysis. In the epithelial cell model, the wound recovered in 36–48 h in controls; wound repair was accelerated by the addition of fetal calf serum (FCS) and hepatocyte growth factor to the medium. In the fibroblast model, repair was accelerated by the addition of bFGF. In these models, the wound was repaired in two steps; an initial cell migration stage and a later proliferation stage. In the epithelial restoration, migration was much more important than proliferation and in the fibroblast model, proliferation was important as well as migration. In conclusion, growth factors modulate wound repair with the induction of both epithelial and mesenchymal cell migration and proliferation.

Keywords: gastric ulcer, growth factor, cytoskeleton, migration, proliferation, wound healing

INTRODUCTION

It has been shown that damage to the gastric surface epithelium is followed by rapid epithelial cell migration called 'restitution' after removal of causative agents [1]. For example, exposure of gastric mucosa to hyperosmolar sodium chloride caused extensive damage to the surface epithelium and epithelial restitution occurred within several minutes after removal of sodium chloride [2]. Silen and his colleagues have extensively investigated the process of restitution and have shown its importance in the initial stage of gastric wound repair [3]. However, many questions remain about the mechanism of gastric mucosal repair. In order to resolve these questions, we recently established a new wound-repair model using primary cultured gastric epithelial cells and fibroblasts. This model allows investigation of cellular capacity for mucosal restoration without the effects of systemic factors. In this paper, we review this wound-repair model and discuss the role of growth factors.

This paper was presented at the Section of IUPHAR GI Pharmacology Symposium on 'Biochemical pharmacology as an approach to gastrointestinal disorders (basic science to clinical perspectives)', October 12–14, 1995, Pécs, Hungary.

PREPARATION AND CULTURE OF PRIMARY CULTURED GASTRIC MUCOSAL CELLS

There are several wound-repair models using cancer cell lines and cloned epithelial cells. Each model has its merits and demerits. In our model, we use primary cultured rabbit gastric epithelial cells which do not transform. Therefore, our model is much more physiological than those using cancer cells and transformed cloned cells. Also, we established a similar model using primary cultured rabbit gastric fibroblasts.

Gastric mucosal cells were isolated from male Japanese white rabbits (body weight 2 kg) according to methods described previously [4] with some modifications. Rabbits were anaesthetized by intraperitoneal administration of nembutal (50 mg/kg). The rabbit stomach was rapidly removed and the fundic mucosa was quickly separated with a razor blade and minced into small pieces (2–3 mm^2). Minced mucosal pieces were incubated in a medium containing 0.07% type I collagenase (Sigma Chemicals Co., St. Louis, MO, USA), 130 mmol/L NaCl, 12 mmol/L $NaHCO_3$, 3 mmol/L NaH_2PO_4, 2 mmol/L $MgSO_4$, 1 mmol/L $CaCl_2$, 0.1% bovine serum albumin and 0.2% glucose for 15 min in a shaker bath at 37°C. After the incubation, minced tissue was washed with Ca^{2+}- and Mg^{2+}-free Hanks balanced salt solution (HBSS) with 1 mmol/L EDTA. These procedures were repeated twice and the cells were filtered through metal mesh (diameter 300 μm). Subsequently, cells were washed in Ca^{2+}- and Mg^{2+}-free HBSS containing 1 mmol/L EDTA and 0.1% bovine serum albumin.

Coon's modified Ham's F-12 medium supplemented with inactivated 10% fetal bovine serum, 100 U/ml of penicillin, 100 μg/ml of streptomycin and 0.25 μg/ml of amphotericin was used for this study. Isolated gastric mucosal cells were inoculated onto collagen (type I)-coated plastic culture dishes (diameter 60 mm, Corning Glass Works, Corning, NY, USA) at a concentration of 5×10^6/dish. Cells were incubated in a 5% CO_2 incubator at 37°C throughout the study.

The viability of isolated gastric mucosal cells was 95% at the time of cell inoculation and 90% 96 h later at the end of the experiment. Inoculated cells attached to culture dishes within 24 h, then spread and grew, becoming a complete monolayer cell sheet 48 h after inoculation.

Histochemical studies indicated that more than 90% of the cells in the monolayer sheet were positive for PAS, indicating that they were mucous cells [4]. Parietal cells and chief cells, assessed by succinic dehydrogenase and Nile blue staining, respectively, were minor components of the monolayer sheet [4]. Four weeks after the epithelial cell culture, all epithelial cells were detached and a complete monolayer cell sheet of fibroblasts was formed.

ARTIFICIAL WOUNDING AND MONITORING OF WOUND REPAIR

Inoculated cultured gastric epithelial cells formed a complete monolayer cell sheet in 48 h. The method of making an artificial wound of constant size in the cell sheet is the key point of this model. An artificial wound was made in the centre of the gastric mucosal cell sheet by cell denudation using a modified pencil type mixer with a rotating silicon tip, resulting in a cell-free area with a constant size (2 mm^2) [4]. It is best to use a silicon tip to make the wound since the silicon tip is too soft to damage the surface coating material of the culture dish. Identical equipment was used for artificial wounding of the fibroblast monolayer. The process of repair was monitored using an inverted phase contrast microscope (Nikon TMD, Nikon, Tokyo, Japan) equipped with a time-lapse videodisc recorder (SONY LVR-3000N, Tokyo, Japan). The recording interval in this model is 1 frame every 90 s from just after wounding until the end of experiment. Using this model, we can analyse the factors affecting the repair process by adding agents to the medium. Therefore, the effects of various concentrations of hepatocyte growth factor (HGF) and basic fibroblast growth factor (bFGF) on the repair process in these models can be assessed (Figure 1).

In the epithelial cell model, in controls, several minutes after artifical wounding by mechanical denudation, the cells at the edge of the wound began to form pseudopodia-like structures (lamellipodia) and to move toward the centre of the wound with a continuous ruffling movement of the lamellipodia (Figure 2). The cell-free area was repopulated gradually with migrated cells. Although the shape of the cells was polygonal before wounding, the cells in the wounded lesion became flat and spindle-shaped and extended toward the centre of the wound as repopulation progressed. The artificial wound was completely repaired 48 h after wounding (Figure 3). The lamellipodia disappeared, and the monolayer cell sheet resembled the original culture by several hours after complete recovery. As expected, addition of fetal calf serum to the medium caused acceleration of wound repair in this model. Therefore, we used serum-free conditions to investigate various factors. Using this model, HGF led to significant acceleration of epithelial restoration [6] but not of fibroblasts.

In the model with fibroblasts, the fashion of wound repair was very different from that of epithelial cells. Although epithelial cells showed sheet migration after wounding, fibroblasts lost their cell contacts around the wound and migrated individually rather than as a sheet. The speed of migration was much slower in fibroblast cultures than in epithelial cultures, with a period of 6 days being required to restore the cell-free area (1.5 mm^2). Basic fibroblast growth factors significantly accelerated this process (Figure 4) [7]; however, HGF did not affect fibroblast wound repair.

ROLE OF CELL PROLIFERATION

In the process of wound repair, cell proliferation plays an important part. Therefore, we investigated the role of cell proliferation in the whole process of gastric mucosal restoration in vitro. DNA-synthesizing cells were detected by indirect immunohistochemical methods using monoclonal anti-5-bromodeoxyuridine (BrdU; Sigma Chemical Co.) [5] antibody. Four groups were compared. In the first group, BrdU was added to the culture medium at a concentration of 10 μg/ml immediately after the artificial wound was made followed by incubation for 12 h (0–12-h group). In the second group, BrdU was added 12 h after wounding and incubation was continued for 12 additional hours (12–24-h group). In the third group, BrdU was added 24 h after wounding and incubation was continued for 12 h (24–36-h group). In the fourth group, BrdU was

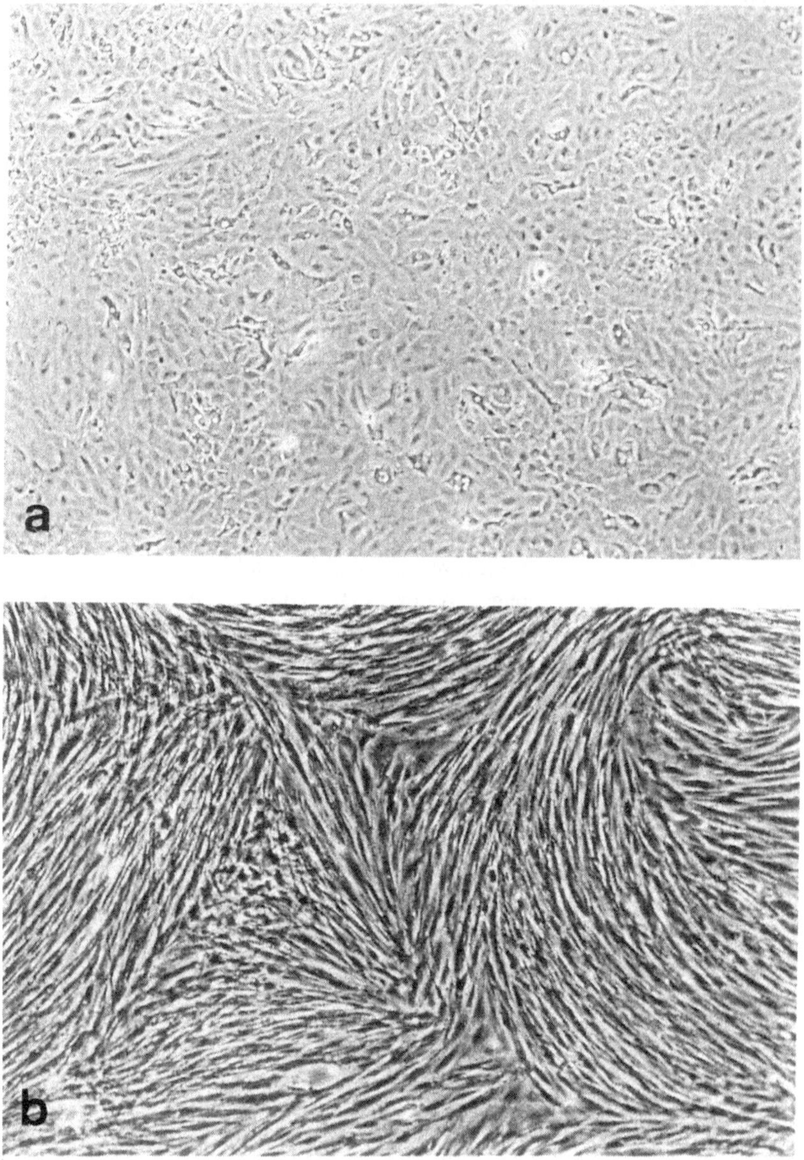

Figure 1. Phase contrast microscopy. (**a**) Monolayer cell sheet of gastric epithelial cells. (**b**) Monolayer cell sheet of gastric fibroblasts

Figure 2. Phase contrast microscopy. After wounding, lamellipodia (arrow heads) showed active ruffling movement

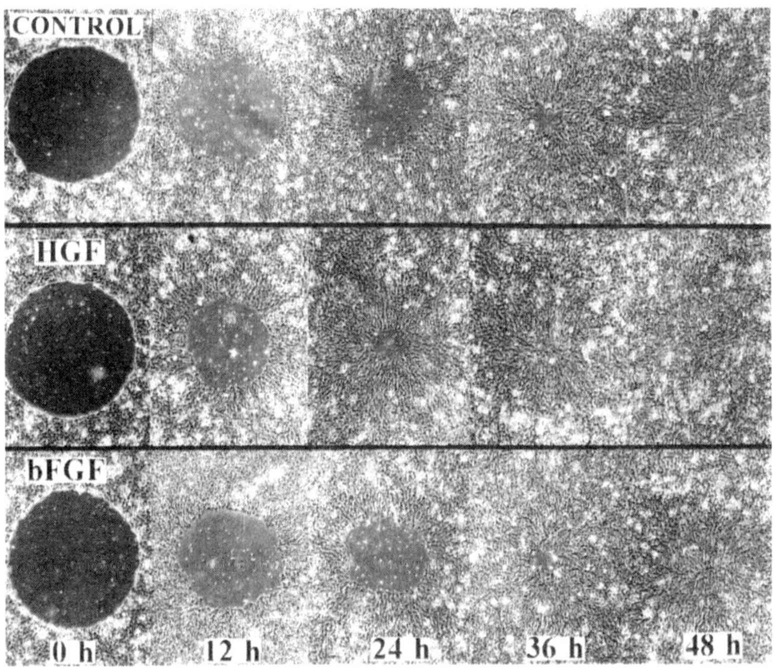

Figure 3. Phase contrast microscopy. The artificial wound in the epithelial cell sheet was completely repaired within 48 h. HGF accelerated wound repair; however, bFGF did not affect the repair process

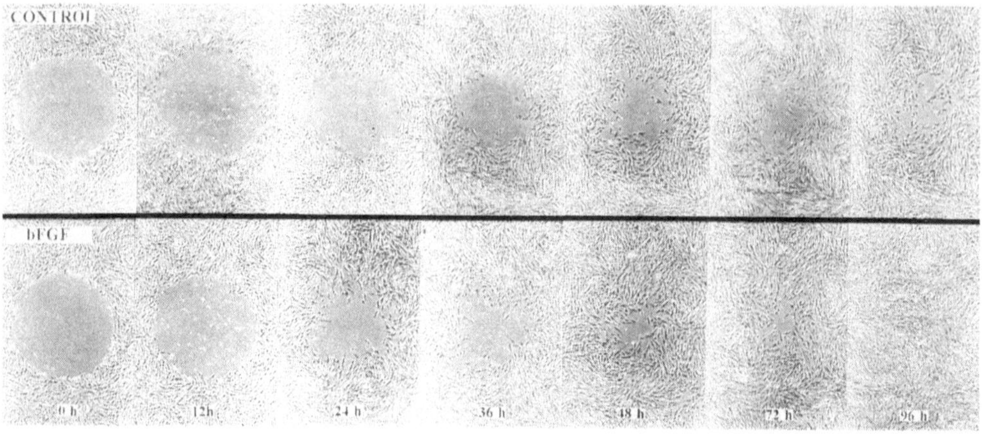

Figure 4. Phase contrast microscopy. Basic fibroblast growth factor accelerated the repair of wounds in fibroblasts

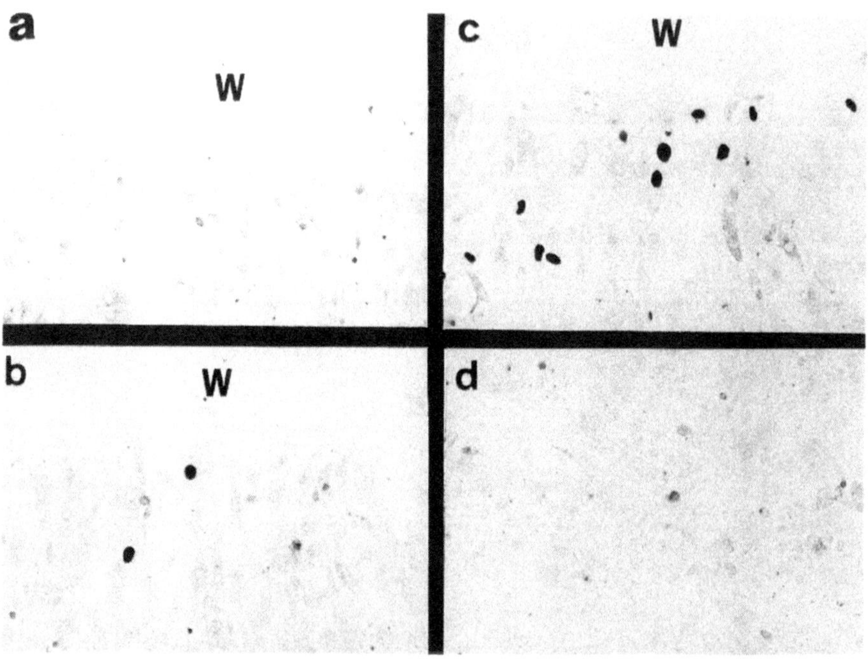

Figure 5. BrdU staining for proliferating cells during the repair process [6]. (**a**) 12 h after wounding, (**b**) 24 h after wounding, (**c**) 36 h after wounding and (**d**) 48 h after wounding, BrdU-positive cells were detected around the wound (**w**)

added 36 h after wounding and incubation was continued for 12 h (36–48-h group). Samples were processed and stained for BrdU by standard techniques, and photomicrographs were taken with a phase contrast microscope. Cell proliferation during the process of wound repair was detected by BrdU staining. BrdU-positive cells were rarely detected in the area far from the wound; however, they were detected around the lesion. BrdU-positive cells were not detectable around the wound in the first 12 h (0–12-h group), and, in the second 12-h period (12–24-h group), they were rarely identified around the wound. However, in the third 12-h period (24–36-h group), the number of BrdU-positive cells increased. Subsequently, the number of BrdU-positive cells decreased as wound recovery occurred and were not detected after the wound was completely repaired (36–48-h) (Figure 5). HGF promoted cell proliferation in this model [6].

The similar sequential staining of proliferating fibroblasts using BrdU showed that cell proliferation was very important in fibroblast restoration. Wound repair and migration was much slower for fibroblasts than for epithelial cells, while the labelling index of proliferative cells around the wounds was much higher in fibroblast cultures than epithelial cell cultures, suggesting an important role for proliferation in restoration by mesenchymal cells. Basic fibroblast growth factor significantly induced cell proliferation fibroblasts as well as wound repair [7].

THE MECHANISM OF MUCOSAL RESTORATION IN THIS MODEL

In the present model, gastric epithelial cells covered the wound within 48 h after wounding without the addition of any growth factors. Therefore, this model may be quite suitable for examining factors which stimulate or retard the process of wound repair in serum-free conditions.

Results of a control study showed that wound repair of gastric mucosal cells in vitro (i.e. the ability of cultured cells to fill the artificially made cell-free area) requires activation of both cell migration and proliferation [4]. However, in this model, the role of cell migration is much more important than that of proliferation because more than three-quarters of wound repair occurred before the detection of BrdU-positive cells. Most of the process, especially the initial stage of repair, is completed by cell migration only and the late stage might include cell proliferation. Factors which might modulate the healing process have been investigated. Addition of hepatocyte growth factor [6] induced wound repair in the monolayer gastric epithelial cell sheet. Takahashi et al. reported the effect of HGF on gastric epithelial cell proliferation [8]. This induction was observed in both the cellular migration and proliferation stages. This effect is thought to be mediated by a direct interaction with the specific receptor for HGF, a transmembrane tyrosine kinase encoded by the *c-met* proto-oncogene [9] because the stimulation was inhibited by the addition of a tyrosine kinase inhibitor to the medium [6].

In a series of experiments, we examined the mechanism of subcellular events during gastric mucosal restoration using the actin inhibitor cytochalasin B [4], the myosin light chain kinase inhibitor wortmannin [10], and the calmodulin inhibitor w-7 [4].

Although, these inhibitors might have some side-effects, these agents were widely used in cell biological experiments. In normal cell migration, the ruffling movement of lamellipodia is a major force for cell movement. Addition of these blockers of cytoskeletal proteins prevented the formation of lamellipodia in cells lining the wound, resulting in inhibition of wound repair [5,10]. We also found that extracellular matrix modulated the speed of restoration [11].

Therefore, the integrity of the cytoskeletal system and the interaction of cytoskeleton and extracellular matrix are essential for gastric epithelial cell migration and gastric mucosal restoration.

A similar phenomenon was observed in mesenchymal cell restoration. And the restoration process of mesenchymal cells was modulated by other growth factors, such as bFGF. As is well documented, each growth factor has its own receptors on target cells and the network system of various growth factors play an important role in the higher quality of ulcer healing in vivo.

REFERENCES

1. Ito S, Lacy ER, Rutten MJ, Critchlow J, Silen W. Rapid repair of injured gastric mucosa. Scand J Gastroenterol. 1984;19(Suppl):87–95.
2. Svanes K, Takeuchi K, Ito S, Silen W. Restitution of the surface epithelium of the in vitro frog gastric mucosa after damage with hyperosmolar sodium chloride. Morphology and physiological characteristics. Gastroenterology. 1982;83:1409–26.
3. Silen W, Ito S. Mechanism for rapid reepithelialization of the gastric mucosal surface. Ann Rev Physiol. 1985;47:217–19.
4. Watanabe S, Hirose M, Yasuda T, Miyazaki A, Sato N. Role of actin and calmodulin in migration and proliferation of rabbit gastric mucosal cells in culture. J Gastroenterol Hepatol. 1994;9:325–33.
5. Gratzner HG. Monoclonal antibody to 5-bromo- and 5-iododeoxyuridine: a new reagent for detection of DNA replication. Science. 1982;218:474–5.
6. Watanabe S, Hirose M, X-E Wang et al. Hepatocyte growth factors accelerates the wound repair of cultured gastric mucosal cells. Biochem Biophys Res Commun. 1994;199:1453–60.
7. Watanabe S, Wang XE, Hirose M et al. Basic fibroblast growth factor accelerates gastric mucosal restoration in vitro by promoting mesenchymal cell migration and proliferation. J Gastroenterol Hepatol. 1995 [in press].
8. Takahashi M, Ota S, Terano A et al. Hepatocyte growth factor induces mitogenic reaction to the rabbit gastric epithelial cells in primary culture. Biochem Biophys Res Commun. 1993;191:528–34.
9. Bottaro DP, Rubin JS, Faletto DL et al. Identification of the hepatocyte growth factor receptor as the c-met proto-oncogene product. Science. 1991;251:802–4.
10. Watanabe S, Wang X-E, Hirose M, Sato N. Effect of myosin light chain kinase inhibitor wortmannin on the wound repair of cultured gastric mucosal cells. Biochem Biophys Res Commun. 1994;199:799–806.
11. Mikami H, Watanabe S, Hirose M, Sato N. Role of extracellular matrix in wound repair by cultured gastric mucosal cells. Biochem Biophys Res Commun. 1994;202:285–92.

Manuscript received 14 Oct. 95.
Accepted for publication 17 Nov. 95.

TS Gaginella et al. (eds.), Biochemical Pharmacology as an Approach to Gastrointestinal Disorders, 269–285

THE EFFECT OF RESINIFERATOXIN ON EXPERIMENTAL GASTRIC ULCER IN RATS

O.M.E. ABDEL-SALAM[1], J. SZOLCSÁNYI[2] AND Gy. MÓZSIK[1*]
[1]First Department of Medicine and [2]Department of Pharmacology, Medical University of Pécs, Ifjúság út, H-7643 Pécs, Hungary
*Correspondence

ABSTRACT

Capsaicin-sensitive sensory nerves are involved in modulation of gastric mucosal integrity. The present study aimed to evaluate the effect of the capsaicin analogue, resiniferatoxin (RTX), on gastric mucosal damage produced by different ulcerogenic agents in the rat. Gastric mucosal damage was evoked in pylorus-ligated rats by the administration of intragastric (ig) HCl (2 ml of 0.6 N), ig ethanol (2 ml of 96% or 50% v/v), ig acidified aspirin (200 mg/kg dissolved in 2 ml of 0.15 HCl), subcutaneous (sc) aspirin (200 mg/kg plus ig 2 ml of 0.15 N HCl) and sc indomethacin (20 mg/kg). Animals were sacrificed at different time intervals after administration of the above ulcerogens, when gastric secretory responses, and the number and severity of mucosal lesions were noted. Intragastric RTX (0.6–2 μg/kg) protected against mucosal injury by 0.6 N HCl in a dose-dependent manner. Resiniferatoxin at 0.4 μg/kg prevented mucosal injury by sc indomethacin or sc aspirin in the 4-h pylorus-ligated rat. Resiniferatoxin (0.6 and 1 μg/kg) co-administered with ethanol reduced mucosal injury caused by 50% ethanol. The protective effect of RTX was more marked if the drug was given 15 min prior to ethanol. Resiniferatoxin protected against damage by 96% ethanol if given 15 min prior to challenge, but, when co-administered with 96% ethanol, RTX aggravated the ethanol-induced mucosal damage. Resiniferatoxin by itself did not produce visible gastric mucosal damage in the saline-treated controls. Data indicated that the capsaicin analogue, resiniferatoxin, exerts potent gastroprotective effects in various experimental ulcer models in the rat.

Keywords: resiniferatoxin, capsaicin, experimental gastric ulcer

INTRODUCTION

Capsaicin (8-methyl-*N*-vanillyl-6-nonenamide), the active ingredient of hot peppers of the plant genus *Capsicum*, is a widely used probe to investigate the participation of afferent sensory nerves in a number of physiological processes. This is due to the remarkable selectivity of the drug in stimulating and subsequently in large doses desensitizing a specific subset of primary afferents with C and Aδ thin fibres [1–3].

Experimental data provided evidence that capsaicin sensitive sensory nerves (CSSN) are involved in the modulation of gastric mucosal defence against ulcerogenic agents [4]. High systemic doses of capsaicin, that induced selective ablation of these sensory nerves, aggravated gastric ulcer induced in the rat by pylorus-ligation, acid distension [4], ethanol [5], cysteamine [6] or indomethacin [6,7]. However, application of the agent in low concentrations into the rat stomach protected the mucosa against mucosal

This paper was presented at the Section of IUPHAR GI Pharmacology Symposium on 'Biochemical pharmacology as an approach to gastrointestinal disorders (basic science to clinical perspectives)', October 12–14, 1995, Pécs, Hungary.

damage produced under different experimental conditions [4,5,7–9]. The release of vasodilator mediators from CSSN endings upon their stimulation with capsaicin in low concentrations and the consequent enhancement of the microcirculation was forwarded as the mechanism underlying these gastroprotective effects of capsaicin [4]. Capsaicin-sensitive sensory nerves containing vasodilator peptides were demonstrated to form a dense plexus around the gastric submucosal arterioles [10,11]. Stimulation of these nerves with capsaicin evoked the release of vasodilator peptides in the stomach [12,13] and enhanced gastric mucosal blood flow as measured by different techniques [14–16] while submucosal application of capsaicin resulted in submucosal arteriolar dilatation [17].

Resiniferatoxin is a phorbol-related diterpene occurring in the latex of plants of the Euphorbia family [18]. The compound has been shown to act as potent analogue of capsaicin, not only at the whole animal and tissue level, but also at the cellular level, and shares the same receptor specificity with capsaicin [19–21]. Resiniferatoxin can thus be considered as a selective probe of capsaicin-sensitive neuronal pathways [20], including those involved in gastric mucosal protection [9]. Resiniferatoxin is used in the present study to evaluate the participation of the vanilloid (capsaicin/RTX)-sensitive neural mechanisms in gastric mucosal protection against noxious injury. This study presents the first systematic study of the acute protective effects of RTX in the rat stomach.

MATERIALS AND METHODS

General

Sprague–Dawley strain rats, of both sexes, 180–200 g body weight, were used throughout the experiments. Animals were housed under standardized conditions for light and temperature and kept in cages with wide-meshed floors to help prevent coprophagy. Animals were fasted for 24 h prior to the experiment but allowed free access to tap water. Pylorus ligation was performed under light ether anaesthesia, care being taken not to interfere with the blood supply to the stomach and duodenum. The antiulcer effect of resiniferatoxin was evaluated in different experimental models of mucosal injury, i.e. ethanol, HCl, aspirin and indomethacin. The ulcerogenic agents were administered immediately after pylorus ligation, either alone or simultaneously with RTX. In some experiments, RTX was given prior to the injurious agents. In certain circumstances, capsaicin or prostacyclin was used to compare its effect with that of RTX. Animals were sacrificed at different time intervals after application of the ulcerogens by cervical dislocation after being lightly anaesthetized with ether. The oesophagus was ligated and the stomach excised. Gastric juice was collected in graduated tubes after removal of the oesophageal ligature and the stomachs were opened along the greater curvature and inspected for the presence of gastric mucosal damage.

Aspirin study

Intragastric aspirin

Acetylsalicylic acid was dissolved in 2 ml of 0.15 N HCl and suspended in 1% methylcellulose solution. Aspirin was given orally in a single dose of 200 mg/kg through a soft orogastric tube immediately after pylorus ligation. Various doses of RTX (0.6, 1.0, 1.4 and 1.8 μg/kg) were given ig together with aspirin. The doses were chosen on the basis of previous studies with the laser Doppler flowmetry technique and were found to produce a highly significant increase in gastric mucosal blood flow in the rat (sent for publication). In order to study the time course of RTX action, animals were sacrificed at 1, 2 and 4 h after its administration. In separate series of experiments, the effect of RTX and capsaicin, both applied at 36 μg/kg, was investigated in the 4-h pylorus-ligated plus aspirin-treated rats. Control rats received the vehicle in an equal volume of saline.

Subcutaneous aspirin

Aspirin was dissolved in 5% sodium bicarbonate, adjusted to pH 7.4 and given sc in a single dose of 200 mg/kg in 0.2 ml volume immediately after pylorus ligation. At the same time, 2 ml of 0.15 N HCl solution was given ig. When the protective effect of RTX was examined, the drug was administered ig at a dose of 0.4 μg/kg together with the 0.15 N HCl while controls received the vehicle in an equal volume of saline. A separate group of rats received only 0.15 N HCl (2 ml) ig after pylorus ligation. Animals were sacrificed 4 h later.

Indomethacin study

Indomethacin was dissolved in 5% sodium bicarbonate and given sc in a single dose of 20 mg/kg immediately after pylorus ligation. At the same time, animals were given 2 ml of physiological saline orally. Resiniferatoxin was given orally at a dose of 0.4 μg/kg with the saline. Controls received the vehicle. Animals were sacrificed 4 h later.

Ethanol study

Immediately after pylorus ligation, 2 ml ethanol (50% or 96% v/v) were given ig either alone or with RTX at 0.6 and 1.0 μg/kg. Animals were sacrificed 1, 2 and 4 h later in order to study the duration of the RTX action. In other animal groups, RTX was administered 15 min prior to pylorus ligation and ethanol. Control rats received the vehicle. Animals were sacrificed 1 h later. The effect of capsaicin on the gastric mucosal damage induced by 96% ethanol was compared with that of RTX.

HCl study

Two ml of 0.6 N HCl were given ig immediately after pylorus ligation. Resiniferatoxin was administered orally at 0.6, 1 and 2 μg/kg 15 min earlier. Controls received the vehicle in saline. Animals were sacrificed 1 h later.

Assessment of gastric mucosal damage

Stomachs were excised, opened along the greater curvature, briefly rinsed with saline and inspected for the presence of gastric mucosal lesions, including haemorrhagic bands, red streaks and mucosal redness. The number and severity of mucosal lesions were noted. Lesions were scaled as follows: petechial lesions = 1; lesions less than 1 mm = 2; lesions between 1 and 2 mm = 3; lesions between 2 and 4 mm = 4; and lesions more than 4 mm = 5 [22].

Histology

The gastroprotective effect of RTX was also evaluated histologically. The 0.6 N HCl and 96% ethanol models were used for this purpose, the first being an HCl-dependent model and the latter a non-HCl-dependent model of gastric mucosal injury [23]. Resiniferatoxin was given orally at doses of 0.6 or 1 μg/kg 15 min prior to ligation and the administration of either 0.6 N HCl (2 ml) or 96% ethanol (2 ml). The effect of RTX was compared with those of prostacyclin (5 μg/kg) or capsaicin (1 μg/kg). Prostacyclin (PGI_2) was also given orally (in 0.5 ml volume) after being dissolved in saline 15 min prior to pylorus ligation and the administration of either 0.6 N HCl or ethanol. Control rats received saline in an equal volume 15 min prior to ligation and HCl or ethanol. After macroscopic evaluation of mucosal lesions, stomachs were pinned flat on cardboard, immersed in 10% formalin solution and later embedded in paraffin. From the paraffin-embedded tissue blocks, haematoxylin- and eosin-stained sections were coded. Sections were evaluated qualitatively under light microscopy in a blinded manner so that the observer was unaware of the treatment group from which each slide came. Sections were evaluated for three grades of histological injury, namely, damage to the surface epithelium, superficial mucosal damage involving the upper one third of the gastric mucosa, and deep mucosal damage extending for more than the upper one third of the mucosa.

Gastric secretory studies

The volume of gastric contents was noted and acid output was determined by titration with 0.1 N NaOH to pH 7 (using a Radelkis pH automatic titrimeter, Budapest, Hungary) and H^+ output expressed in μEq/rat. Gastric H^+ back-diffusion was calculated as follows: net ion flux = [ions recovered] – [(ions instilled) – (initial ions)], i.e. net ion flux = [the amount of H^+ recovered at the end of the experimental period at 1 or 2 h in the HCl or acidified salicylate-treated groups] – [(the acid instilled into the stomach; 2 ml of 0.15 N HCl) – (the initial amount of H^+ in the stomach)]. Positive values indicate a net gain of ions, while negative values indicate loss of ions from the lumen (H^+ back-diffusion) [24]. Results are expressed in μEq/rat; values are mean ± SEM.

Drugs

Indomethacin, aspirin (acetylsalicylic acid; Chinoin, Hungary), resiniferatoxin, capsaicin (Sigma, USA) and methylcellulose (Sigma, USA) were used. Stock solutions of resiniferatoxin (0.5 mg/ml) and capsaicin (10 mg/ml) contained 10% ethanol, 10% Tween 80 and 80% saline solution. Resiniferatoxin or capsaicin was freshly dissolved in isotonic NaCl immediately before the experiments to obtain the necessary doses.

Statistical analysis

The results were expressed as mean ± SEM. Data were analysed by unpaired Student's *t*-test and values of $p < 0.05$ were regarded as significant. The Mann–Whitney's U-test was applied for mathematical analysis of non-parametric results (ulcer severity).

RESULTS

Aspirin-induced gastric lesions

Intragastric aspirin

Resiniferatoxin (0.6–1.8 μg/kg) co-administered with topical acidified aspirin prevented in a dose-dependent manner the development of gastric mucosal damage by aspirin. The protection by RTX in this dose range lasted for 1 h; no significant protective effect of the drug was seen in the 2-h or 4-h pylorus-ligated plus aspirin-treated rats (Figure 1). Resiniferatoxin in a dose of 1.8 μg/kg produced a 69.1% inhibition of lesion severity caused by aspirin in the 1-h pylorus-ligated rat. A twenty-times higher dose of RTX, however, significantly reduced the aspirin-induced injury in the 4-h pylorus-ligated rat by 36.7% ($p < 0.01$). Similar protective action of capsaicin was seen but did not reach statistical significance (Figures 2 and 3).

Subcutaneous aspirin

Aspirin given sc together with the ig application of 0.15 N HCl resulted in a minor degree of gastric mucosal damage in the 4-h pylorus-ligated rat. The number and severity of gastric mucosal lesions were 1.2 ± 0.6 and 2.0 ± 1.2, respectively ($n = 6$),

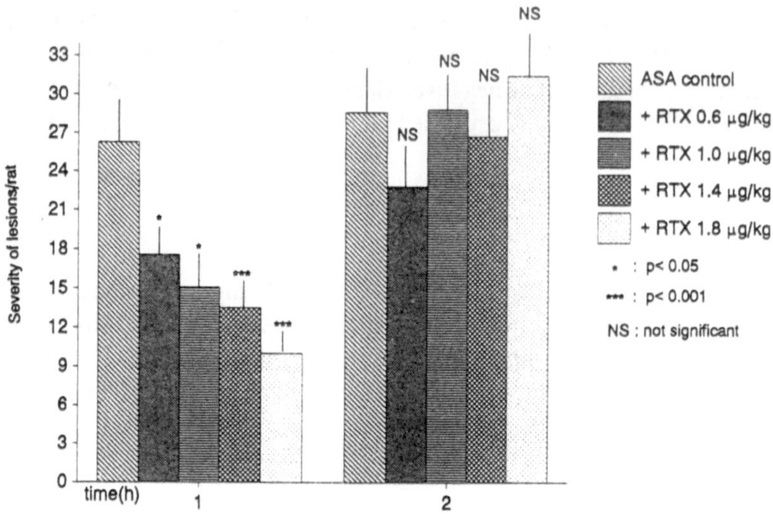

Figure 1. The effect of graded doses of resiniferatoxin (RTX) on the severity of gastric mucosal injury produced by topical acidified aspirin (ASA, 200 mg/kg in 2 ml of 0.15 N HCl) in the 1-h and 2-h pylorus-ligated rat. RTX was given ig together with aspirin immediately after pylorus ligation and animals were sacrificed 1 or 2 h later. Control rats received the vehicle. Results are mean ± SEM; $n = 6–8$ per group. Asterisks indicate significant change from control values in the corresponding time period: * = $p < 0.05$; *** = $p < 0.001$ relative to their controls. Abdel-Salam et al. [25]

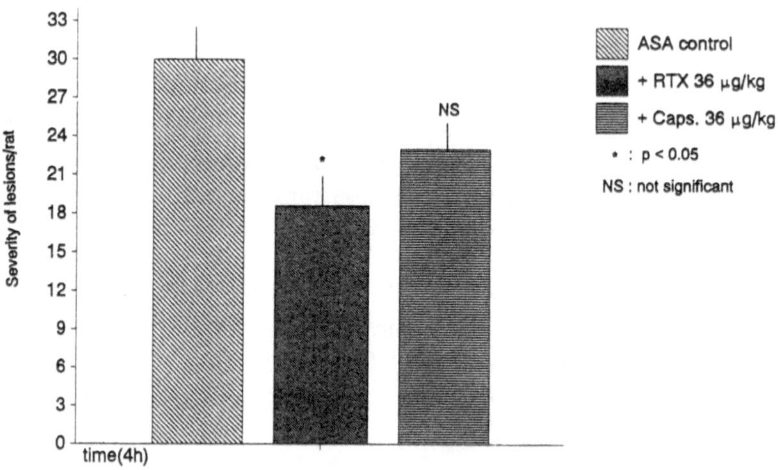

Figure 2. The effect of resiniferatoxin (RTX; 36 µg/kg) or capsaicin (36 µg/kg) on the severity of the gastric mucosal injury produced by topical acidified aspirin (200 mg.kg in 2 ml of 0.15 N HCl) in the 4-h pylorus-ligated rat. RTX or capsaicin were given ig together with aspirin immediately after ligation and animals sacrificed 4 h later. Control rats received the vehicle. Results are mean ± SEM; $n = 6$ per group; * = $p < 0.05$; NS = not significant compared with control values

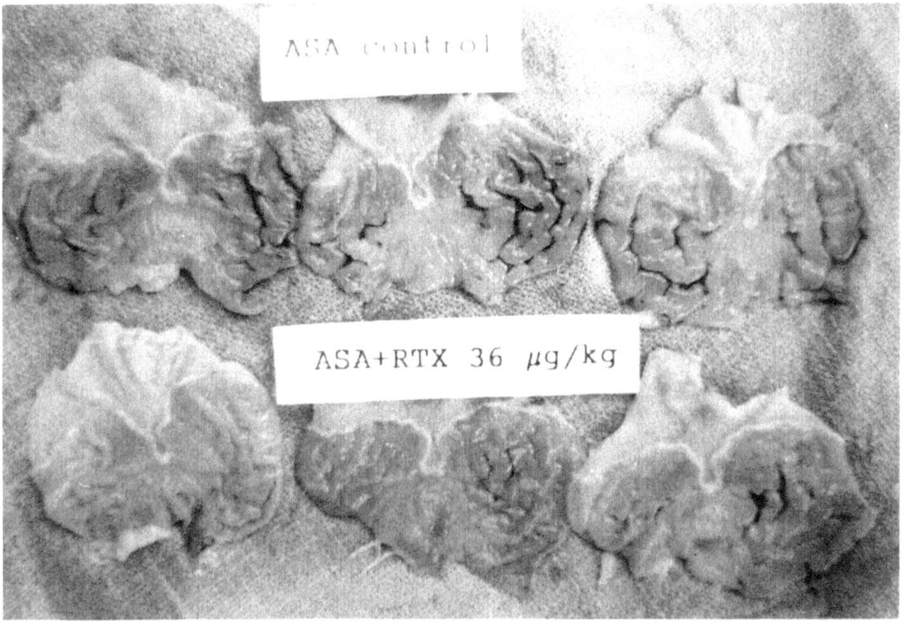

Figure 3. Gross appearance of the rat gastric mucosa 4 h after exposure to acidified aspirin (ASA) showing control rat stomachs (above) and stomachs from rats treated with resiniferatoxin (RTX) 36 μg/kg (below). Aspirin was given in a single dose of 200 mg/kg in 2 ml of 0.15 N HCl immediately after pylorus ligation with or without RTX. Control rats received the vehicle. Rats were sacrificed 4 h later

while the incidence of lesions was 50%. This was not significantly different from gastric mucosal lesions seen in rats given 0.15 N HCl only (the number and severity of mucosal lesions corresponded to 1.8 ± 0.8 and 2.3 ± 1.2, respectively, and the incidence of lesions was 50%; $n = 5$). No lesions were seen in the systemic aspirin-treated group that received RTX in 0.4 μg/kg ($n = 6$). The effect of sc aspirin plus ig acid contrasted markedly with the severe gastric mucosal damage caused by topical acidified aspirin in the 4-h pylorus-ligated rats (the number and severity of mucosal lesions corresponded to 10.8 ± 1.0 and 22.2 ± 3.0, respectively, with 100% incidence of lesions; $n = 17$). Aspirin given by both routes, however, resulted in a highly significant and nearly equal disappearance of intraluminal acid for the 4-h period (Table 1).

Indomethacin-induced gastric lesions

Resiniferatoxin at 0.4 μg/kg prevented the development of gastric mucosal lesions by sc indomethacin for a 4-h period. The number and severity of gastric mucosal lesions were reduced from control values of 3.2 ± 1.4 and 5.6 ± 0.5 ($n = 7$), respectively, to 0.2 ± 0.2 and 0.6 ± 0.5, respectively ($n = 6$). The above dose of RTX had no significant

TABLE 1
Comparison of intragastric (ig) and subcutaneous (sc) aspirin administration in the 4 h pylorus-ligated rat

Parameter	Aspirin (ig)	Aspirin (sc)	p value
Number of lesions/rat/4 h	10.8 ± 1.0	1.2 ± 0.6	<0.001
Severity of lesions/rat/4 h	22.2 ± 3.0	2.0 ± 1.2	<0.001
Gastric secretory volume (ml/rat/4 h)	6.8 ± 0.5	3.6 ± 0.2	<0.001
Gastric acid output (μEq/rat/4 h)	427.7 ± 30.0	296.7 ± 22.0	<0.01
Extent of H^+ back-diffusion (μEq/rat/4 h)	-788.0 ± 65.0	-919.6 ± 56.0	NS

Values are means ± SEM. For calculation of H^+ back-diffusion see Methods.
p value = the statistical significance of the difference between ig and sc aspirin-treated groups
NS = $p > 0.05$

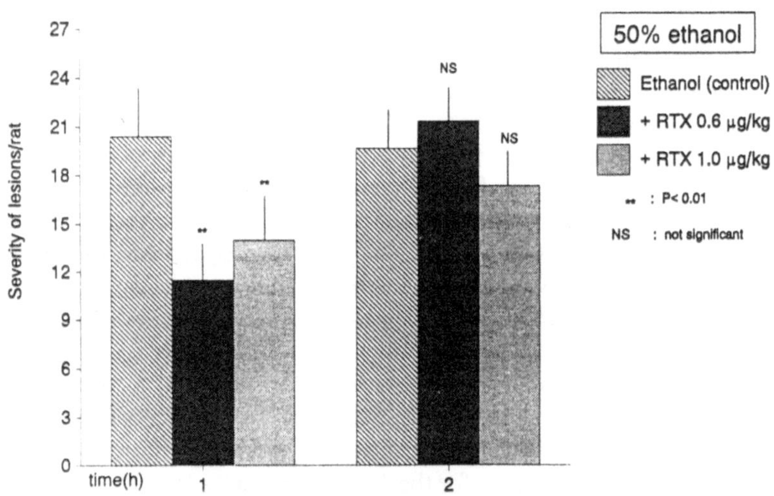

Figure 4. The effect of resiniferatoxin (RTX) on the severity of gastric mucosal lesions induced in the rat by ig ethanol (50% v/v, 2 ml). RTX (in doses of 0.6 and 1.0 μg/kg) was given ig together with ethanol immediately after pylorus ligation and animals sacrificed 1 and 2 h later. Control rats received the vehicle. Results are mean ± SEM; $n = 6$–7 per group. Asterisks indicate significant change from control values in the corresponding time period: ** = $p < 0.01$, NS = not significant relative to their controls. From Abdel-Salam et al. [25]

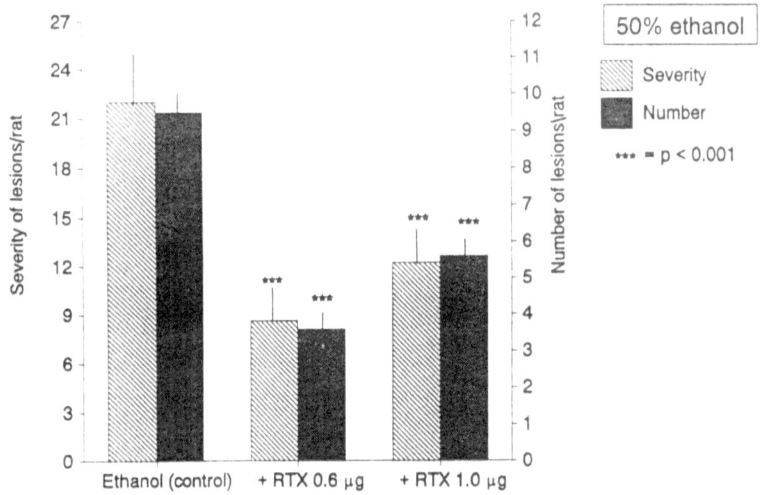

Figure 5. The effect of resiniferatoxin (RTX) on the severity and the number of gastric mucosal lesions induced in the rat by ig ethanol (50% v/v, 2 ml). RTX at doses of 0.6 and 1 µg/kg was given ig 15 min before pylorus ligation and ethanol administration and rats were sacrificed 1 h later. Control rats received the vehicle. Results are mean $\pm$ SEM; $n = 6$–7 per group. Asterisks indicate significant change from control values: *** $= p < 0.001$ compared with their control values. From Abdel-Salam et al. [25]

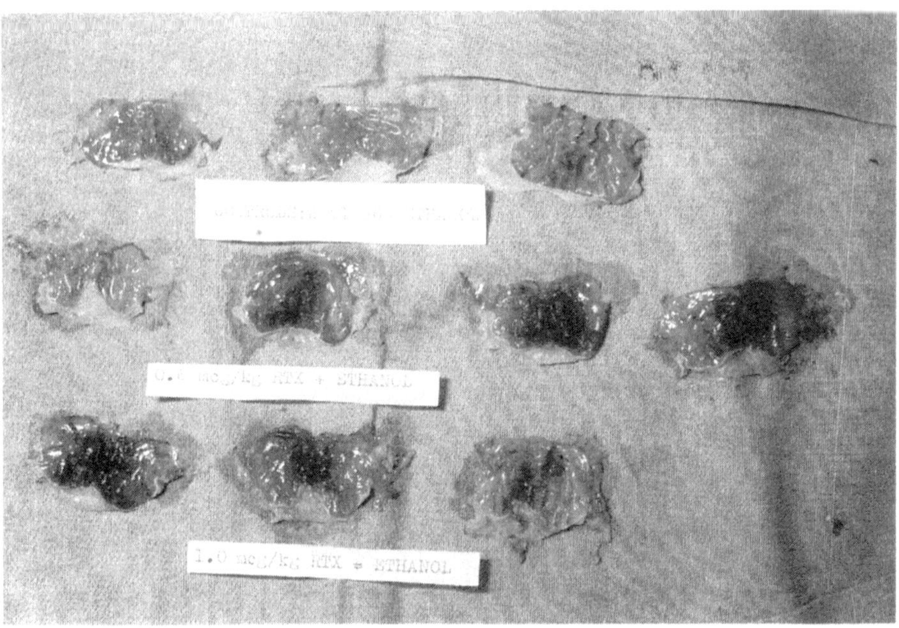

Figure 6. Gross appearance of the gastric mucosa exposed to 96% ethanol with or without the simultaneous administration of resiniferatoxin (RTX) (0.6 and 1 µg/kg). Ethanol (2 ml), with or without RTX, was given immediately after pylorus ligation and animals were sacrificed 1 h later. Control rats received the vehicle

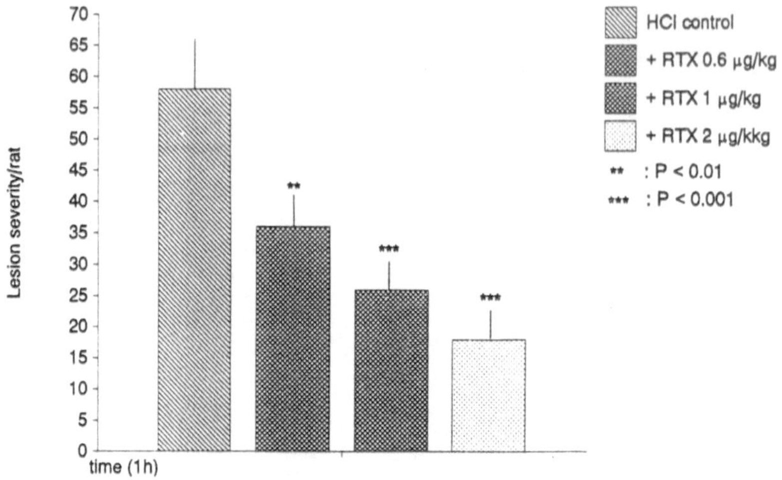

Figure 7. The protective effect of resiniferatoxin (0.6–2 µg/kg) on the severity of gastric mucosal damage produced by 0.6 N HCl in the rat. Resiniferatoxin was given ig in 0.5 ml volume 15 min prior to pylorus ligation and HCl administration. Control rats received the vehicle in an equal volume of saline. Rats were sacrificed 1 h later

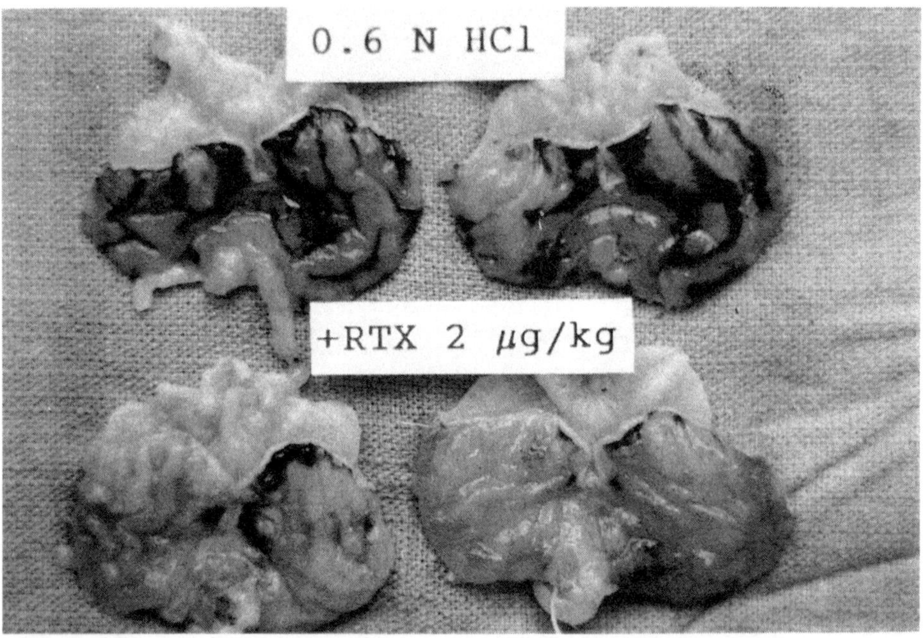

Figure 8. Gross appearance of rat gastric mucosa exposed to 0.6 N HCl for 1 h showing stomachs from control rats (above) and rats pretreated with resiniferatoxin (RTX) at 2 µg/kg (below). Resiniferatoxin was given orally 15 min prior to pylorus ligation and HCl administration. Controls received the vehicle. Rats were sacrificed 1 h after HCl

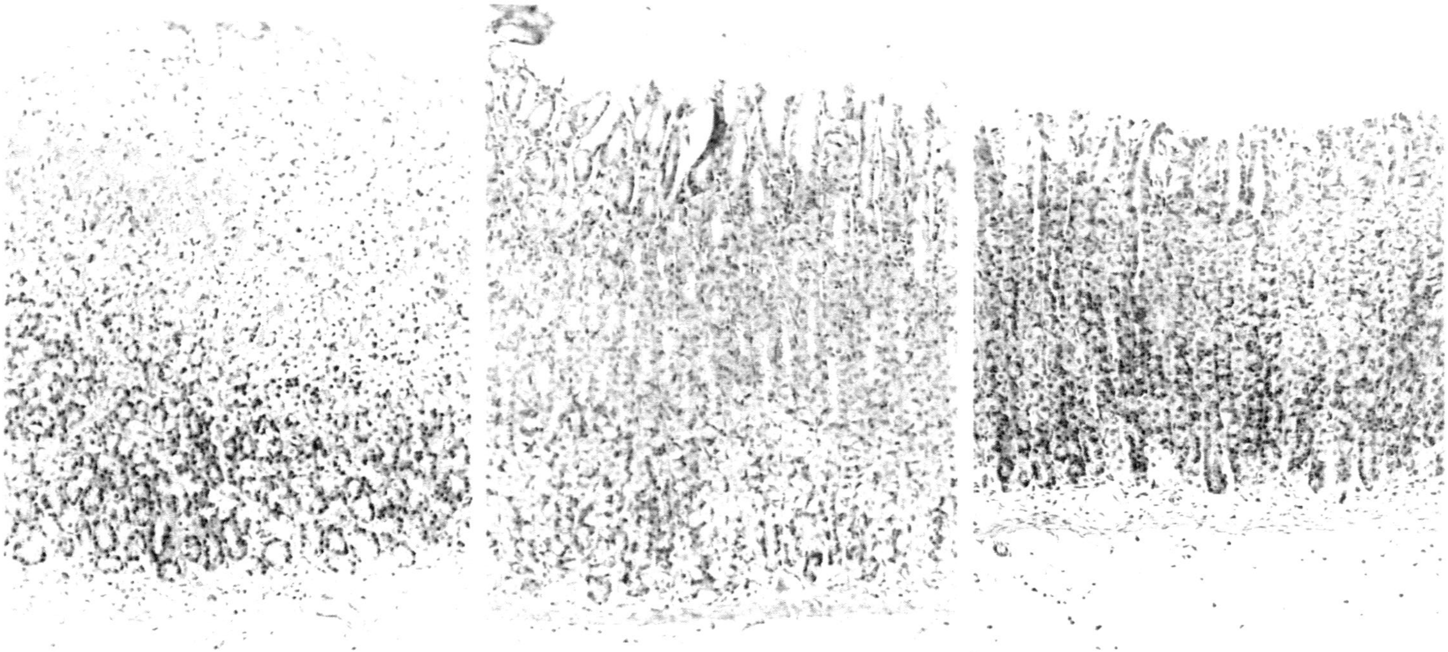

(A) (B) (C)

Figure 9. Histological sections of rat gastric mucosa 1 h after being exposed to 96% ethanol, stained with haematoxylin and eosin. Ethanol (2 ml) was given orally immediately after pylorus ligation and animals were sacrificed 1 h later. **(A)** A control rat (received saline 15 min before ligation). The section shows desquamation of the epithelium and widespread haemorrhagic necrosis (× 60). **(B)** Rat gastric mucosa pretreated with resiniferatoxin (RTX) at 1 μg/kg 15 min before pylorus ligation and administration of ethanol. Note near normal appearance of the mucosa (× 60). **(C)** Rat gastric mucosa pretreated with prostacyclin PGI_2 at 5 μg/kg 15 min prior to pylorus ligation and administration of ethanol. Some disruption to the surface epithelium is seen and the mucosa is near normal (× 80)

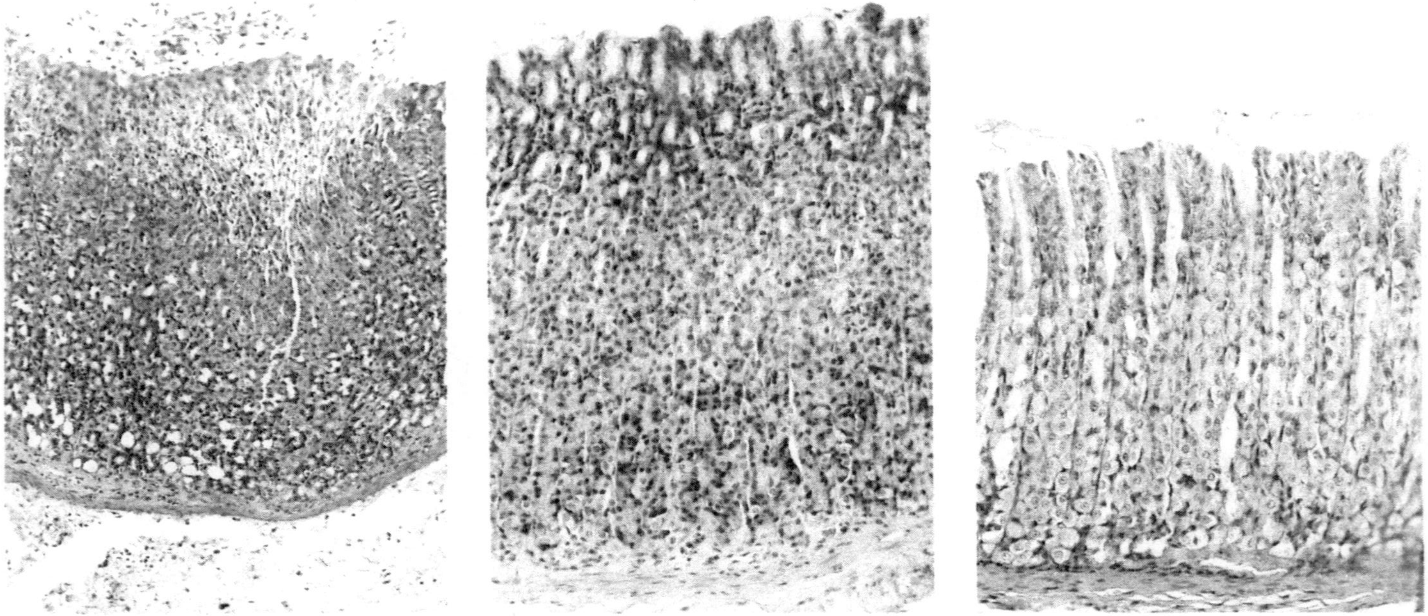

(A) (B) (C)

Figure 10. Histological sections of rat gastric mucosa 1 h after being exposed to 0.6 N HCl stained with haematoxylin and eosin. HCl (2 ml) was given orally immediately after pylorus ligation and animals were sacrificed 1 h later. (**A**) Control rat (received saline 15 min before ligation and HCl administration). Note the widespread haemorrhage and necrosis (× 50). (**B**) Rat gastric mucosa pretreated with resiniferatoxin (RTX) at 0.6 μg/kg 15 min before pylorus ligation and administration of HCl (× 50). (**C**) Rat gastric mucosa pretreated with capsaicin at 1 μg/kg 15 min prior to pylorus ligation and the administration of HCl (× 80)

effect on gastric acid output in the 2-h [24] or 4-h [25] pylorus-ligated rat given ig saline (2 ml) and did not change the gastric acid output in the 4-h pylorus-ligated plus indomethacin-treated rats in the present study.

Ethanol-induced gastric lesions

When RTX (0.6 and 1 μg/kg) was given simultaneously with 50% ethanol, the drug reduced both the number and severity of the gastric mucosal lesions compared with the control group. The lesion-preventive effect of RTX was evident for 1 h (Figure 4). The protective effect of RTX was most marked when the compound was administered 15 min prior to ethanol (Figure 5). Resiniferatoxin (0.6 and 1 μg/kg) given 15 min prior to 96% ethanol similarly reduced the ethanol-induced damage for 1 h. On the other hand, when RTX was given simultaneously with 96% ethanol, the degree of macroscopic damage was significantly greater than that in the control group in the first hour after its administration (Figure 6). Capsaicin (1 μg/kg) given simultaneously with 96% ethanol, however, did not aggravate gastric mucosal damage by ethanol. The severity and number of gastric mucosal lesions in the ethanol control group were 32.5 ± 4.2 and 16.5 ± 2.5 vs. 34.7 ± 5 and 14.5 ± 2.7 in the ethanol plus capsaicin group.

HCl-induced gastric lesions

Resiniferatoxin, at 0.6, 1 and 2 μg/kg, significantly prevented the development of HCl damage in a dose-dependent manner. Resiniferatoxin at 2 μg/kg reduced the severity of gastric mucosal damage caused by 0.6 N HCl in the 1-h pylorus-ligated rat by 68.9% (Figures 7 and 8).

The histological study

Histological sections from the gastric wall of the ethanol control rats (which received saline 15 min before being exposed to 2 ml of 96% ethanol, $n = 5$) showed diffuse or multiple desquamation of the surface epithelium and deep multifocal necrotic lesions extending into more than two thirds (3/5) or involving the entire thickness of the gastric mucosa (2/5). Haemorrhage was evident in all cases (Figure 9A). Histological sections from the gastric wall of the HCl control rats (which received saline 15 min before being exposed to 2 ml of 0.6 N HCl, $n = 4$) revealed desquamation of the surface epithelium, deep necrotic lesions of focal character involving more than two thirds of the gastric mucosa and focal interstitial haemorrhage (Figure 10A).

In both models of gastric mucosal injury, pretreatment with RTX (0.6 or 1 μg/kg), capsaicin (1 μg/kg) or PGI_2 (5 μg/kg) prevented the development of deep haemorrhagic lesions. Superficial epithelial disruption, however, was not prevented, although in some cases the gastric mucosa exhibited normal appearance (Figures 9B and 9C and 10B and 10C).

DISCUSSION

The present study provided the evidence that the capsaicin analogue RTX administered in very low concentrations to the rat stomach exerts antiulcer effects in different models of gastric mucosal injury. The protective effect of RTX was evident in both acid-dependent (e.g. HCl and acidified aspirin) and non-acid-dependent (e.g. ethanol) [23] models of gastric mucosal damage. Resiniferatoxin thus possesses the same mucosal protective properties previously described for capsaicin in the rat stomach [4,5–9]. The degree and duration of protection by RTX varied, however, depending on the model used. Resiniferatoxin at the very low concentration of 40 ng/ml (0.4 μg/kg) was able to prevent mucosal injury by sc indomethacin or aspirin for 4 h, while much higher concentrations of 3.6 μg/ml (36 μg/kg) were needed to protect against injury by acidified aspirin in the 4-h ligated rat. Further, the ethanol-induced gastric lesions differed from the HCl-induced lesions regarding the protective effect of RTX. Resiniferatoxin was a potent protective agent against HCl-induced damage, although, if given simultaneously with 96% ethanol, the result is potentiation of the ethanol-damaging effect.

In recent years, experimental evidence has emphasized the important role of microcirculatory events in the pathogenesis of gastric mucosal injury. Severe gastric mucosal damage ensues under conditions of reduced mucosal blood flow [26,27]. The microcirculation was shown to be the initial site of damage following challenge with absolute ethanol and the site where prostaglandins are likely to exert their cytoprotective effects by maintaining blood flow at appropriate levels [28–32]. Aspirin [33–35] and indomethacin [36–38] were found to reduce gastric mucosal blood flow (GMBF) under different experimental conditions and vascular endothelial injury was an early event following their application [39,40]. Non-steroidal anti-inflammatory drugs (NSAIDs) inhibit cyclo-oxygenase, the key enzyme in prostaglandin synthesis [41]. Prostaglandins, especially prostacyclin, exert potent vasodilatory effects on the gastric mucosa [42] and prostacyclin at non-antisecretory doses inhibited the development of acute gastric mucosal lesions by aspirin [41]. Administration of prostaglandins increased GMBF and protected against damage caused by indomethacin in the rat stomach [36,37].

The mechanisms underlying the gastroprotective effects of sensory nerve stimulation are thought to primarily involve an increase in GMBF through the local release of vasodilator peptides contained in sensory nerve endings [4,12,15]. In our studies with the laser Doppler flowmetry technique, RTX has also been found to produce a pronounced and dose-dependent increase in gastric blood flow in the rat (sent for publication). In addition, we have demonstrated that capsaicin or RTX inhibit gastric acid secretion in pylorus-ligated rats [43]. An inhibitory effect on gastric acid secretion might, therefore, be an important additional mechanism underlying the mucosal protective effect of sensory nerve stimulation [25]. Administration of these compounds, at very low concentrations, to the stomach thus not only enhances defence mechanisms in the stomach but reduces the aggressive side of the balance. Although, in the present study, it is difficult to correlate the protective action of RTX against topical acidified aspirin with inhibition of gastric acid secretion since acid was given exogenously (in which the aspirin was dissolved), it remains likely that the antisecretory effect of ig RTX contributes to its ulcer preventive properties. As remarked by Guth et al. [44] "it might be acid in the depth of glands which is more important in pathogenesis of gastric mucosal injury".

Concentrated ethanol rapidly penetrates the gastric mucosa and is associated with a complete blockade of blood flow in the damaged area due to submucosal venular constriction [45]. Severe segmental constriction of the large submucosal venules by 52% of its original diameter occurred 22 s after exposing the mucosa to absolute ethanol [32]. The ethanol-induced microcirculatory derangement is thus too rapid to be prevented by co-administration of protective agents. Resiniferatoxin stimulates the sensory nerve ending and evokes the release of their neuropeptide content [20]. It has been proposed that calcitonin gene-related peptide (CGRP), as a consequence of its potent vasodilator activity, can act in synergy with mediators of increased microvascular permeability or neutrophil accumulation to promote the inflammatory response [46–48]. The secondary vascular reaction and the increase in vascular permeability after 96% ethanol are thus increased by the simultaneous administration of RTX, with enhanced mucosal damage as seen in the present work.

ACKNOWLEDGEMENTS

This study was supported by grants from the Hungarian National Research Fund (OTKA No. T 020098 and T 016945) and Ministry of Health and Welfare (ETT-03 660/93 and ETT-T 563).

REFERENCES

1. Szolcśanyi J. Capsaicin, irritation, and desensitization: Neurophysiological basis and future perspectives. In: Green BG, Mason JR, Kare MR, eds. Chemical Senses. Irritation. Vol. 2. New York: Marcel Dekker; 1989:141–69.
2. Szolcśanyi J. Actions of capsaicin on sensory receptors. In: Wood JN, ed. Capsaicin in the Study of Pain. Neuroscience Perspectives. London: Academic Press; 1993:1–23.
3. Holzer P. Capsaicin, cellular targets, mechanisms of action, and selectivity for thin sensory neurons. Pharmacol Rev. 1991;43:143–201.
4. Szolcśanyi J, Barthó L. Impaired defense mechanism to peptic ulcer in the capsaicin-desensitized rat. In: Mózsik Gy, Hänninen O, Jávor T, eds. Gastrointestinal Defense Mechanisms. Oxford and Budapest: Pergamon Press and Akademiai Kiadó; 1980:39–51.
5. Holzer P, Lippe IT. Stimulation of afferent nerve endings by intragastric capsaicin protects against ethanol-induced damage of gastric mucosa. Neuroscience. 1988;27:981–7.
6. Holzer P, Sametz W. Gastric mucosal protection against ulcerogenic factors in the rat mediated by capsaicin-sensitive neurons. Gastroenterology. 1986;91:975–81.
7. Gray JL, Bunnett NW, Orloff SL, Mulvihill SJ, Debas HT. Role of calcitonin gene-related peptide in protection against gastric ulceration. Ann Surg. 1994;219:58–64.
8. Holzer P, Pabst MA, Lippe IT. Intragastric capsaicin protects against aspirin-induced lesion formation and bleeding in the rat gastric mucosa. Gastroenterology. 1989;96:1425–33.
9. Szolcśanyi J. Effect of capsaicin, resiniferatoxin and piperine on ethanol-induced gastric ulcer of the rat. Acta Physiol Hung. 1990;75(Suppl):267–8.

10. Sternini C, Reeve JR, Brecha N. Distribution and characterization of calcitonin gene-related peptide immunoreactivity in the digestive system of normal and capsaicin-treated rats. Gastroenterology. 1987;93:852–862.
11. Green T, Dockray GJ. Characterization of the peptidergic afferent innervation of the stomach in the rat, mouse and guinea pig. Neuroscience. 1988;25:181–93.
12. Holzer P, Peskar BM, Peskar BA, Amann R. Release of calcitonin gene-related peptide induced by capsaicin in the vascularly perfused rat stomach. Neurosci Lett. 1990;108:195–200.
13. Renzi D, Santicioli P, Maggi CA, Surrenti C, Pradelles P, Meli A. Capsaicin-induced release of substance P-like immunoreactivity from guinea pig stomach in vitro and in vivo. Neurosci Lett. 1988;92:254–8.
14. Lippe IT, Pabst MA, Holzer P. Intragastric capsaicin enhances rat gastric acid elimination and mucosal blood flow by afferent nerve stimulation. Br J Pharmacol. 1989;96:91–100.
15. Holzer P, Livingstone EH, Saria A, Guth PH. Sensory neurons mediate protective vasodilatation in rat gastric mucosa. Am J Physiol. 1991;260:G363–70.
16. Li DS, Raybould HE, Quintero E, Guth PH. Role of calcitonin gene-related peptide in the gastric hyperemic response to intragastric capsaicin. Am J Physiol. 1991;261:G657–61.
17. Chen RYZ, Li DS, Guth PH. Role of calcitonin gene-related peptide in capsaicin-induced gastric submucosal arteriolar dilatation. Am J Physiol. 1992;262LH1350–5.
18. Schmidt RJ, Evans FJ. A new aromatic ester diterpene from Eurphorbia poisonii. Phytochemistry. 1976;15:1778-9.
19. Szallasi A, Blumberg PM. Specific binding of resiniferatoxin, an ultrapotent capsaicin analog, by dorsal root ganglion membranes. Brain Res. 1990;524:109–11.
20. Szolcśanyi J, Szallasi A, Szallasi Z, Joo F, Blumberg PM. Resiniferatoxin: an ultrapotent selective modulator of capsaicin-sensitive primary afferent neurons. J Pharmacol Exp Ther. 1990;255:923–8.
21. Szallasi A, Blumberg PM. Mechanisms and therapeutic potential of vanilloids (capsaicin-like molecules). Adv Pharmacol. 1992;24:123–55.
22. Mózsik Gy, Móron F, Jávor T. Cellular mechanisms of the development of gastric mucosal damage and of gastric cytoprotection induced by prostacyclin in rats. A pharmacological study. Prostagl Leukotrienes Med. 1982;9:71–84.
23. Davenport HW. Ethanol damage to canine oxyntic glandular mucosa. Proc Soc Exp Biol Med. 1967;126:657–62.
24. Abdel-Salam OME, Bódis B, Karádi O, Nagy L, Szolcśanyi J, Mózsik Gy. Stimulation of capsaicin-sensitive sensory peripheral nerves with topically applied resiniferatoxin decreases salicylate-induced gastric H^+ back-diffusion in the rat. Inflammopharmacology. 1995;3:121–33.
25. Abdel-Salam OME, Bódis B, Karádi O, Szolcsányi J, Mózsik Gy. Modification of aspirin and ethanol-induced mucosal damage in rats by intragastric application of resiniferatoxin. Inflammopharmacology. 1995;3:135–47.
26. Ritchie WP Jr. Acute gastric mucosal damage induced by bile salts, acid and ischaemia. Gastroenterology. 1975;68:699–707.
27. Leung FW, Itoh M, Hirabayashi K, Guth PH. Role of blood flow in gastric and duodenal injury in the rat. Gastroenterology. 1985;88:281–9.
28. Guth PH, Paulsen G, Nagata H. Histologic and microcirculatory changes in alcohol-induced gastric lesions in the rat: effect of prostaglandin cytoprotection. Gastroenterology. 1984;87:1083–90.
29. Ohya Y, Guth PH. Ethanol-induced gastric mucosal blood flow and vascular permeability changes in the rat. Dig Dis Sci. 1988;33:883–8.
30. Trier JS, Szabó S, Allan CH. Ethanol-induced damage to mucosal capillaries of rat stomach. Ultrastructural features and effect of prostaglandin $F_{2\beta}$ and cysteamine. Gastroenterology. 1987;92:13–22.
31. Oates PJ, Hakkinen JP. Studies on the mechanism of ethanol-induced gastric damage in rats. Gastroenterology. 1988;94:10–21.
32. Bou-Abboud CF, Wayland H, Paulsen G, Guth PH. Microcirculatory stasis precedes tissue necrosis in ethanol-induced gastric mucosal injury in the rat. Dig Dis Sci. 1988;33:872–7.
33. Kauffman GL, Aures Jr D, Grossman MI. Intravenous indomethacin and aspirin reduce basal gastric mucosal blood flow in dogs. Am J Physiol. 1980;238:G131–4.
34. Ashley SW, Sonnenschein LA, Leung LY. Focal gastric mucosal blood flow at the site of aspirin-induced ulceration. Am J Surg. 1985;149:53–9.
35. Kitahora T, Guth PH. Effect of aspirin plus hydrochloric acid on the gastric mucosal microcirculation. Gastroenterology. 1987;93:810–17.
36. Whittle BJR. Mechanisms underlying gastric mucosal damage induced by indomethacin and bile salts, and the actions of prostaglandins. Br J Pharmacol. 1977;60:455–60.

37. Hirose H, Takeuchi K, Okabe S. Effect of indomethacin on gastric mucosal blood flow around acetic acid-induced gastric ulcers in rats. Gastroenterology. 1991;100:1259–65.
38. Shorrock CJ, Rees WSW. Mucosal adaptation to indomethacin induced gastric damage in man – studies on morphology, blood flow, and prostaglandin metabolism. Gut. 1992;33:164–9.
39. Tarnawski A, Stachura J, Gergely H, Hollander D. Gastric mucosal epithelium: a major target for aspirin-induced injury and arachidonic acid protection, and ultrastructural analysis in the rat. Eur J Chem Invest. 1990;20:432–40.
40. Wallace IL, Keenan CM, Granger DN. Gastric ulceration induced by nonsteroid anti-inflammatory drugs is a neutrophil dependent mechanism. Am J Physiol. 1990;259:G462–7.
41. Whittle BJR, Higgs GA, Eakins KE, Moncada S, Vane JR. Selective inhibition of prostaglandin production in inflammatory exudates and gastric mucosa. Nature. 1980;284:271–3.
42. Main IHM, Whittle BJR. Investigation of the vasodilator and antisecretory role of prostaglandins in the rat gastric mucosa by use of non-steroidal anti-inflammatory drugs. Br J Pharmacol. 1977;60:455–60.
43. Abdel-Salam OME, Szolcśanyi J, Mózsik Gy. Effect of resiniferatoxin on stimulated gastric acid secretory responses in the rat. J Physiology (Paris). 1995;88:353–8.
44. Guth PH, Aures D, Paulsen G. Topical aspirin plus HCl gastric lesions in the rat. Gastroenterology. 1977;76:88–93.
45. Szabó S, Goldberg I. Experimental pathogenesis: drugs and chemical lesions in the gastric mucosa. Scand J Gastroenterol. 1990;25(Suppl 174):1–8.
46. Brain SD, Williams TJ. Inflammatory oedema induced by synergism between calcitonin gene-related peptide (CGRP) and mediators of increased microvascular permeability. Br J Pharmacol. 1985;86:855–900.
47. Buckley TL, Brain SD, Rampart M, Williams TJ. Time-dependent synergistic interactions between the vasodilator neuropeptide, calcitonin gene-related peptide (CGRP) and mediators of inflammation. Br J Pharmacol. 1991;103:1515–19.
48. Newbold P, Brain SD. The modulation of inflammatory oedema by calcitonin gene-related peptide. Br J Pharmacol. 1993;108:705–10.

Manuscript received 6 Nov. 95.
Accepted for publication 19 Nov. 95.

TS Gaginella et al. (eds.), Biochemical Pharmacology as an Approach to Gastrointestinal Disorders, 287–295

AIDS TREATMENT AND THE HEAT SHOCK PROTEIN LEVEL IN THE GASTROINTESTINAL TRACT

P. CSERE[1], G. VARBIRO[1], B. SUMEGI[2] AND Gy. MÓZSIK[1*]
[1]First Department of Medicine and [2]Department of Biochemistry, Medical University of Pécs, Pécs, Hungary
*Correspondence

This paper was first published in: Inflammopharmacology. 1997;5:83–91.

ABSTRACT

AIDS has several manifestations in the gastrointestinal tract – 2′,3′-dideoxycytidine (ddC) as an anti-AIDS drug will also produce some effects on the alimentary tract: it causes inflammation. The analysis of the expression of the heat shock proteins (hsp60 and hsp70) is a new marker of the inflammation caused by external stress. The hsp60 is located mainly in the mitochondria; hsp70 is found in both cytoplasm and the mitochondria. The aim of the present study was to reveal whether ddC can produce any expressive biochemical changes in the oral cavity or generally in the gastrointestinal tract.

Methods

The rats were treated with intraperitoneal administration of 1 mg ddC/day for two weeks. The animals were killed by cervical dislocation, then the buccal, lingual, oesophageal, gastric, duodenal and colon mucosae were removed, and frozen in liquid nitrogen. Protein extract was obtained and separated by SDS–PAGE, followed by the Western blotting of the proteins to the nitrocellulose membrane. After binding the first antibody (mouse-derived anti-heat shock protein), a second antibody was administered (anti-mouse IgG, labelled with peroxidase). The antigen–antibody reaction was detected by 3,3′-diaminobenzidine tetrahydrochloride dihydrate.

Results

1. In the control and in the treated groups, the hsp60 monoclonal antibody binding was visible in the oesophageal, gastric, duodenal and colon mucosae, but, in the buccal and lingual mucosae, it was not detectable in the treated group.
2. The hsp70 was detectable in every tissue of both treated and non-treated groups. To verify whether the cause was indirect oxidative damage, the NADH-dihydrogenase (complex I), cytochrome-oxidoreductase (complex III) and cytochrome-oxidase (complex IV), members of the respiratory chain, were examined but no alterations were found. Our results indicate that the disappearance of hsp60 in the oral cavity is a unique phenomenon following ddC treatment. This damage might be caused by the ddC interaction with hsp60; however, the exact mechanism is not yet known.

Keywords: AIDS, dideoxycytidine, inflammation, heat shock protein

---

This paper was presented at the Section of IUPHAR GI Pharmacology Symposium on 'Biochemical pharmacology as an approach to gastrointestinal disorders (basic science to clinical perspectives)', October 12–14, 1995, Pécs, Hungary.

INTRODUCTION

AIDS is a widely examined disease: much is known about the replication of the virus from the cell attachment to the final step, to the release of the infectious virions. However, it is not clear whether the anti-AIDS therapy can alone produce deleterious side-effects. The first agent developed for the treatment of AIDS was 3′-azido-3′-deoxythimidine (AZT) which causes myopathy and cardiomyopathy, showing maternal inheritance (personal communication from Sumegi et al.). This effect is due to the inhibition of mitochondrial DNA replication and mutation in mitochondrial DNA [1–4]. Like other nucleotide inhibitors, ddC requires intracellular activation to an active triphosphate for activity, basing its effect on blocking viral reverse transcriptase enzyme [5]. The inhibition of cellular DNA polymerase, particularly in the mitochondria, is another site of action of nucleotide analogues; this is an important site due to the lack of a mitochondrial DNA-repair mechanism. Thus, this could lead to mitochondrial DNA damage, leading to inappropriate respiratory complexes and deterioration of terminal oxidation [1,2]. Furthermore, ddC treatment is associated with peripheral neuropathy, rash, pancreatitis and inflammation, e.g. stomatitis in the early stages of AIDS therapy [5]. These inflammatory effects could lead to cellular stress, altering the levels of stress-responsive heat shock proteins (hsp) [6–10]. The rapid synthesis of a number of such proteins is a nearly universal cellular response to a variety of exogenous, environmental stresses (heat, ethanol, amino acids, steroid hormones, toxic chemicals, oxidative stress due to anoxia) [11]. A wide variety of ‘stress’ occurs in the life of the cell. Induction of extremely high levels of hsps has been observed for a number of diseases, infections, fever, inflammation, trauma and cancer [8,10,12,13]. The hsps protect the cell from developmental defects and lethality [12,13]. It is commonly accepted that the function of the hsps is to protect the organism from subsequent heat stress or to enhance the ability of organism to recover from the toxic effects of heat or other stress [10,13,14]. The induction of hsp is involved in preventing the denaturation of proteins; they assist in the refolding of damaged proteins or facilitate proteolytic degradation of protein too damaged to refold. The hsps have also been identified as molecular chaperons, involved directly in the process of protein biogenesis. The hsps are grouped on the basis of their molecular weight and amino acid sequence homologies into families (hsp20, hsp60, hsp70, hsp90, hsp100). The hsps are abundant proteins in the cell, i.e. they do not exist only in an inducible form. Mostly, hsp60 are present under non-stress conditions; however, hsp70 proteins have stress-inducible and constitutive forms. The hsp70 are involved in protein synthesis, folding, assembly and degradation. They stabilize unfolded precursor proteins, and they enter pathways for protein translocation into subcellular organelles. The hsp60 play a centrol role in folding of protein assembly mechanisms [12–17].

Therefore, our aim was to reveal whether:

1. ddC expresses biochemical effects in the tissues of the oral cavity due to the inflammatory side-effects – stomatitis,, or

2. ddC causes cellular stress and thus alters hsp levels generally in the whole gastro-intestinal tract

3. A further aim of recent observations was to reveal whether the above effect is due to indirect oxidative damage.

The analysis of the expression of the hsp, mainly hsp60 and hsp70, might be a new marker of inflammatory conditions, obtaining information about the inflammation–protective cascade mechanism within the cell at the same time. It would give more information about the protective cascade than the analysis of the levels of prostaglandins (PGs) because these PGs themselves induce the synthesis of hsp70 [18].

To protect the cell from suspected secondary oxidative damage induced by ddC, one can treat the animal with various types of antioxidant agents – vitamin C, vitamin E, dihydrolipoamide. The first has a strong acid character; vitamin E shows differences in in-vitro and in-vivo administration. Lipoamide is converted to dihydrolipoamide by cellular enzyme lipoamide dehydrogenase, and the dihydrolipoamide is a very effective antioxidant agent, penetrates through membrane unhindered, and does not have an acid character [19].

MATERIALS AND METHODS

Young Wistar rats weighing 80–100 g were treated with intraperitoneal administration of 1–2 mg kg^{-1} day^{-1} ddC for two weeks; a group of animals also received dihydrolipoamide (150 mg kg^{-1} day^{-1}). Rats were sacrificed by cervical dislocation then the buccal, lingual, oesophageal, gastric, duodenal and colon tissues were removed; the mucosal layer was dissected off the muscularis propria layer and frozen in liquid nitrogen. Cell extracts were made in Laemmli buffer containing β-mercaptoethanol from about 50 mg of each tissue. Aliquots (20 μl) of these extracts were subjected to electrophoresis in 12% sodium-dodecyl-sulphate polyacrylamide gel, using 120 V DC. The protein extracts were transferred onto a nitrocellulose sheet using 30 V DC for 2 h. The non-specific binding sites of the blot were blocked with 2% (w/v) powdered low-fat milk in Tris-buffered saline (TBS, 20 mmol/L Tris-HCl and 150 mmol/L NaCl, pH 7.5) for 3 h at room temperature. Primary mouse-derived monoclonal antibodies against hsp60 were used at 1:400 and hsp70 at 1:1000 dilution (supplied by Sigma-Aldrich) [20,21] rabbit-derived polyclonal anti-complex-I in 1:500, anti-complex-IV (own product) at 1:500 dilution for overnight at 4°C and subsequently treated with second antibodies peroxidase conjugated with anti-rabbit IgG at 1:1000 dilution for 3 h at 4°C. Binding of the conjugates was visualized by using 3,3′-diaminobenzidine tetrahydrochloride dihydrate (supplied by Fluka) in Tris-buffered saline (50 mmol/L Tris, pH=7.5) and hydrogen peroxide 0.7% containing $NiSO_4$. Complex-I and complex-IV were detected using alkaline-phosphate conjugated goat anti-rabbit IgG (supplied by Sigma–Aldrich)) at 1:1000 dilution, developed in alkaline buffer (100 mmol/L Tris–HCl, 100 mmol/L $MgCl_2$, pH=9.5) containing the substrates, nitroblue tetrazolium and 5-bromo-4-chloro-3-indolylphosphate (supplied by

Sigma–Aldrich). The reactions were quenched by washing with distilled water.

The complex-I-III and complex-IV enzyme activity was measured using 50 mg of each tissue which was homogenized in 0.5 ml Na-phosphate buffer (50 mmol/L, pH=7.4). The complex-IV enzyme activity was measured at 555 nm, using the samples at 1:50 dilution with Na-phosphate buffer with 0.04% (v/v) cytochrome c; in the case of complex-I-III, at 1:50 dilution in Na-phosphate buffer containing 1 mmol/L sodium azide and 0.1% (w/v) NADH. The data, obtained by photometric measurements, were statistically analysed.

At the time of sacrificing the animals, we examined the buccal, lingual, oesophageal, gastric, duodenal and colon tissues for macroscopic and microscopic traces of inflammation.

RESULTS

No macroscopic or histological signs of inflammation were detected at the time of sacrificing the animals; however, we examined whether ddC can cause alterations at the molecular level.

We examined the expression of hsp60 and hsp70 in the buccal mucosa at first. We found a considerable quantity of hsp60 in buccal mucosa derived from liver and male and female controls, but we were not able to detect it in the buccal mucosa of ddC-treated male or female rats or in ddC plus dihydrolipoamide-treated male or female rats (Figure 1A).

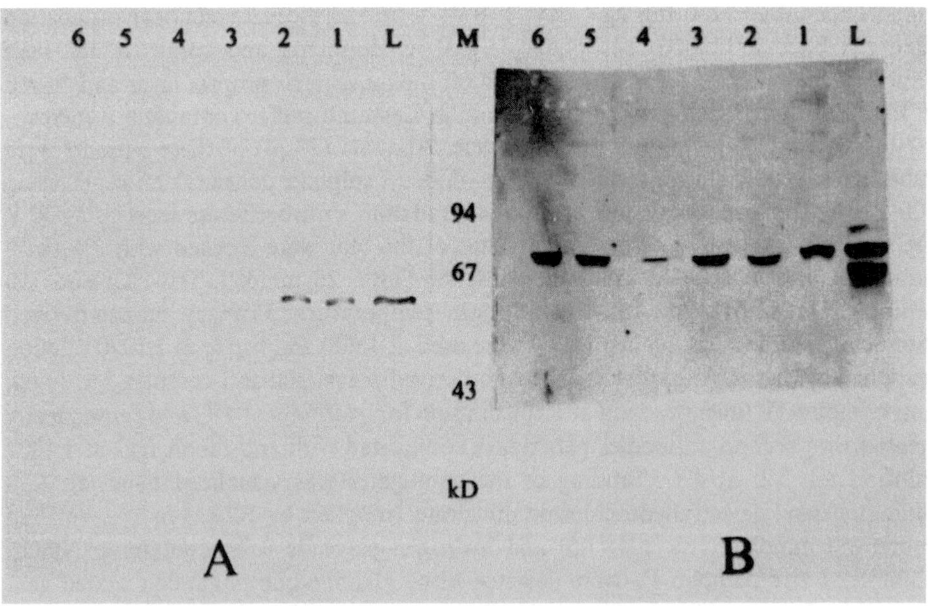

Figure 1. **A.** Immunoblot of the level of hsp60 in the buccal musoca. **B.** Immunoblot of the level of hsp70 in the buccal mucosa. L: liver control; 1: male control; 2: female control; 3: ddC-treated male; 4: ddC-treated female; 5: ddC plus dihydrolipoamide-treated male; 6: ddC plus dihydrolipoamide-treated female

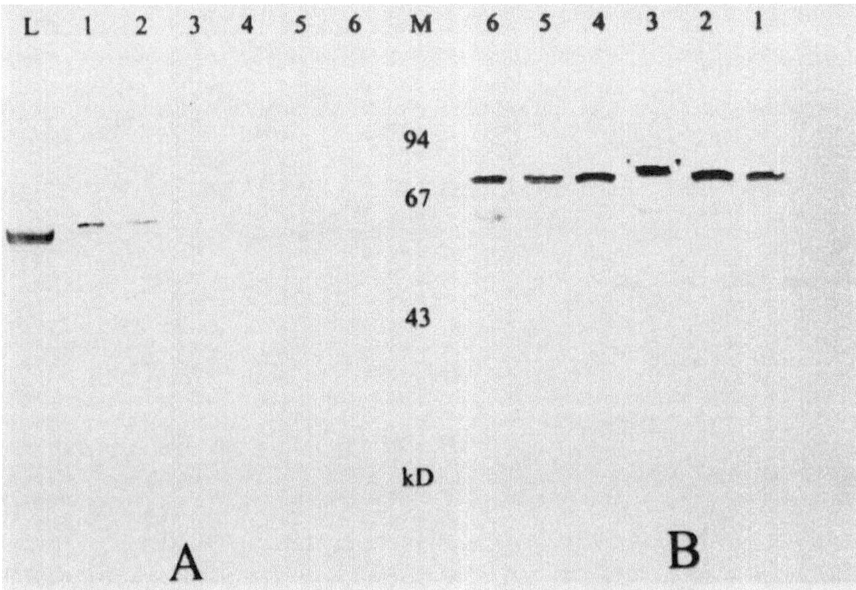

Figure 2. **A**. Immunoblot of the level of hsp60 in the lingual mucosa. **B**. Immunoblot of the level of hsp70 in the lingual mucosa. L: liver control; 1: male control; 2: female control; 3: ddC-treated male; 4: ddC-treated female; 5: ddC plus dihydrolipoamide-treated male; 6: ddC plus dihydrolipoamide-treated female

The hsp70 level was the same in the buccal mucosa of the untreated, the ddC-treated and the ddC plus dihydrolipoamide-treated animals (Figure 1B). We could not see any alterations in the expression of hsp70 with this technique.

We found no differences in the enzyme activity of the respiratory chain, and no alterations were detected on the blots of complex-I or complex-IV (results not shown).

We also found similar results in lingual mucosa. The hsp60 level was detectable in the liver and male and female controls, but hsp60 could not be detected in the ddC-treated male or female or in the ddC plus dihydrolipoamide-treated male or female rats (Figure 2A).

However, there were no differences in the level of hsp70 between the controls and treated groups (Figure 2B) and no differences between the blots of complex-I and complex-IV. There were no differences in respiratory enzyme activity between the control and treated groups.

The results from other parts of the gastrointestinal tract were surprising. There were no differences in the hsps examined or enzyme activity in the mucosa of treated and untreated animals. In the oesophageal mucosa, we did not detect any alterations in the levels of hsp60, hsp70, complex-I or complex-IV, and the same enzyme activity was measured in the different groups (Figure 3). Similar results were obtained from the gastric mucosa – no changes in the expression of hsp60 or hsp70 (Figure 4). The

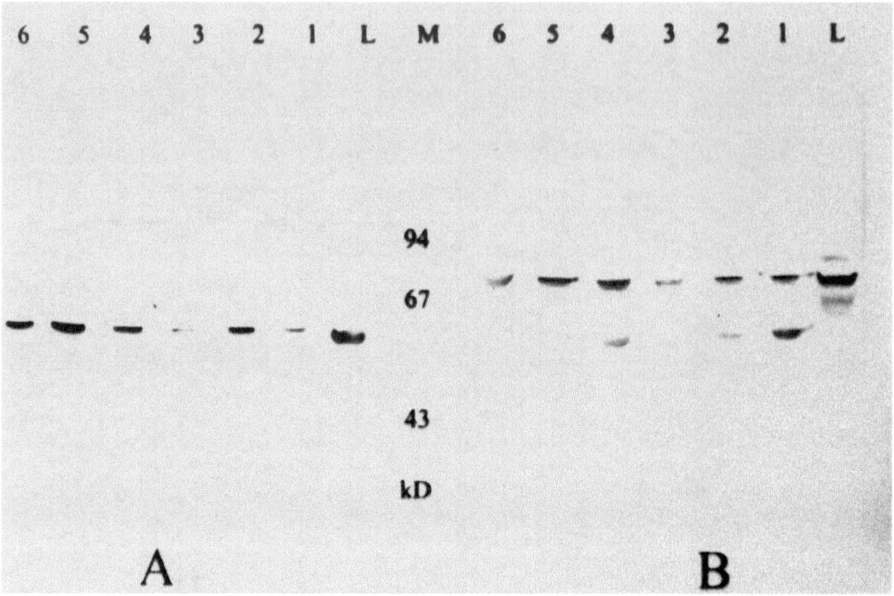

Figure 3. A. Immunoblot of the level of hsp60 in the oesophageal mucosa. B. Immunoblot of the level of hsp70 in the oesophageal mucosa. L: liver control; 1: male control; 2: female control; 3: ddC-treated male; 4: ddC-treated female; 5: ddC plus dihydrolipoamide-treated male; 6: ddC plus dihydrolipoamide-treated female

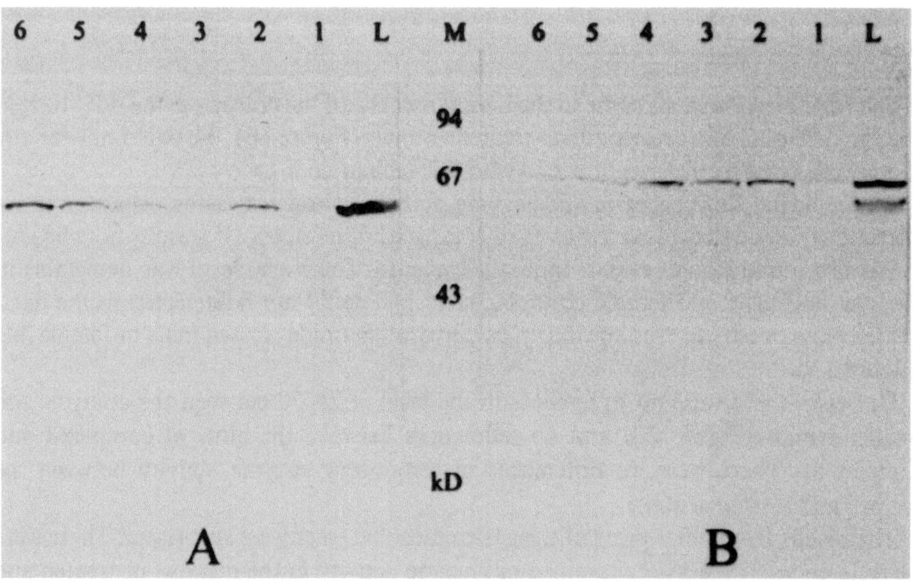

Figure 4. A. Immunoblot of the level of hsp60 in the gastric mucosa. B. Immunoblot of the level of hsp70 in the gastric mucosa. L: liver control; 1: male control; 2: female control; 3: ddC-treated male; 4: ddC-treated female; 5: ddC plus dihydrolipoamide-treated male; 6: ddC plus dihydrolipoamide-treated female

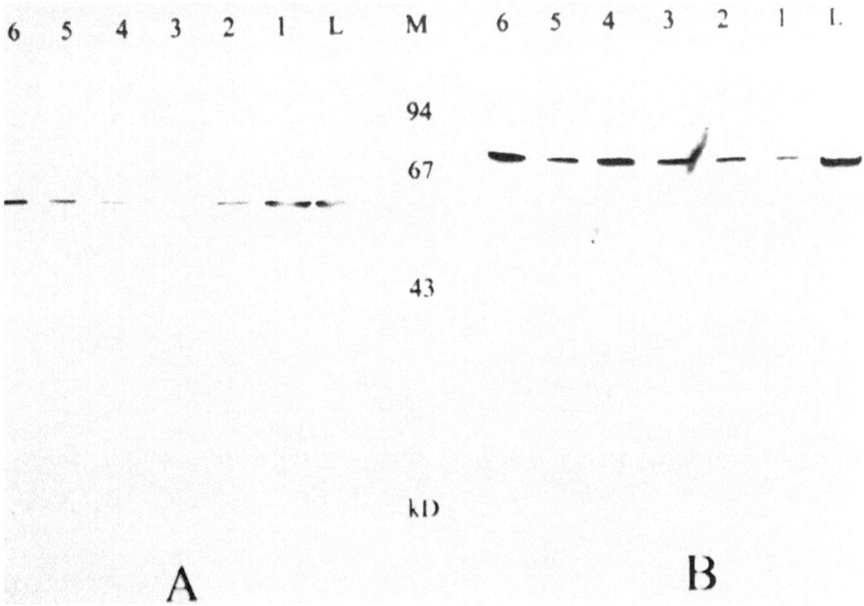

Figure 5. **A**. Immunoblot of the level of hsp60 in the duodenal mucosa. **B**. Immunoblot of the level of hsp70 in the duodenal mucosa. L: liver control; 1: male control; 2: female control; 3: ddC-treated male; 4: ddC-treated female; 5: ddC plus dihydrolipoamide-treated male; 6: ddC plus dihydrolipoamide-treated female

duodenal and colonic mucosa also gave these results – no differences in hsp60 or hsp70 between untreated controls (liver, male, female) and ddC-treated males and females or ddC plus dihydrolipoamide-treated males and females (Figures 5 and 6).

DISCUSSION

Our results show that ddC treatment has no effect on the hsp levels in the oesophageal, gastric, duodenal and colonic mucosa, but the results obtained from the tissues of the oral cavity are the opposite of those expected. The hsp60 level decreases considerably in rat buccal and lingual mucosa following ddC treatment. This decrease of hsp60 in the buccal and in the lingual mucosa is, to our knowledge, a unique phenomenon. The proper mechanism is not known but it is not due to a secondary oxidative effect of ddC because the antioxidant agent, dihydrolipoamide, does not have a protective effect on the decrease in hsp60 level. If there had been an oxidative effect, the enzyme activity of the respiratory chain would have been altered. However, these results were the same from both treated and untreated groups.

In our view, the deterioration might be caused by an interaction between the ddC and the hsp60, resulting from the peculiar environment of the oral cavity; the O_2

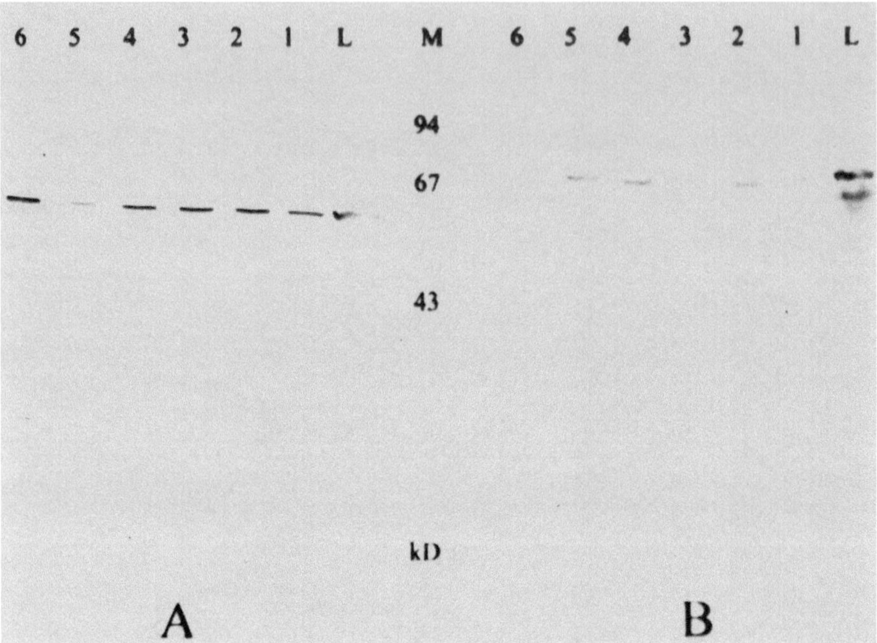

Figure 6. A. Immunoblot of the level of hsp60 in the colon mucosa. B. Immunoblot of the level of hsp70 in the colon mucosa. L: liver control; 1: male control; 2: female control; 3: ddC-treated male; 4: ddC-treated female; 5: ddC plus dihydrolipoamide-treated male; 6: ddC plus dihydrolipoamide-treated female

tension is higher in the cells here. The suppression of hsp60 gene expression could also cause these results.

Higher hsp levels were expected after ddC treatment to protect the cell from the cellular stress. However, such results were not found [8,10,11]. Perhaps the inflammatory effects of ddC contribute to the decrease in hsp60 level, missing a protective mechanism.

Analysis of the hsp level highlights deeper molecular interaction not yet completely known. Whether the decrease in hsp60 is permanent or whether it returns to the normal level is yet to be examined. Maybe when the proper mechanism is known this phenomenon will be understood and treatment or prevention of the inflammatory effects of different agents will be possible.

ACKNOWLEDGEMENTS

This study was supported by a Hungarian National Research Fund (OTKA No. TO20098) and the Ministry of Health and Welfare (ETT-03660/93).

REFERENCES

1. De Vivo DC. The expanding clinical spectrum of mitochondrial diseases. Brain Devel. 1993;15:1.
2. Zeviani M, Gellera C, Antozzi C et al. Maternally inherited myopathy and cardiomyopathy: association with mutation in mitochondrial DNA tRNA. Lancet. 1991;338:143–7.
3. Helbert M, Fletcher T, Peddle B, Harris JR, Pinching AJ. Zidovudine-associated myopathy. Lancet. 1988;2(8612):689–90.
4. Herskowitz A, Willoughby SB, Baughman KL, Schulman SP, Bartlett JD. Cardiomyopathy associated with antiretroviral therapy in patients with HIV infection: A report of six cases. Ann Intern Med. 1992;116:311–13.
5. Hirsch MS, D'Aquila RT. Therapy for human immunodeficiency virus infection. N Engl J Med. 1993;328:1686–95.
6. Carper SW, Duffy JJ, Gerner EW. Heat shock proteins in thermotolerance and other cellular processes. Cancer Res. 1987;47:5249–55.
7. Bhattacharyya T, Karnezis A, Murphy SP et al. Cloning and subcellular localisation of human mitochondrial hsp70. J Biol Chem. 1995;270:1705–10.
8. Knowlton AA. Heat shock proteins, stress, and the heart. Ann NY Acad Sci. 1994;723:128–37.
9. Pelham H. Activation of heat-shock genes in eukaryotes. Trends Genet. 1985;1:31–5.
10. Jacquier-Sarlin MR, Fuller K, Dinh-Xuan AT, Richard M-J, Polla BS. Protective effect of hsp70 in inflammation. Experientia. 1994;50:1031–8.
11. Hall TJ. Role of hsp70 in cytokine production. Experientia. 1994;50:1048–53.
12. Feige U, Polla BS. Heat shock proteins: the hsp70 family. Experientia. 1994;50:979–86.
13. Wynn RM, Davie JR, Cox RP, Chuang DT. Molecular chaperons: Heat shock proteins, foldases and matchmakers. J Lab Clin Med. 1994;124:31–6.
14. Burel C, Mezger V, Pinto M, Rallu M, Trigon S, Morange N. Mammalian heat shock protein families. Expression and function. Experientia. 1992;48:629–33.
15. Becker J, Craig EA. Heat shock proteins as molecular chaperones. Eur J Biochem. 1994;219:11–23.
16. Craig EA, Gambill BD, Nelson RJ. Heat shock proteins: Molecular chaperons of protein biogenesis. Microbiol Rev. 1993;57:402–14.
17. Stuart RA, Cyr DM, Neupert W. Hsp70 in mitochondrial biogenesis: From chaperoning nascent polypeptide chains to facilitation of protein degradation. Experientia. 1994;50:1002–11
18. Santoro GM. Heat shock proteins and virus replication: hsp70s as mediators of the antiviral effects of prostaglandins. Experientia. 1994;50:1039–47.
19. Sumegi B, Butwell NB, Malloy CR, Sherry AD. Lipoamide influences substrate selection in post-ischaemic perfused rat hearts. Biochem J. 1992;297:109–13.
20. Boog CJP, de Graeff-Meeder ER, Voorhorst-Ogink M, van Kooten PJS, Geuze HJ, van Eden W. Two monoclonal antibodies generated against human hsp60 show reactivity with synovial membranes of patients with juvenile chronic arthritis. J Exp Med. 1992;175:1805–10.
21. Velez-Granell CS, Arias AE, Torres-Ruiz JA, Bendayan M. Molecular chaperons in pancreatic tissue: the presence of cpn10, cpn60 and hsp70 in distinct compartments along the secretory pathway of the acinar cells. J Cell Sci. 1994;107;539–49.

Manuscript received 31 Oct. 95.
Accepted for publication 18 Dec. 95.

Anti-AIDS Consultation on the use of the [illegible]

REFERENCES

1. De Vivo DC. The expanding clinical spectrum of mitochondrial diseases. Brain Dev 1993;15: [illegible]
2. Zeviani M, Gellera C, [illegible] Maternally inherited myopathy and cardiomyopathy: association with mutation in mitochondrial DNA tRNA Leu(UUR). Lancet 1991;338:143.
3. [illegible]

TS Gaginella et al. (eds.), Biochemical Pharmacology as an Approach to Gastrointestinal Disorders, 297–301

ELISA AND WESTERN BLOT STUDIES WITH BASIC FIBROBLAST GROWTH FACTOR (bFGF) AND PLATELET-DERIVED GROWTH FACTOR (PDGF) IN EXPERIMENTAL DUODENAL ULCERATION AND HEALING

Á. VINCZE[1], M. NAGATA[1], Zs. SANDOR[1] AND S. SZABÓ[2]*
[1]Department of Pathology, Brigham & Women's Hospital, Harvard Medical School, Boston, MA; [2]Pathology and Laboratory Medicine Service, VA Medical Center, 5901 East 7th St., Long Beach, CA 90822, USA
*Correspondence

This paper was first published in: Inflammopharmacology. 1996;4:261–265.

ABSTRACT

Time-dependent changes of duodenal and gastric mucosal levels of bFGF and PDGF were examined in rats after oral administration of the duodenal ulcerogen cysteamine-HCl. The animals were killed at 12 h, 24 h, 48 h, 7 days or 14 days after the first dose of cysteamine and the duodenal ulcers were evaluated. The gastric and duodenal mucosa was scraped and homogenized for Western blot and ELISA studies. The ulcer formation was macroscopically detectable at 12 h while the largest ulcers were seen at 48 h. In parallel, the duodenal mucosal concentration of bFGF increased at 12 and 24 h and reached its maximum at 48 h, while the PDGF concentration was slightly elevated at 12 and 48 h, and a more than 3-fold peak was seen at 24 h. The gastric mucosal level of bFGF and PDGF did not change during the development and healing of duodenal ulcers.

Conclusions
1. The early (24–48 h) elevation of duodenal mucosal bFGF and PDGF might be a tissue-specific response to duodenal ulceration.
2. These high endogenous levels of growth factors are not sufficient to prevent the ulcer formation and are not maintained in the spontaneous healing phase (7–14 days)
3. Thus, bFGF and PDGF may have a role in the natural history of duodenal ulcer disease.

Keywords: basic fibroblast growth factor, platelet-derived growth factor, cysteamine, duodenal ulcer, ulcer development and healing

INTRODUCTION

Growth factors stimulate virtually all the cellular responses of ulcer healing such as angiogenesis, granulation tissue production and re-epithelialization, but their specificity and potency vary. Epidermal growth factor (EGF) which inhibits acid secretion was first found to exert antiulcer activity [1,2]. Subsequently, basic fibroblast growth factor (bFGF) was also found to have anti-ulcerogenic effect in rats [3,4] as well as in

---

This paper was presented at the Section of IUPHAR GI Pharmacology Symposium on 'Biochemical pharmacology as an approach to gastrointestinal disorders (basic science to clinical perspectives)', October 12–14, 1995, Pécs, Hungary.

humans [5]. More recently, platelet-derived growth factor (PDGF) was also shown to exert a strong healing effect, both in experimental chronic duodenal ulcers and chronic gastritis [6,7].

Cysteamine causes severe duodenal ulcers with perforation within 24–48 h after its administration in rats. This animal model resembles the human duodenal ulcer disease by several morphological and functional parameters [8–10]. Because of its simplicity and reproducibility, this animal model offers a good opportunity to examine the biochemical changes in the duodenal mucosa during the early pre-ulcerogenic as well as the later healing phase.

In addition to the pharmacological use of exogenous bFGF and PDGF, we recently tested the hypothesis that endogenous bFGF and PDGF play a role in the healing of gastric and duodenal ulcers, e.g. that neutralizing antibodies would delay the healing of experimental ulcers [11]. The results demonstrated that the anti-bFGF and anti-PDGF neutralizing antibodies delayed the healing of duodenal ulcers both in the 7- and 14-day experiments. The size of the ulcer craters was more than doubled after the decreased availability of bFGF and PDGF while the non-neutralizing antibodies were ineffective [11]. These observations indicate that endogenous growth factors may have a role in the natural history and pathogenesis of gastrointestinal ulceration.

As a follow-up to these pharmacological studies, we performed biochemical experiments to assess the possible time-dependent changes in duodenal and gastric mucosal levels of bFGF and PDGF during experimental duodenal ulceration and healing. We used ELISA methods to actually measure the concentrations of these growth factors, in addition to Western blotting which allows the characterization of molecular forms of these peptides.

DUODENAL ULCER DEVELOPMENT

For these studies, Sprague–Dawley (Harlan Sprague–Dawley, San Diego, CA) female rats were maintained on Purina laboratory chow and tap water ad libitum. Every group consisted of 3–5 rats and the experiments were repeated at least once, the results being pooled.

Duodenal ulcers were induced by oral administration of cysteamine-HCl at 25 mg/100 g intragastrically 3 times, with about 4-h intervals, in the first day. The rats were killed at 12, 24 and 48 h (acute ulcers) and 7 and 14 days (chronic or healed ulcers) after the first dose of cysteamine. The stomach and duodenum were rapidly removed (within 1 min), the diameters of duodenal ulcers were measured and the severity of ulcers was scored [14].

Morphological studies revealed that duodenal ulcer formation was macroscopically detectable from 12 h after the first dose of cysteamine. Ulcers in the proximal duodenum were barely visible at 12 h, about 3 mm^2 at 24 h and about 20 mm^2 at 48 h when they peaked. Ulcers began to heal spontaneously and decreased in size in a time-dependent manner at 7 and 14 days. Similar changes were seen in the case of ulcer severity using a semiquantitative scale system (Table 1).

TABLE 1
Duodenal ulcer development and changes in duodenal mucosal concentration of bFGF and PDGF after cysteamine administration in rats

	Duodenal ulcer			
Time of autopsy	Severity (Scale:0–3)	Size (mm^2)	bFGF (pg/mg protein)	PDGF
Controls	0 ± 0	0 ± 0	442 ± 178	26 ± 6
12 h	0.1 ± 0.1	0.02 ± 0.02	587 ± 91	46 ± 16
24 h	0.9 ± 0.3	1.7 ± 0.6	748 ± 277	107 ± 29*
48 h	2.1 ± 0.3	18.0 ± 11.0	978 ± 98*	28 ± 8
7 d	1.5 ± 0.2	4.9 ± 2.2	862 ± 149	12 ± 8
14 d	0.9 ± 0.1	1.8 ± 0.3	514 ± 159	11 ± 5

$p < 0.05$. The statistical significance of differences of the group means were calculated (for parametric data) by two-tailed Student's *t*-test or (for non-parametric statistics) by the Mann–Whitney U-test

ELISA

The glandular stomach and proximal duodenum were scraped and frozen in liquid nitrogen and stored at –80°C until assay. The samples were homogenized for 2–3 × 15 s on ice with an ultrasonic homogenizer in a 1:3 ratio lysis buffer (2 mol/L NaCl, 10 mmol) TRIS buffer (pH 7.4) with protease inhibitors (100 μg/ml phenylmethylsulphonyl fluoride, 1 μg/ml leupeptin, 1 μg/ml aprotinin)). After homogenization, the samples were centrifuged at 4°C (14 000 rpm, 10 min) to obtain a supernatant, which was used for Western blot and ELISA assays. Protein concentration was measured by the Bradford microassay [12].

The Fibroblast Growth Factor, basic and Platelet-derived Growth Factor AB Quantikine Immunoassays (R&D Systems, Minneapolis, MN) were used for the ELISA. The supernatant was diluted in phosphate-buffered saline (PBS, pH 7.4) at 1:2 ratio for the PDGF and 1:100 ratio for the bFGF measurement. The assays were carried out in duplicate for each sample. The plates were covered by monoclonal anti-bFGF or anti-PDGF-AA antibody. The secondary antibodies were polyclonal against bFGF or PDGF-BB conjugated to horseradish peroxidase. The optical density of each well was determined after the colour development, using a Microplate Autoreader (Bio-Tek Instruments, Inc., Winooski, VT) at 450 nm wavelength. The final concentrations were determined by extrapolation from the standard curve and expressed as pg/mg protein [13,14].

The endogenous levels of duodenal mucosal bFGF started to increase from 12 h and reached maximal values at 48 h when they were significantly higher than the basal value (Table 1). Similarly, the duodenal mucosal PDGF-AB concentration showed some elevation at 12 h and reached its peak at 24 h. It decreased to the control value at 48 h after the first dose of cysteamine and decreased further during the healing phase of experimental duodenal ulcer (Table 1).

The bFGF and PDGF-AB concentrations in the gastric mucosa did not change during the entire induction and healing of duodenal ulcers, despite the intragastric administration of the duodenal ulcerogen, cysteamine (Figure 1). This indicates a high degree of specificity of changes in the availability of growth factors in the proximal duodenum where the lesions occur.

WESTERN BLOT

For Western blot studies, Hoefer's gel electrophoresis unit was used: 10% acrylamide gel was prepared and 100 μl supernatant plus 100 μl 2 × treatment buffer (Hoefer Pharmacia Biotech, San Francisco, CA) placed into the gel and 25 mA current was applied for each gel. A tank electro-transfer unit (Transphor, Hoefer Pharmacia Biotech, San Francisco, CA) was used for transferring the protein to nitrocellulose membrane (0.45 μm pore). The primary antibodies, bFGF rabbit polyclonal antibody (Sigma, St. Louis, MO), PDGF-BB monoclonal rabbit antibody (Creative Biomolecules, Hopkinton, MA) was applied at 1:1000–1:2000 dilution. For secondary antibody, anti-rabbit IgG alkaline phosphatase conjugate (Sigma, St. Louis, MO) was used at 1:5000 dilution [15].

Western blot studies confirmed the presence of duodenal mucosal bFGF and PDGF. The results were in agreement with ELISA studies, i.e. showing prominent bands at 18 kDa and 30 kDa, respectively, at 24–48 h after initiation of experimental duodenal ulceration. The corresponding bands were barely visible in the duodenum of control rats and in animals with partially or completely healed duodenal ulcers.

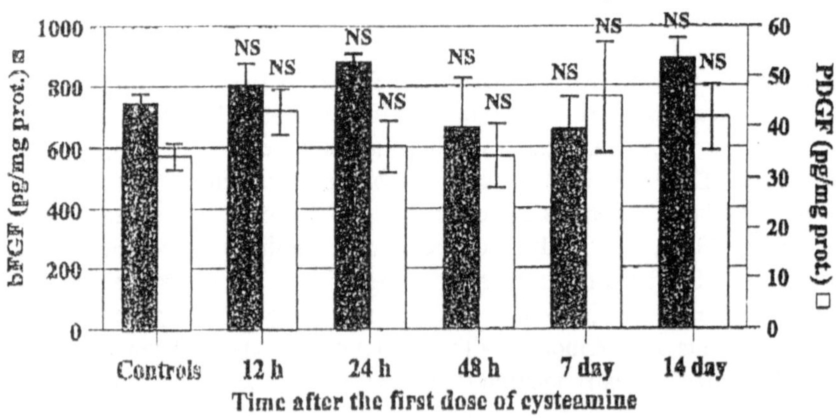

Figure 1. Gastric mucosal bFGF and PDGF concentrations after intragastric administration of the duodenal ulcerogen cysteamine. NS = not significant

The time-course studies revealed that the duodenal mucosal concentrations of bFGF and PDGF correlated with the severity of duodenal ulcers and they returned to normal as the ulcers healed. It is important that, during the entire natural history of duodenal ulcers, the levels of gastric mucosal bFGF and PDGF did not change, suggesting a local pathogenetic role of growth factors in duodenal ulceration.

Taken together, endogenous bFGF and PDGF play an important role in the natural history and spontaneous healing of duodenal ulcers.

REFERENCES

1. Poulsen SS, Olsen PS, Kirkegaard P. Healing of cysteamine-induced duodenal ulcers in the rat. Dig Dis Sci. 1985;30:161–7.
2. Konturek SJ, Brzozowski T, Dembinski A et al. Gastric protective and ulcer-healing action of epidermal growth factor. In: Garner A, Whittle BJR, eds. Advances in Drug Therapy of Gastrointestinal Ulceration. New York: John Wiley and Sons; 1989:261–73.
3. Szabó S, Folkman J, Vattay P et al. Duodenal ulcerogens: The effect of FGF on cysteamine-induced duodenal ulcer. In: Halter F, Garner A, Tytgat GNJ, eds. Mechanisms of Peptic Ulcer Healing. London: Kluwer Academic Publishers; 1991:139–50.
4. Szabó S, Folkman J, Vattay P, Morales RE, Pinkus GE, Kato K. Accelerated healing of duodenal ulcers by oral administration of a mutein of fibroblast growth factor in rats. Gastroenterology. 1994;106:1106–11.
5. Wolfe MM, Bynum TE, Parsons WG et al. Safety and efficacy of an angiogenic peptide, basic fibroblast growth factor (bFGF), in the treatment of gastroduodenal ulcers: A preliminary report. Gastroenterology. 1994;106:A212.
6. Vattay P, Gyömbér E, Morales RE et al. Effect of orally administered platelet-derived growth factor (PDGF) on healing of chronic duodenal ulcers and gastric secretion in rats. Gastroenterology. 1991;100:A180.
7. Kusstatscher S, Szabó S. Effect of platelet-derived growth factor (PDGF) on the healing of chronic gastritis in rats. Gastroenterology. 1993;104:A125.
8. Selye H, Szabó S. Experimental model for production of perforating duodenal ulcers by cysteamine in the rat. Nature. 1973;244:458–9.
9. Szabó S. Animal model of human disease: duodenal ulcer diseases. Animal model: cysteamine-induced acute and chronic duodenal ulcer in the rat. Am J Pathol. 1978;93:273–6.
10. Szabó S, Cho CH. From cysteine to MPTP: structure–activity studies with duodenal ulcerogens. Toxicol Pathol. 1988;16:205–12.
11. Kusstatscher S, Sandor Z, Satoh H et al. Inhibition of endogenous basic fibroblast growth factor (bFGF) delays duodenal ulcer healing in rats: Implication for a physiologic role of bFGF. Gastroenterology. 1994;106:A113.
12. Bradford MM. A rapid and sensitive method for quantitation of microgram quantities of protein utilizing the principle of protein-dye binding. Anal Biochem. 1976;72:248–54.
13. Watanabe H, Hori A, Seno M et al. A sensitive enzyme immunoassay for human basic fibroblast growth factor. Biochem Biophys Res Commun. 1991;175:229–35.
14. Harrison AA, Dunbar PR, Neale TJ. Immunoassay of platelet-derived growth factor in the blood of patients with diabetes mellitus. Diabetologia. 1994;37:1142–6.
15. Sasahara M, Fries JWU, Raines EW et al. PDGF B-chain in neurons of the central nervous system, posterior pituitary, and in a transgenic model. Cell. 1991;64:217–21.

Manuscript received 25 Nov. 95.
Accepted for publication 25 Nov. 95

The time course studies revealed that the duodenal mucosal concentrations of [illegible] and PDGF correlated with the severity of duodenal ulcers and they returned to normal as the ulcers healed. It is important that, during the entire natural history of duodenal ulcers, the levels of gastric mucosal bFGF and PDGF did not change, [illegible]

[illegible]

REFERENCES

[illegible]

TS Gaginella et al. (eds.), Biochemical Pharmacology as an Approach to Gastrointestinal Disorders, 303–311

BIOLOGICAL OXIDANTS AS INTESTINAL SECRETAGOGUES

T.S. GAGINELLA
School of Pharmacy, University of Wisconsin, 425 N. Charter Street, Madison, WI 53705, USA

ABSTRACT

Inflammatory bowel disease (IBD) is associated with the release by granulocytes of a variety of oxidants. These oxidants include hydrogen peroxide, hypochlorous acid, superoxide radicals and nitrogen-containing compounds, such as *N*-chloramines and nitric oxide and its metabolites. In-vivo experiments and clinical observations suggest that some or all of these oxidants may be involved in the pathophysiology of the diarrhoea that is a hallmark symptom of IBD. In vitro, all of these oxidants stimulate to varying degrees small intestinal and/or colonic electrolyte secretion. This chapter will focus principally on the action of monochloramine (formed from hypochlorous acid and ammonia) and nitric oxide (NO). Evidence is presented to support the idea that these oxidants act through direct and indirect mechanisms in the mucosa to stimulate electrolyte secretion. This may contribute to the accumulation of fluid in the intestine of patients with IBD and contribute to diarrhoea. NO is intriguing because it may physiologically stimulate absorption yet, at higher concentrations, stimulate secretion (as in IBD) and be involved in the diarrhoeagenic action of several laxatives.

Keywords: diarrhoea, electrolyte secretion, oxidants, free radicals, nitric oxide, monochloramine, inflammatory bowel disease, laxatives, short-circuit current

INTRODUCTION

Inflammatory bowel disease (IBD) is accompanied by the generation of a complex array of mediators capable of directly or indirectly causing mucosal injury. Secretory diarrhoea is a common symptom associated with IBD. Free radicals and other oxidants originating oxygen and nitrogen metabolism in inflammatory cells are implicated in the pathogenesis of the diarrhoea associated with IBD [1]. The focus of this review will be on one group of these inflammatory mediators – biochemical oxidants. These include reactive oxygen and nitrogen metabolites produced by activated neutrophils and macrophages. Some of these labile but highly reactive molecules yield other, more stable and/or more potent biological oxidants. In turn, these evoke changes in mucosal electrolyte transport, resulting in luminal fluid accumulation and clinically significant diarrhoea.

Mucosal inflammation can arise from a variety of causes, including Crohn's disease, ulcerative colitis, acute enteric infections (e.g. *Salmonella*, *Shigella*, *E. coli*/O157:H57), food allergy (eosinophilic enteritis) and pelvic irradiation [1]. A common feature of these conditions is secretory diarrhoea. Patients with ulcerative colitis can excrete up to 1500 g/day faecal water, far exceeding the volume that defines secretory diarrhoea

This paper was presented at the Section of IUPHAR GI Pharmacology Symposium on 'Biochemical pharmacology as an approach to gastrointestinal disorders (basic science to clinical perspectives)', October 12–14, 1995, Pécs, Hungary.

clinically [2–4]. Compared with healthy volunteers, patients with Crohn's disease [5] and proctocolitis [6] absorb fluid from the intestine at a lower rate, resulting in more luminal fluid than in normal individuals. Whether this result is due to stimulation of plasma-to-lumen flux or inhibition of lumen-to-plasma ion transport in IBD is not precisely known. It is likely that factors such as increased mucosal permeability [7–9] and inhibition of sodium/potassium-ATPase [10] contribute to the 'secretory' diarrhoea. Indeed, the response of inflamed mucosa in experimental studies is actually less than the response in normal tissue [11–13], indicating a possible defect in signal transduction for secretory stimuli rather than enhanced sensitivity to secretagogues.

GRANULOCYTE-DERIVED OXIDANTS

Reactive oxygen metabolites (ROM) include superoxide, hydrogen peroxide (H_2O_2) and hypochlorous acid (HOCl). Subsequent reaction of HOCl with ammonia and proteins yields monochloramine (NH_2Cl) and *N*-chloramines, respectively [14]. NH_2Cl is a lipophilic molecule that can readily penetrate cell membranes. This ROM can react with components of extracellular membranes and at many intracellular sites, possibly effecting changes in membrane-associated receptors and cell metabolism.

Nitric oxide (NO) is derived from arginine, through the action of NO synthase, and is thus a reactive nitrogen metabolite; as a free radical it is highly reactive and capable of oxidizing enzymes (e.g. guanylyl cyclase) and other cell components [14]. NO can have functionally opposite effects, being either beneficial or detrimental, depending upon whether it is derived from constitutive (cNOS) or inducible (iNOS) nitric oxide synthesis [15]. Superoxide and NO can react to form peroxynitrite which is believed to produce cellular injury, either through its own action or indirectly via its potent free radical metabolites, OH and NO_2 [16–19] (Figure 1).

ROM and NO have direct and indirect effects that can contribute to their secretory action on the intestinal mucosa. The effects may be indirect due to injury to mesenchymal and mast cells and myenteric neurons. Such an effect may evoke the release of eicosanoids, histamine/5-HT, kinins, acetylcholine and substance P – all of which are intestinal secretagogues [20–22] (Figure 2).

ROM AS SECRETAGOGUES: NEURAL VERSUS DIRECT EFFECTS

Hydrogen peroxide, HOCl and NH_2Cl increase short-circuit current (Isc) and evoke net anion secretion in rat colon, rat ileum and human T_{84} cells in culture [23]. Indirect and direct effects on ion transport thus have been demonstrated. The indirect component involves neural and non-neural aspects. The response to ROM, particularly NH_2Cl in the colon is biphasic. A portion of the Isc response to H_2O_2 and NH_2Cl can be blocked by tetrodotoxin and atropine [24–26], indicating that cholinergic (and perhaps other) nerves are involved. This finding is supported by results showing that NH_2Cl stimulates the release of acetylcholine from a cholinergically innervated preparation of mucosa/submucosa of rat colon [27].

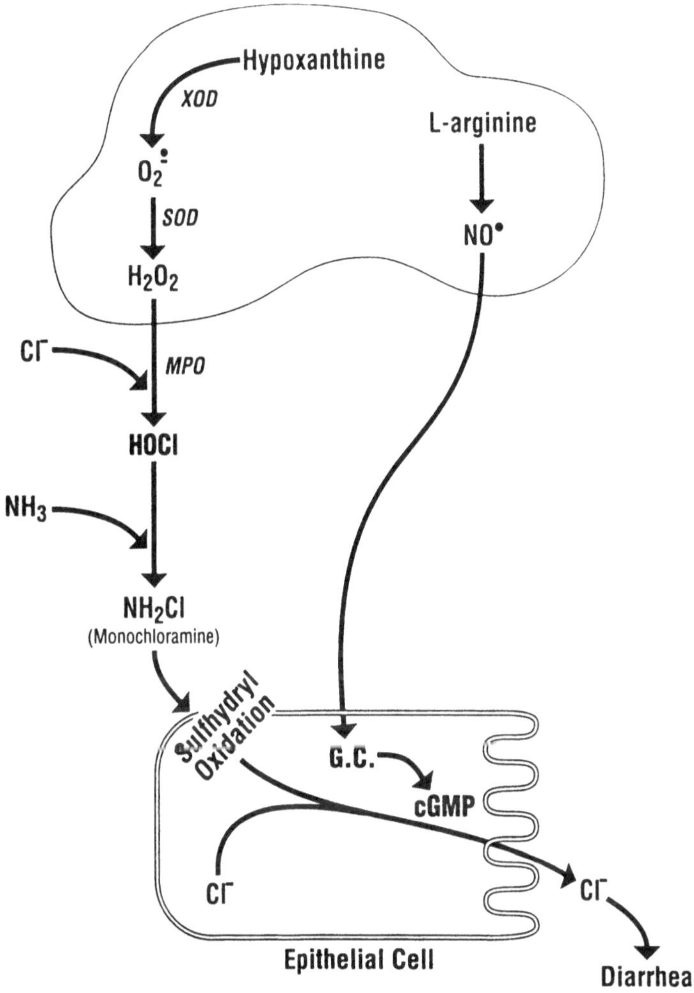

Figure 1. The formation of superoxide from hypoxanthine in a granulocyte, such as a neutrophil. Superoxide dismutase (SOD) forms hydrogen peroxide from the superoxide radical. In the presence of granulocyte myeloperoxidase (MPO) and halide (here chloride) ions, hypochlorous acid (HOCl) is formed. Subsequent reaction with ammonia yields monochloramine, a stable, lipophilic and potent biological oxidant. The monochloramine can oxidize extracellular and intracellular sulphydryl moieties to alter metabolism and possibly perturb calcium homeostasis, leading to calcium-evoked chloride secretion. Nitric oxide (NO) is produced from L-arginine by constitutive and inducible forms of NO synthase. The former is calcium dependent and exists primarily in neurons, endothelial and epithelial cells; the latter is independent of calcium modulation and is present in granulocytes, macrophages, nerves, epithelia and smooth muscle cells. The NO free radical can activate soluble guanylyl cyclase and guanylin, an endogenous activator of guanylyl cyclase

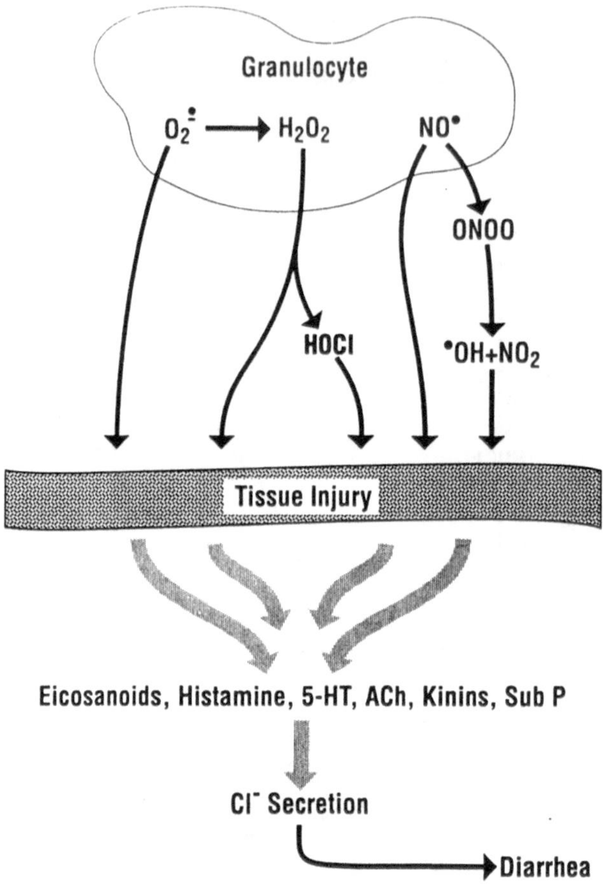

Figure 2. Illustration of how superoxide, hydrogen peroxide, hypochlorous acid and nitric oxide might release other mediators of intestinal secretion upon injury to subepithelial tissue, including nerves, mast cells and mesenchymal cells. NO and superoxide can react to form peroxynitrite (ONOO), which may produce oxidation of tissue components. In addition, this labile radical can yield hydroxyl and the nitrogen dioxide radicals, which are potent oxidants

The neural component of the response is also associated with the release of E-type prostaglandins [24–27]. These findings fit with the observations that there are abnormalities in enteric nerve structure and/or function and prostaglandins are released to a greater extent (than normal) in tissue obtained from patients with IBD [28]. The extent to which these are epiphenomena is not known. Based on partial inhibition of the ROM-induced response by inhibitors of cyclo-oxygenase, the data support a connection between the increased tissue levels of prostaglandins and the neural component of the Isc response. Because prostaglandins stimulate anion secretion through direct interaction with epithelial cells [22,28], some of the Isc response is undoubtedly due to direct effects of the prostaglandins. This may arise from a direct effect of ROM on epithelial cell membranes.

Verification of the direct effects of ROM on epithelial cells comes from the data showing stimulation of Isc in non-innervated monolayers of T_{84} cells [29]. In this preparation, NH_2Cl increased Isc without increasing intracellular levels of cyclic AMP or cyclic GMP; nor was there evidence for increased phosphatidylcholine turnover or cytotoxicity. There was an increase in intracellular calcium (believed to arise from intra- and extracellular sources). The mechanism was speculated to involve ROM-induced lipoprotein oxidation and aberrations in the epithelial cell membranes. Consistent with this, but on a more macroscopic scale, are the findings that ROM, including NH_2Cl, increase mucosal permeability when perfused through the lumen of the rat ileum at concentrations from 0.1 mmol/L to 1.0 mmol/L [30]. Oxidation of intracellular thiols also seems to be involved in the action of NH_2Cl [31] (see Figure 1).

The biological effects of the ROM are related to a great extent to their stability and oxidizing potential. In aqueous media, superoxide anion radical has a half-life of 10–20 s, hydroxyl radical about 1 ns, and hydroxyperoxyl radical about 7 s. NH_2Cl (and other chloramines), HOCl and H_2O_2 are 'stable' [14]. However, NH_2Cl is more lipophilic than H_2O_2, which is believed to be, at least in part, responsible for its greater potency than H_2O_2 as a secretagogue [29,30]. In vitro, NH_2Cl produces maximal effects at <100 μmol/L (generally 50 μmol/L), whereas H_2O_2 requires concentrations 10-fold higher than this [24–26]. It is estimated that it is possible to achieve a concentration of 50 μmol/L NH_2Cl in inflamed tissue [30].

NITRIC OXIDE AS A SECRETAGOGUE

Mucosal NO synthesis is increased and nitrite, a major metabolite of NO, is elevated in the lumen of patients with active ulcerative colitis (see Reference 15 for review). As early as 1982, it was noted that nitroprusside (0.5 mmol/L) evoked fluid secretion into tied-off intestinal loops of mice [32]. Subsequently, this NO donor was shown to produce secretion in the rat colon [33] and guinea-pig ileum [34]. Through the use of synthesis inhibitors and antagonists, the effect of nitroprusside was found to be partially neurally mediated, dependent to some extent on prostaglandins and possibly associated with increases in intracellular cAMP levels; nitrite and nitrate were not responsible for the effect of nitroprusside on the Isc [33]. *E. coli*-stable toxin-a (STa) stimulates chloride ion secretion in the rat ileum by activating reflex myenteric neural activity involving NO [see Reference 15]. It is possible that the NO is released by the nerves in response to the toxin (followed by effects of the NO on neighbouring mesenchymal, epithelial and mast cells) to directly or indirectly cause the secretory response.

As a follow-up to the NO donor studies, Tamai and Gaginella [35] added NO gas to the fluid bathing rat colon in Ussing chambers, and demonstrated that NO itself causes an increase in Isc (bumetanide inhibitable, net chloride secretion). The comparative response to the NO donor sodium nitroprusside in the same study was delayed slightly and the sodium nitroprusside was of lower apparent potency than NO itself. Thus, the effects of sodium nitroprusside in earlier studies were not likely to be due to intrinsic activity of the nitroprusside molecule. The response to NO gas was also inhibited by tetrodotoxin, confirming the neural involvement in the secretory effect of NO, as shown for the ROM hydrogen peroxide and NH_2Cl (see above).

Laxatives (e.g. castor oil, phenolphthalein, bisacodyl, bile acids and magnesium sulphate) stimulate fluid accumulation in the lumen of experimental animals and humans. In vitro, those laxatives that have been tested for effects on Isc and anion secretion cause a net movement of chloride ions in the serosal-to-mucosal direction. Castor oil, bile salts, phenolphthalein and bisacodyl cause 'diarrhoea', net fluid secretion and mucosal injury in vivo. Based upon studies with L-NAME and other inhibitors of NO synthase (including dexamethasone, an inhibitor of iNOS synthesis), and in some instances measurements of NOS activity, this response is proposed to be partly due to NO [36–39]. The laxative effect begins in about three hours, which is enough time for iNOS synthesis [14,15]. Surprisingly, the effect of magnesium sulphate (a so-called osmotic laxative) on luminal fluid accumulation is associated with increases in NO [40]. This seems reasonable if one assumes a primary effect of magnesium sulphate on enteric nerves.

The final mediator of NO-induced secretion is unknown, but guanylyl cyclase is an inescapable choice as a candidate. NO activates soluble guanylyl cyclase [41–43] in the intestine, but the source of the enzyme is probably nerves or cells, rather than the epithelial cells. The intestinal epithelial cells contain only about 5% soluble guanylyl cyclase [44,45]. Othe components (nerves, smooth muscle, blood vessels) could be the source of the particulate form of the enzyme, which when activated by NO generates cAMP that diffuses to the epithelial cells. An alternative explanation is that guanylin is responsible for generating the cGMP subsequent to activation of soluble guanylyl cyclase. Guanylin is an endogenous stimulant of STa/epithelial-cell-responsive particulate guanylyl cyclase, and the enzyme requires oxidation for its activation [46]. Studies have confirmed that guanylin stimulates intestinal chloride secretion in vitro [47,48]. It seems reasonable, therefore, that activation of guanylin by NO could elevate intracellular levels of cGMP, a proven second messenger for certain secretagogues [49,50].

NO AS A PHYSIOLOGICAL REGULATOR OF ABSORPTION

Although NO is a secretagogue under some conditions, it also tends to enhance absorption of water and electrolytes in some situations. In anaesthetized rats, L-NAME (25 mg/kg iv) reversed jejunal fluid absorption to secretion [51]. NO synthase inhibitors are "secretagogues" in some instances in guinea-pig [52], rabbit [53], mouse [54] and rat [55] small intestine. Furthermore, L-NAME increased prostaglandin- and STa-induced jejunal fluid secretion in the rat, suggesting that NO promotes absorption and is an antagonist of secretion in the small intestine [51]. L-NAME also increases pancreatic and gastric secretion [56,57].

Together the studies present the possibility that, physiologically, NO promotes absorption, possibly by an effect on mucosal blood flow or selective activation of noradrenergic myenteric neurons. Pathophysiologically, at higher concentrations NO may have the opposite effect. NO generated in response to endotoxin application to rat enterocytes is associated with cytotoxicity to the epithelial cells [58]. This would impair absorption, cause intraluminal accumulation of fluid and would be observed as net secretion in experiments performed in vivo.

CONCLUSION

ROM and NO are undoubtedly involved in mucosal pathology and pathophysiology in IBD. There is not just one mechanism or mediator responsible for the pathogenic effects of NO and ROM.

NO is intriguing because of its duplicity of action. Its potential to act as a secretagogue is revealed during mucosal injury. On the one hand, NO can increase absorption. The complexity of action of NO is illustrated by the example of dissociation of the mucosal injury and diarrhoea produced by castor oil: L-NAME ameliorates the diarrhoea but exacerbates the mucosal injury produced by oral dosing of castor oil [38]. It is probable that the 'protective' tissue level of NO generated normally by cNOS is masked in the presence of a higher concentration of NO produced in response to castor-oil-induced mucosal injury.

New approaches to therapy for mucosal injury and/or diarrhoea associated with ROM and NO will focus on more effective antioxidants and free radical scavengers, as well as selective inhibitors of iNOS. Further research will certainly enlighten our understanding of the dual role of NO and other biological oxidants in mucosal function. Hopefully this will lead to safe and more effective therapy for the diarrhoea and other sequelae of IBD.

REFERENCES

1. Gaginella TS, Kachur JF, Tamai H, Keshavarzian A. Reactive oxygen and nitrogen metabolites as mediators of secretory diarrhea. Gastroenterology. 1995;109:2019–28.
2. Caprilli R, Sopranzi N, Colaneri O. Salt losing diarrhea in idiopathic proctocolitis. Scand J Gastroenterol. 1978;13:331–5.
3. Schilli R, Brueur RI, Klein F. A comparison of the composition of fecal fluid in Crohn's disease and ulcerative colitis. Gut. 1982;23:326–32.
4. Smiddy FG, Gregory SD, Smith IB, Goligher JC. Faecal loss of fluid, electrolytes and nitrogen in colitis before and after ileostomy. Lancet. 1960;1:14–19.
5. Harris J, Shields R. Absorption and secretion of water and electrolytes by the intact human colon in diffuse untreated proctocolitis. Gut. 1970;11:27–33.
6. Head LH, Heaton JW Jr, Kivel RM. Absorption of water and electrolytes in Crohn's disease of the colon. Gastroenterology. 1969;56:571–9.
7. Jenkins RT, Goodacre RL, Rooney PJ, Bienenstock J, Sivakumaran J, Walker WHC. Studies of intestinal permeability in inflammatory diseases using polyethylene glycol 400. Clin Biochem. 1986;19:298–302.
8. Ukabam SO, Clamp JR, Cooper BT. Abnormal small intestinal permeability to sugars in patients with Crohn's disease of the terminal ileum and colon. Digestion. 1982;27:70–4.

9. Bjarnasson I, O'Morain C, Levi AJ, Peters AJ. Absorption of ^{51}chromium-labeled ethylenediaminetetraacetate in inflammatory bowel disease. Gastroenterology. 1983;85:318–22.
10. Rachmilewitz D, Karmeli F, Sharon P. Decreased colonic Na–K–ATPase activity in active ulcerative colitis. Israel J Med Sci. 1984;20:681–4.
11. Kachur JF, Keshavarzian A, Sundaresan R et al. Colitis reduces the short-circuit response to inflammatory mediators in rat colonic mucosa. Inflammation. 1995;19:245–59.
12. Goldhill J, Zhao L, Xu Y, Donovan V, Burakoff R. Defective stimulation of cyclic AMP by prostaglandin E_2 in colonic epithelial cells in colitis. Eur J Pharmacol. 1993;238:387–90.
13. Goldhill JM, Burakoff R, Donovan V, Rose K, Percy WH. Defective modulation of colonic secretamotor neurons in a rabbit model of colitis. Am J Physiol. 1993;264:G671–7.
14. Yamada T, Grisham MB. Pathogenesis of tissue injury: role of reactive metabolites of oxygen and nitrogen. In: Targan SR, Shanahan F, eds. Inflammatory Bowel Disease from Bench to Bedside. Baltimore: Williams and Wilkins; 1994:133–50.
15. Miller MJS, Gaginella TS. Nitric oxide as a mediator of mucosal function. In: Gaginella TS, ed. Regulatory Mechanisms in Gastrointestinal Pharmacology. Boca Raton: CRC Press. 1995:199–218.
16. Rachmilewitz D, Stamler JSJ, Karmeli F et al. Peroxynitrite-induced rat colitis – a new model of colonic inflammation. Gastroenterology. 1993;105:1681–8.
17. Beckman JSJ, Beckman TW, Chen J, Marshall PA, Freeman BA. Apparent hydroxyl radical production by peroxynitrite: implications for endothelial injury from nitric oxide and superoxide. Proc Natl Acad Sci USA. 1990;87:1620–4.
18. Halliwell B. Free radicals, antioxidants, and human disease: curiosity, cause, or consequence? Lancet. 1994;344:721–4.
19. Radi R, Beckman JS, Bush KM, Freeman BA. Peroxynitrite-induced membrane lipid peroxidation: the cytotoxic potential of superoxide and nitric oxide. Arch Biochem Biophys. 1991;288:481–7.
20. Gaginella TS. Receptor pharmacology of intestinal secretion. In: Lebenthal E, Duffey M, eds. Secretory Diarrhea. New York, NY: Raven Press; 1990:163–78.
21. Gaginella TS, Kachur JF. Kinins as mediators of intestinal secretion. Am J Physiol. 1989;256:G1–G15.
22. Gaginella TS. Eicosanoid-mediated intestinal secretion. In: Lebenthal E, Duffey M, eds. Secretory Diarrhea. New York, NY: Raven Press; 1990:15–30.
23. Gaginella TS. Absorption and secretion in the colon. Curr Opin Gastroenterol. 1995;11:2–8.
24. Karayalcin SS, Sturbaum CW, Wachsman JT, Cha J-H, Powell DW. Hydrogen peroxide stimulates rat colonic prostaglandin production and alters electrolyte transport. Clin Invest. 1990;86:60–8.
25. Tamai H, Kachur JF, Baron DA, Grisham MB, Gaginella TS. Monochloramine, a neutrophil-derived oxidant, stimulates rat colonic secretion. J Pharmacol Exp Ther. 1991;257:887–94.
26. Bern MJ, Ssturbaum CW, Karayalcin SS, Bernschneider HM, Wachsman JT, Powell DW. Immune system control of rat and rabbit colonic electrolyte transport: Role of prostaglandins and enteric nervous system. J Clin Invest. 1988;83:1810–20.
27. Gaginella TS, Grisham MB, Thomas DB, Walsh R, Moummi C. Oxidant-evoked release of acetylcholine from enteric neurons of the rat colon. J Pharmacol Exp Ther. 1992;263:1068–73.
28. Donowitz M. Arachidonic acid metabolites and their role in inflammatory bowel disease: An update requiring addition of a pathway. Gastroenterology. 1985;85:50–587.
29. Tamai H, Gaginella TS, Kachur JF, Musch MW, Chang EB. Ca-mediated stimulation of Cl secretion by reactive oxygen metabolites in human colonic T84 cells. J Clin Invest. 1992;89:301–7.
30. Grisham MB, Gaginella TS, von Ritter C, Tamai H, Be RM, Granger DN. Effects of neutrophil-derived oxidants on intestinal permeability, electrolyte transport, and epithelial cell viability. Inflammation. 1990;14:531–42.
31. Tamai H, Kachur JF, Grisham MB, Musch MW, Chang EB, Gaginella TS. Effect of the thiol-oxidizing agent diamide on NH_2Cl-induced rat colonic electrolyte secretion. Am J Physiol. 1993;265:C166–70.
32. Thomas DD, Knoop FC. The effect of calcium and prostaglandin inhibitors on the intestinal fluid response to heat-stable enterotoxin of *Escherichia coli*. J Infect Dis. 1982;145:141–5.
33. Wilson KT, Xie Y, Musch MW, Chang EB. Sodium nitroprusside stimulates anion secretion and inhibits sodium chloride absorption in rat colon. J Pharmacol Exp Ther. 1993;266:224–30.
34. MacNaughton WK. Nitric oxide-donating compounds stimulate electrolyte transport in the guinea pig intestine in vitro. Life Sci. 1993;53:585–93.
35. Tamai H, Gaginella TS. Direct evidence for nitric oxide stimulation of electrolyte secretion in the rat colon. Free Rad Res Commun. 1993;19:229–39.
36. Mascolo N, Izzo AA, Barbato F, Capasso F. Inhibitors of nitric oxide synthetase prevent castor-oil-induced diarrhoea in the rat. Br J Pharmacol. 1993;108:861–4.
37. Mascolo N, Gaginella TS, Izzo AA, DiCarlo G, Capasso F. Nitric oxide involvement in sodium choleate-induced fluid secretion and diarrhoea in rats. Eur J Pharmacol. 1994;264:21–6.

38. Capasso F, Mascolo N, Izzo AA, Gaginella TS. Dissociation of castor-oil-induced diarrhea and intestinal mucosal injury in rat: effect of N^G-nitro-L-arginine methylester. Br J Pharmacol. 1994;113:1127–30.
39. Gaginella TS, Mascolo N, Izzo AA, Autore G, Capasso F. Nitric oxide as a mediator of bisacodyl and phenolphthalein laxative action: induction of nitric oxide synthase. J Pharmacol Exp Ther. 1994;270:1239–45.
40. Izzo A, Gaginella TS, Mascolo N, Caspasso F. Nitric oxide as a mediator of the laxative action of magnesium sulphate. 1994;113:228–32.
41. Murad F, Mittal CK, Arnold WP, Katsuki S, Kimura H. Guanylate cyclase: activation by azide, nitro compounds, nitric oxide, and hydroxyl radical and inhibition by hemoglobin and myoglobin. In: George WJ, Ignarro LJ, eds. Advances in Cyclic Nucleotide Research. New York: Raven Press, 1978.
42. Schmidt HHHW. NO·, CO and ·OH endogenous soluble guanylate cyclase-activating factors. Fed Eur Biochem Soc. 1992;307:102–7.
43. Arnold WP, Mittal CK, Katsuki S, Murad F. Nitric oxide activates guanylate cyclase and increases guanosine 3′:5′-cyclic monophosphate levels in various tissue preparations. Proc Natl Acad Sci USA. 1977;74:3203–7.
44. DeJonge HR. The localization of guanylate cyclases in rat small intestinal epithelium. FEBS Lett. 1975;53:237–42.
45. Craven PA, DeRubertis FR. Cyclic nucleotide metabolism in rat colonic epithelial cells with different proliferative activities. Biochem Biophys Acta. 1981;676:155–69.
46. Currie MG, Fok KF, Kato J et al. Guanylin: an endogenous activator of intestinal guanylate cyclase. Proc Natl Acad Sci USA. 1992;89:947–51.
47. Forte LR, Eber SL, Turner JT, Freeman RH, Fok KF, Currie MG. Guanylin stimulation of Cl^- secretion in human intestinal T_{84} cells via cyclic guanosine monophosphate. J Clin Invest. 1993;91:2423–8.
48. Wiegand RC, Kato J, Huang MD, Fok KF, Kachur JF, Currie MG. Human guanylin: cDNA isolation, structure and activity. FEBS Lett. 1992;311:150-154.
49. Guandalini S, Migliavacca M, de Campora E, Rubino A. Cyclic guanosine monophosphate effects on nutrient and electrolyte transport in rabbit ileum. Gastroenterology. 1982;83:15–21.
50. Brasitus TA, Field M, Kimberg DV. Intestinal mucosal cyclic GMP: regulation and relation to ion transport. Am J Physiol. 1976;231:G275–82.
51. Schirgi-Degen A, Beubler E. Significance of nitric oxide in the regulation of intestinal fluid transport in the rat jejunum in vivo. Gastroenterology. 1992;106:A269.
52. Miller MJS, Sadowska-Krowicka H, Chotinaruemol S, Kakkis JL, Clark DA. Amelioration of chronic ileitis by nitric oxide synthase inhibition. J Pharmacol Exp Ther. 1993;264:11–16.
53. Barry MK, Aloisi JD, Pickering SP, Yeo CJ. Nitric oxide modulates water and electrolyte transport in the ileum. Ann Surg. 1994;219:382–8.
54. Rao RK, Riviere PJM, Pascaud X, Junien JL, Porreca F. Tonic regulation of mouse ileal ion transport by nitric oxide. J Pharmacol Exp Ther. 1984;269:626–31.
55. Mailman D. Differential effects of lumenal L-arginine and N^G-nitro L-arginine on blood flow and water fluxes in rat ileum. Br J Pharmacol. 1994;112:304–10.
56. Takeuchi K, Ohuchi T, Miyake H, Niki S, Okabe S. Effects of nitric oxide synthase inhibitors on duodenal alkaline secretion in anesthetized rats. Eur J Pharmacol. 1993;231:135–9.
57. Konturek SJ, Bilski J, Konturek PK, Cieszkowski M, Pawlik W. Role of endogenous nitric oxide in the control of canine pancreatic secretion and blood flow. Gastroenterology. 1993;104:896–902.
58. Tepperman BL, Brown JF, Whittle BJR. Nitric oxide synthase induction and intestinal epithelial cell viability in rats. Am J Physiol. 1993;93:G214–18.

Manuscript received 14 Oct. 95.
Accepted for publication 24 Nov. 95.

TS Gaginella et al. (eds.), Biochemical Pharmacology as an Approach to Gastrointestinal Disorders, 313–334

A NEW UNIFORM BIOCHEMICAL EXPLANATION FOR THE DEVELOPMENT AND LOCATION OF 'GENUINE' GASTRIC, DUODENAL AND JEJUNAL ULCERS IN PATIENTS

Gy. MÓZSIK*, B. BÓDIS, I. JURICSKAY, O. KARÁDI, Cs. KÖVESDY AND L. NAGY
First Department of Medicine, Medical University of Pécs, H-7643 Pécs, Hungary
*Correspondence

ABSTRACT

Tissue metabolism was studied in the corpus, antral, duodenal and jejunal mucosa and musculature in patients with decreased, normal and increased gastric acid output, with and without the presence of a 'genuine' ulcer. The term 'genuine' means that no clinically detectable reason was found for ulcer development in the antrum, duodenum and jejunum.

The tissue levels of ATP, ADP, AMP, RNA and DNA were measured and Mg^{2+}-Na^{+}-K^{+}-dependent ATPase prepared and its activity measured in vitro, with and without the administration of various drugs.

It has been found that:

1. Energy and biochemical gradients exist between corpus vs. antral, antral vs. duodenal (jejunal) and corpus vs. duodenal (jejunal) mucosa in patients, dependent on their gastric acid secretions;
2. Energy and biochemical gradients exist between non-ulcerated and ulcerated mucosal tissues of the antrum, duodenum and jejunum (with 'genuine' ulcers);
3. The membrane ATPase activity is proportional to the amount of ATP–ADP transformation.

It has been concluded that:

1. Energy turnover is much higher in human gastric corpus mucosa than in antral or duodenal (jejunal) mucosa, and its extent depends on gastric acid secretion;
2. Energy turnover is 2–3 times higher in ulcerated antral, duodenal and jejunal mucosa than in non-ulcerated specimens;
3. The appearance of 'genuine' ulcers in the antral, duodenal and jejunal mucosa is a consequence of exhaustion of metabolic adaptation.

A uniform biochemical explanation can be found for the development of 'genuine' gastric, duodenal and jejunal ulcers and their location in patients.

Keywords: 'genuine' antral, duodenal and jejunal ulcer; mucosal biochemistry

---

This paper was presented at the Section of IUPHAR GI Pharmacology Symposium on 'Biochemical pharmacology as an approach to gastrointestinal disorders (basic science to clinical perspectives)', October 12–14, 1995, Pécs, Hungary.

INTRODUCTION

Peptic ulcer disease is very common, appearing in about 10% of the inhabitants of Hungary.

The definition of peptic ulcer disease (PUD) suggests the presence of injury to the muscularis mucosa histologically. Many drugs (non-steroidal anti-inflammatory drugs, steroids, etc.) produce mucosal damage in the gastrointestinal (GI) tract, but no typical histological picture occurs due to ulcer. Furthermore, the symptoms of patients with non-ulcer dyspepsia (NUD) are typical of those of patients with ulcer disease. However, no endoscopic evidence supports the findings.

Clinicians frequently observe patients with histologically proven GI ulcer but no clinically detectable reason(s) for the presence of the 'classical' ulcer. Aetiological roles of drugs, alcohol and other diseases (like liver, pulmonary, circulatory or endocrine diseases) can be clinically excluded. Under these circumstances, we use the term 'genuine' ulcer, which is located in the gastric (usually antral), duodenal and jejunal (after Billroth II type of partial gastrectomy) mucosa.

The exact ratio of unidentified ('genuine') to identified factor(s) inducing PUD is unknown, the estimated value being approximately 80% (i.e. 4:1 ratio) in Hungary.

Theories about the impaired balance between the aggressive (HCl, pepsin) and the defensive (mucus secretion, blood flow, biochemical background) factors causing development of mucosal damage are very attractive; however, the details are still unclear in human beings [1–6].

We have applied biochemical–pharmacological approaches to ulcer disease in the past [7–10], and recently a shift towards a biochemical–pharmacological approach has been observed internationally [11]. Studies performed in animals can improve our understanding of the details of GI mucosal damage and help in prevention. However, extending these experimental observations to make assumptions about human pathology is quite difficult.

There are many unresolved contradictions in the theories accepted as 'classical' impaired balance between the aggressive and defensive factors located in the upper part of the GI tract of patients (stomach, duodenum, jejunum), like:

1. GI mucosal ulceration does not represent a specific injury to a particular type of cell (thus, the appearance of an ulcer is a result of an unspecific reaction of the GI mucosa);

2. There is no generally accepted explanation for the location of PUD in the stomach, duodenum and jejunum;

3. The biochemical reactions of GI mucosal tissues cannot be separated according only to ulcer development (aggressive functions, e.g. HCl, pepsin secretion) or to ulcer healing (blood flow, mucus production, mucosal biochemistry, etc.);

4. Early published observations described only fractions of the whole phenomenon; however, these appeared at different levels of tissue reactions (GI functions, morphology, biochemistry, blood flow, oxygen free radicals etc.);

5. Surprisingly, we can apply the metabolic blocking compounds (anticholinergic, antimuscarinic agents, H_2-blockers, H^+-K^+-ATPase blockers) in the treatment of patients with PUD.

We used biochemical pharmacology as an approach to study the GI mucosa in the event of gastric acid secretion [12] and ulcer development in patients with 'genuine' PUD. The biochemical measurement of adenosine triphosphate (ATP), diphosphate (ADP), monophosphate (AMP), adenine–adenosine and the calculation of different ratios (like ATP/ADP, 'energy charge') could provide a good and general information on tissue metabolism. Tissue metabolism represents the actual energy state of the GI mucosa (and musculature), which gives us information on possible mechanisms existing in the tissues. The tissue level of ATP informs us of the actual equilibrium of ATP breakdown and resynthesis (Figure 1). Intact oxidative phosphorylation is necessary for the resynthesis of ATP. The 'energy charge' [(ATP+0.5ADP)/(ATP+ADP+AMP)] gives more information on the cells [13]: this value is theoretically 1 when all adenosine compounds are phosphorylated, while its value is 0 when all adenosine compounds are dephosphorylated. By measuring the substrate (ATP), the substrate-splitting (membrane-bound) ATP-dependent enzymes and the results of the enzyme activities (ADP, AMP) at the same time, we obtain a possible dynamic approach to studying the equilibrium (balance) between the adenosine compounds (ATP, ADP, AMP).

We used these methods widely in animal experiments, where it was possible to alter only one (or a few) circumstances in the processes of mucosal damage and prevention [14,15].

In this paper we aimed:

1. To characterize biochemically the tissue metabolism around 'genuine' gastric, duodenal and jejunal ulcers in patients;
2. To obtain biochemical evidence for the existence of biochemical and energy gradients between:
   a. Corpus vs. antral, corpus vs. duodenal and antral vs. duodenal mucosa in patients with gastric hyperacidity;
   b. Corpus (antral) vs. duodenal mucosa in patients with normal gastric secretory responses;
   c. No difference between corpus vs. antral vs. duodenal mucosa in hypoacid patients;
3. To give a brief summary of the regulation of membrane-bound ATP-dependent enzymes; and
4. To create a uniform biochemical explanation for the development of 'genuine' ulcer and its location in human antral, duodenal and jejunal mucosa.

MATERIALS AND METHODS

The experiments were carried out on resecata of stomach and small intestine (duodenum and jejunum) of patients who underwent gastric surgery. All patients suffered from 'genuine' gastric or small intestinal ulcer. Those patients who suffered from jejunal ulcer underwent earlier Billroth II type gastric resection.

The patients had been treated with different drugs (mostly with different generations of H_2-blocking compounds) at least for 4–6 weeks. The patients did not heal over this time period, and requests for gastric surgery were given by physicians or by the patients themselves.

The gastric secretory responses (basal acid output and maximal acid output) were measured one or two days before surgery (the patients received higher doses of antacids for a one-week period before the operation).

The tissue specimens were obtained immediately in the operation room, where the 'genuine' ulcers were cut into two parts (for histological and biochemical examinations). There was no suspicion of malignancy before the operation in these patients. The histological examination indicated a typical microscopic picture of PUD in all patients included in the present study. The corpus, the antral and duodenal parts as well as the mucosa and the musculature were separated and put into liquid nitrogen immediately.

The adenosine compounds were measured chromatographically or enzymatically (Boehringer, Ingelheim, Germany) [see details in Reference 7]. The ribonucleic acid (RNA) and deoxyribonucleic acid (DNA) were measured with the method of Thannhauser [16]. The substrates were expressed as nmol (ATP, ADP, AMP) or mmol (adenine–adenosine) corresponding to 1.0 mg DNA. Two or three parallel measurements were obtained simultaneously from one tissue sample. All biochemical measurements were made simultaneously on all tissue specimens obtained from one patient (ulcerated and non-ulcerated GI mucosa, corpus, antral, duodenal mucosa and musculature). The ratio of ATP/ADP, adenylate pool (ATP+ADP+AMP) and 'energy charge' [(ATP+0.5ADP)/(ATP+ADP+AMP)] were calculated. Results were taken as the average of two or three biochemical measurements.

The membrane ATPase was prepared according to the method published earlier [17,18]. Membrane ATPase activity was measured by the liberation of inorganic phosphate (P_i) from ATP. The protein content of the membrane was assayed by the method of Lowry et al. [19]. The enzyme activity was expressed as μmol of P_i (mg protein)$^{-1}$ h^{-1}.

Acetylcholine (acetylcholine chloride, Fluka), pentagastrin (Peptavlon, ICI, UK), histamine (Perermin, Chinoin, Hungary), PGE_1 and PGE_2 (Chinoin, Hungary), atropine (EGYS, Hungary) and cAMP (Sigma Chemical Co., St Louis) were dissolved and diluted in the aliquot for membrane ATPase determination. The effects of the drugs were expressed as percent values of ATPase activity (obtained without drugs).

The results were expressed as mean ± SEM. The unpaired Student's *t*-test was used for statistical analyses. Fisher's U-test was applied for correlation calculation, when the regression equation, *r* and *p* values were calculated for the patients [20].

The biochemical results were expressed as mean ± SEM in the same patients (mucosal and musculature specimens). It was of course, not possible to carry out all measurements in one patient, so the results were compared with the relevant measurements in the same group of patients.

RESULTS

Changes in the membrane-bound ATP-dependent energy systems in ulcerated antral, duodenal and jejunal mucosa around the 'genuine' ulcer

The results of biochemical measurements in the control group (non-ulcerated mucosa 2 cm from the ulcer) were taken to be 100%, and the results obtained in the ulcerated mucosa (location up to 2 cm from the ulcer) were expressed as percentage values of their controls.

The tissue levels of ATP (Figure 1), ADP (Figure 2) and AMP (Figure 3) increased significantly around the ulcerated antral, duodenal and jejunal mucosa.

The ratio of ATP/ADP slightly decreased in the ulcerated antral mucosa ($p<0.05$), while it was significantly higher in the ulcerated duodenal ($p<0.001$) and jejunal ($p<0.001$) mucosa.

Adenylate pool (ATP+ADP+AMP) increased significantly around antral, duodenal and jejunal tissues (Figure 5).

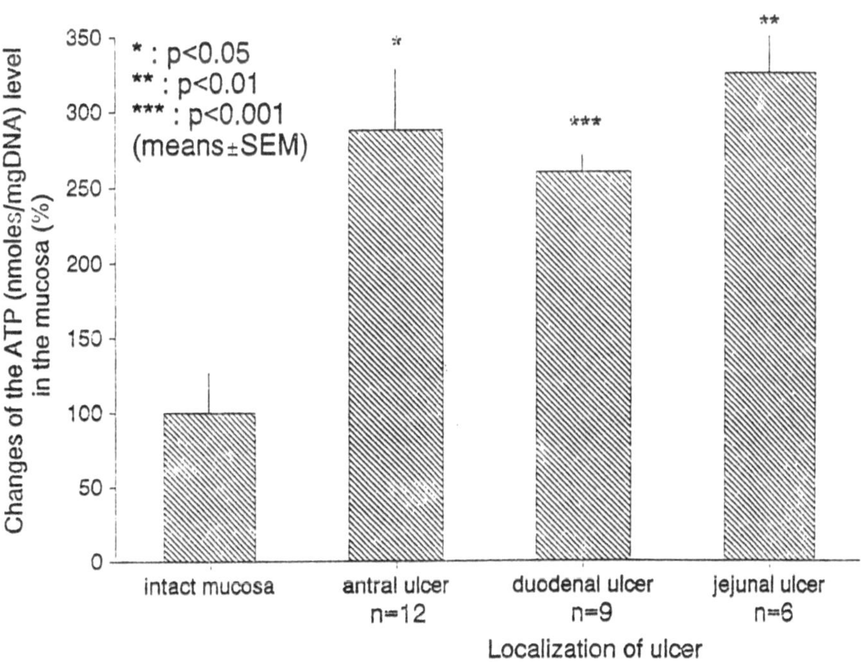

Figure 1. Changes in the ATP level of ulcerated mucosa in patients with antral, duodenal and jejunal ulcers compared with patients with intact mucosa in the same places

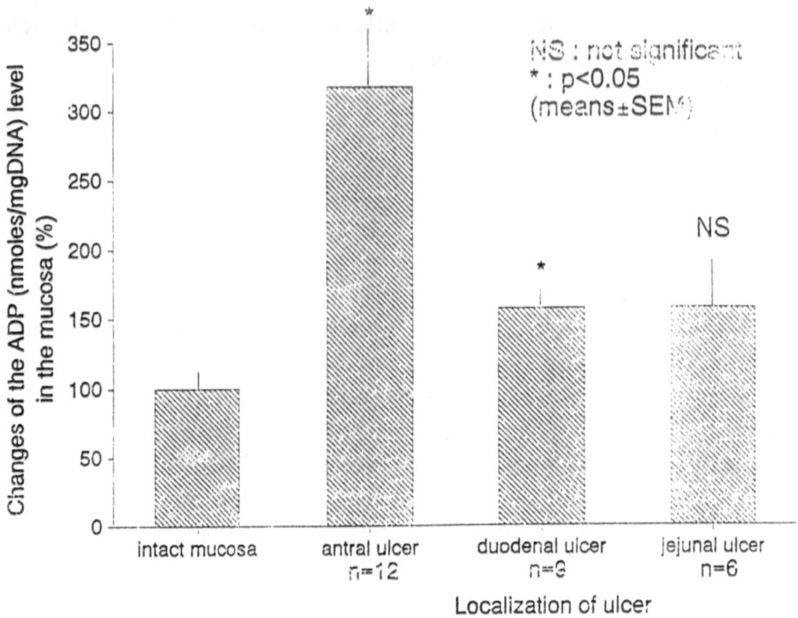

Figure 2. Changes in the ADP level of ulcerated mucosa in patients with antral, duodenal and jejunal ulcers compared with patients with intact mucosa in the same places

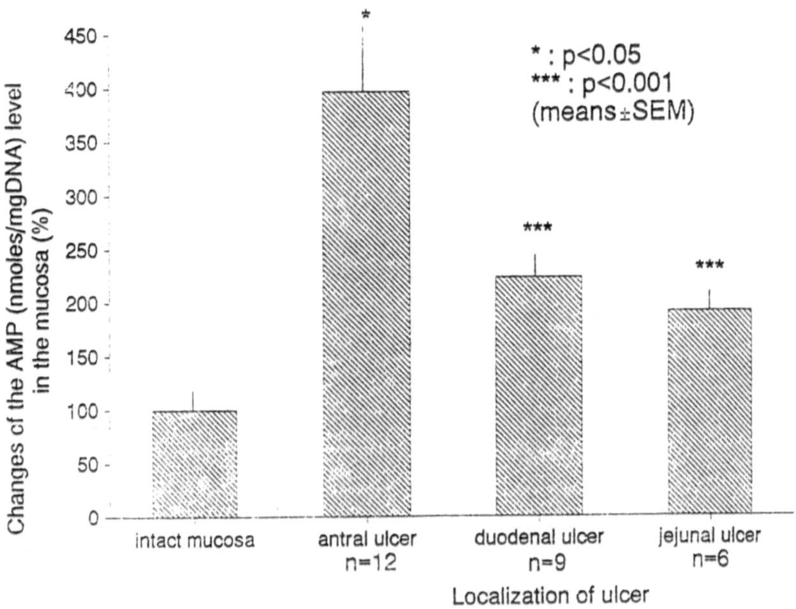

Figure 3. Changes in the AMP level of ulcerated mucosa in patients with antral, duodenal and jejunal ulcers compared with patients with intact mucosa in the same places

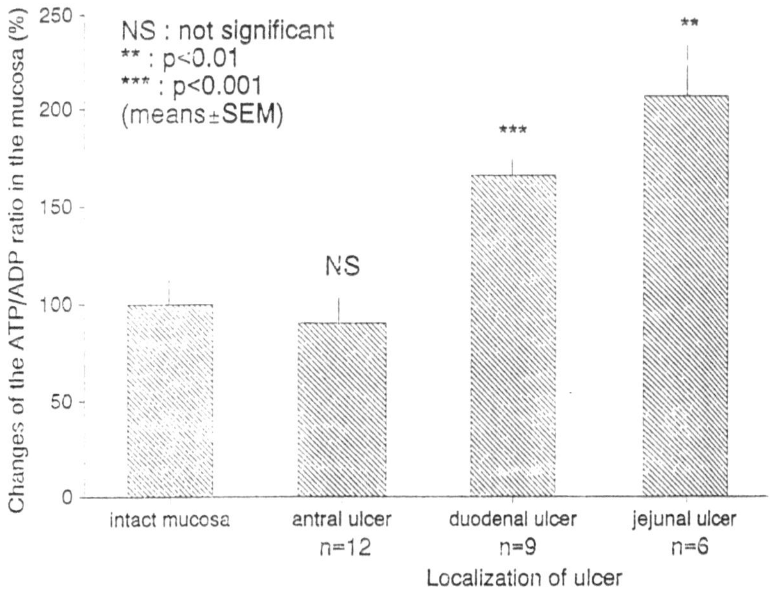

Figure 4. Changes in the ATP/ADP ratio of ulcerated mucosa in patients with antral, duodenal and jejunal ulcers compared with patients with intact mucosa in the same places

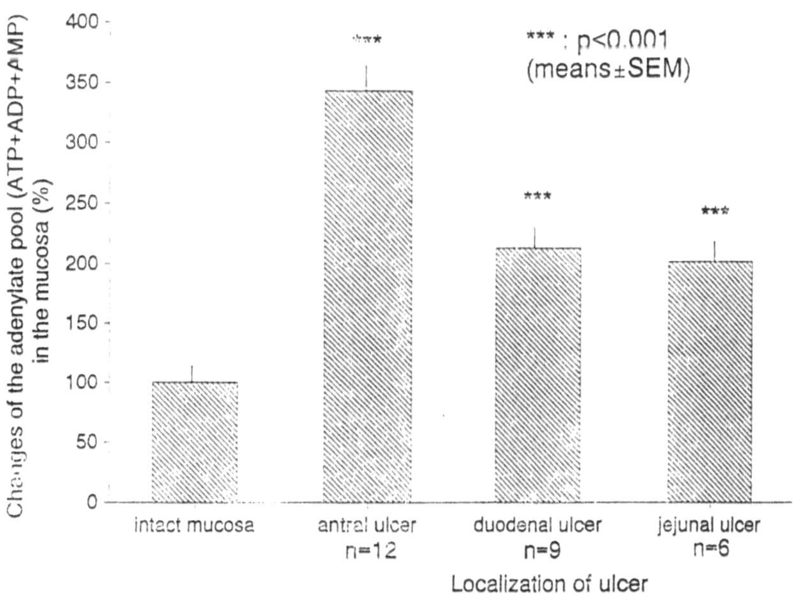

Figure 5. Changes in the adenylate pool (ATP+ADP+AMP) of ulcerated mucosa in patients with antral, duodenal and jejunal ulcers compared with patients with intact mucosa in the same places

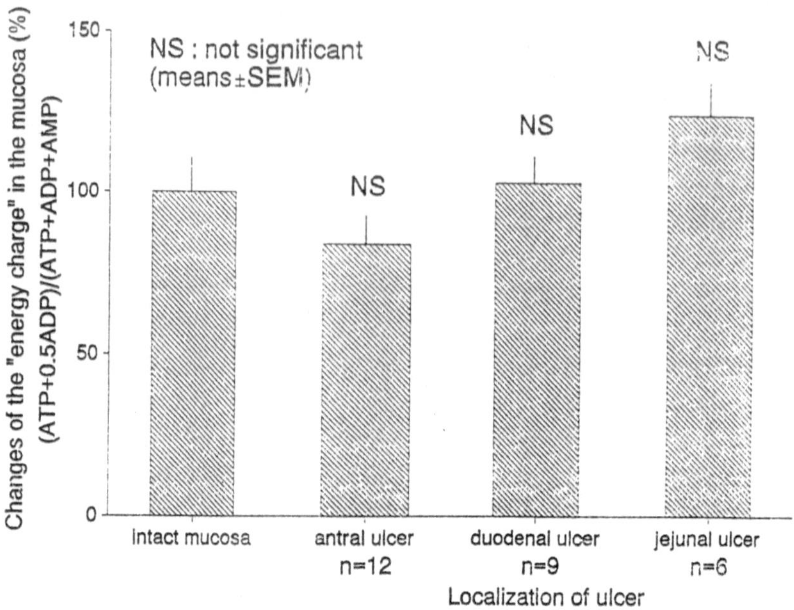

Figure 6. Changes in the 'energy charge' (ATP+0.5ADP)/(ATP+ADP+AMP) of ulcerated mucosa in patients with antral, duodenal and jejunal ulcers compared with patients with intact mucosa in the same places

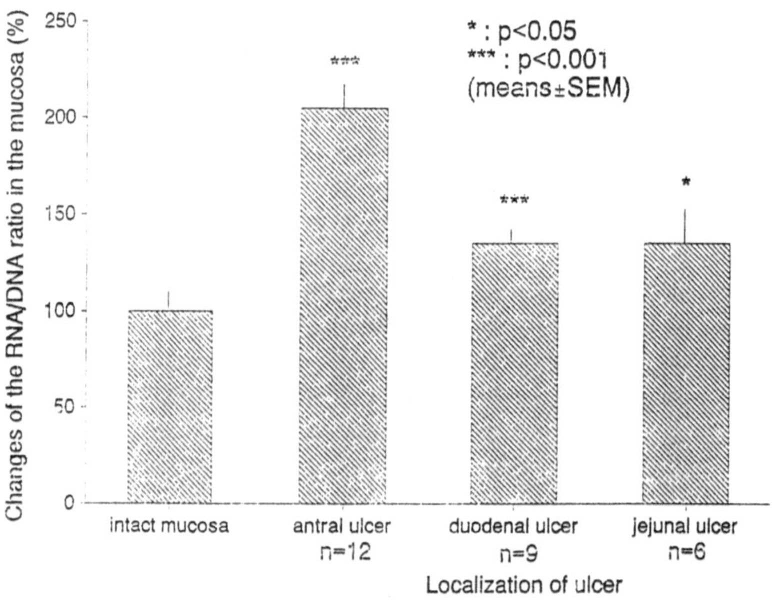

Figure 7. Changes in the RNA/DNA ratio in ulcerated mucosa of patients with antral, duodenal and jejunal ulcers compared with patients with intact mucosa in the same places

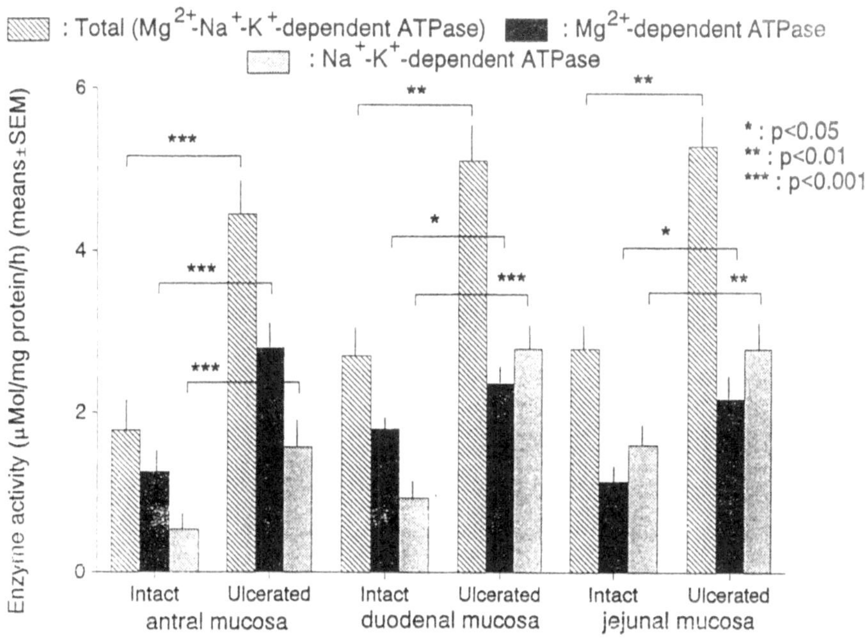

Figure 8. Changes in membrane-bound (Mg^{2+}-Na^{+}-K^{+}-dependent, Na^{+}-K^{+}-dependent and only Mg^{2+}-dependent) ATPases prepared from the non-ulcerated and ulcerated antral, duodenal and jejunal mucosa

Surprisingly, no significant differences was obtained in values (extents) or 'energy charge' in these types of ulcerated and non-ulcerated antral, duodenal and jejunal mucosa (Figure 6). However, the absolute values of biochemical parameters were higher in the non-ulcerated antral mucosa than in the duodenum and jejunum.

The changes in the ratio of RNA/DNA also increased in the tissues around antral, duodenal and jejunal ulcers (Figure 7).

When measuring the membrane (total, Mg^{2+}-dependent and Na^{+}-K^{+}-dependent) ATPase activity, we found a significant increase in the ulcerated mucosal specimens (Figure 8).

Adenosine phosphate compounds in the gastric (corpus, antral) and duodenal mucosa and musculature

The adenosine triphosphate (ATP), diphosphate (ADP), monophosphate (AMP), ratio of ATP/ADP, adenylate pool (ATP+ADP+AMP) and 'energy charge' were measured simultaneously from the gastric (corpus and antral) and duodenal mucosa and musculature in 41 patients with different gastric BAO and MAO values (Figures 9–14).

Significant amounts of ATP (Figure 9), ADP (Figure 10), AMP (Figure 11), adenylate pool (Figure 12) were measured in the corpus compared with antral and

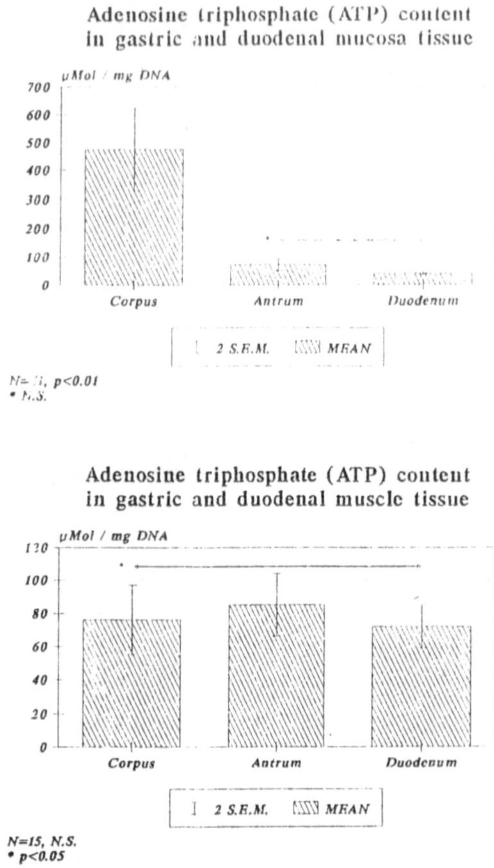

0 < Basal acid output < 6.5 mmol/h
0 < Maximal acid output < 22.5 mmol/h

Figure 9. ATP content in gastric (corpus and antral) and duodenal mucosal and muscle tissue of the corpus, antrum and duodenum in patients

duodenal mucosa. Smaller (but mathematically significant) differences were obtained in the antral vs. duodenal mucosa.

The ratio of ATP/ADP indicated a similar tendency in the gastric (corpus) vs. duodenal mucosa (Figure 13), while no difference was obtained in 'energy charge' (Figure 14).

The tissue content of adenine–adenosine was higher in corpus vs. antral vs. duodenal mucosa than in the musculature (Figure 15). However, no significant alteration was detected between the musculature specimens.

The average values of BAO (2.68 ± 0.33 mmol/h) and MAO (14.75 ± 1.04 mmol/h) indicated normal acidity in the examined 41 patients.

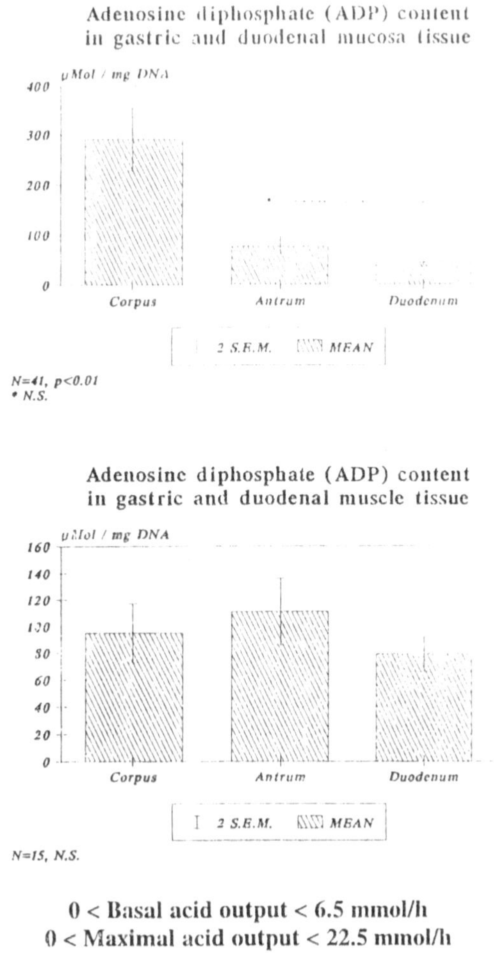

Figure 10. ADP content in gastric (corpus and antral) and duodenal mucosal and muscle tissue of the corpus, antrum and duodenum in patients

After sorting the patients into hyperacidic, normacidic and hypocidic groups, the following results were obtained:

1. The biochemical contents were significantly higher in corpus vs. antral vs. duodenal mucosa in hyperacidic patients (Figure 16);

2. The biochemical results showed similarities in the antral and duodenal mucosa, and were significantly higher in the corpus mucosa of the patients with normacidity (Figure 17);

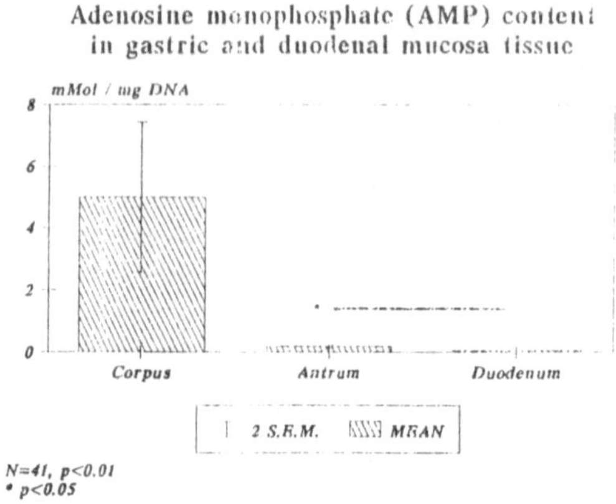

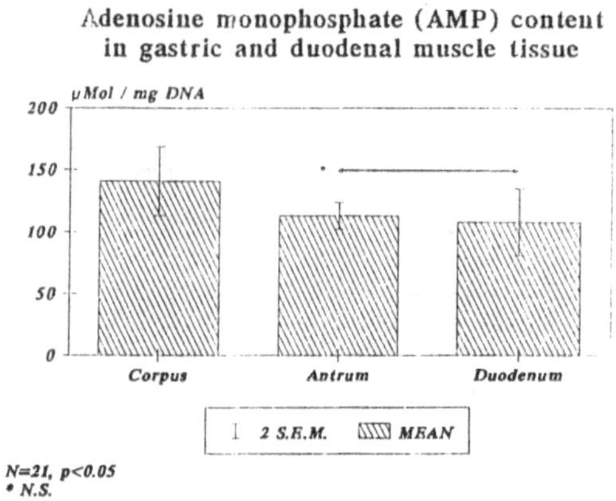

0 < Basal acid output < 6.5 mmol/h
0 < Maximal acid output < 22.5 mmol/h

Figure 11. AMP content in gastric (corpus and antral) and duodenal mucosal and muscle tissue of the corpus, antrum and duodenum in patients

3. No differences were obtained in the biochemical parameters of the gastric vs. duodenal mucosa of patients with decreased gastric BAO and MAO values (Figure 18).

Interestingly, the values of ATP/ADP and of 'energy charge' were practically the same in the corpus, antral and duodenal mucosal specimens of the different groups.

The membrane ATPase (including total, Mg^{2+}-dependent and Na^{+}-K^{+}-dependent) activities indicated a close correlation between the tissue levels of ATP and ADP.

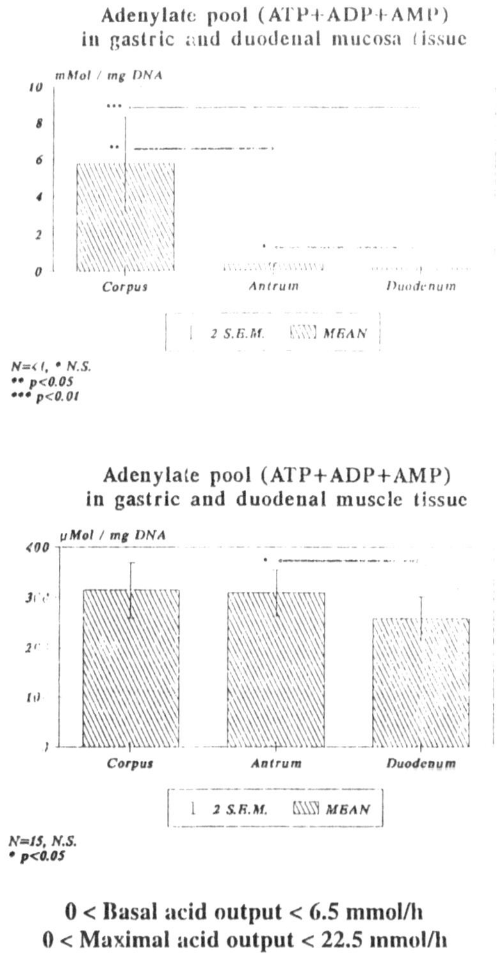

Figure 12. Adenylate pool (ATP+ADP+AMP) in gastric (corpus and antral) and duodenal mucosal and muscle tissue of the corpus, antrum and duodenun in patients

Molecular–pharmacological regulations of membrane-bound ATP-dependent energy systems in GI mucosal and musculature tissue specimens in patients

Many drugs, hormones and mediators regulate the activities of membrane-bound ATP-dependent energy systems [10,13]. The ATP–ADP transformation is more sensitive to the agents mentioned above than the ATP–cAMP transformation.

The affinity and intrinsic activity curves (and furthermore the pA_2, pD_2 and α values) of these compounds were determined. The possible physiological or pharmacological regulation due to these compounds and the causal interrelationships between the two energy systems were revealed by the results of these observations.

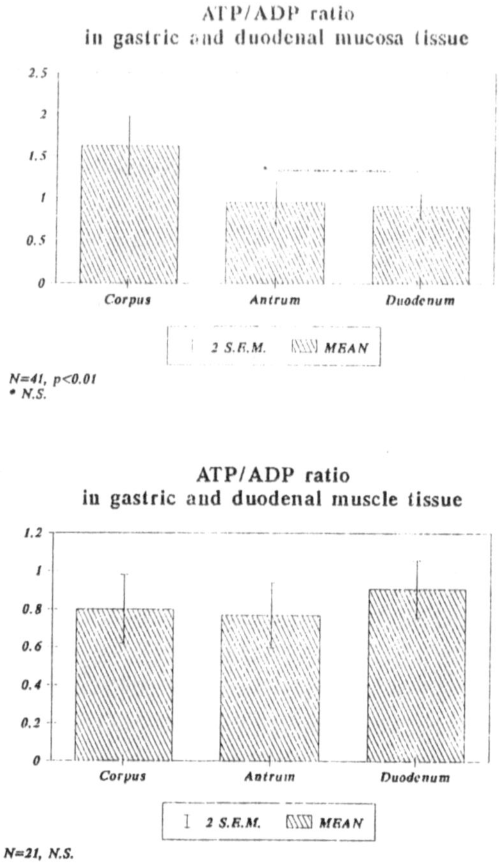

$0 <$ Basal acid output < 6.5 mmol/h
$0 <$ Maximal acid output < 22.5 mmol/h

Figure 13. ATP/ADP ratio in gastric (corpus and antral) and duodenal mucosal and muscle tissue of the corpus, antrum and duodenum in patients

The results were the same as those published in other papers [12]. Furthermore, the magnitudes of the effects of these drugs, mediators and hormones were dependent on the original magnitudes of the enzyme activities [see Reference 12].

DISCUSSION

The goals of this work were approached in several different ways:

1. By the biochemical evaluation of the ulcerated tissues located in the stomach, duodenum and jejunum;

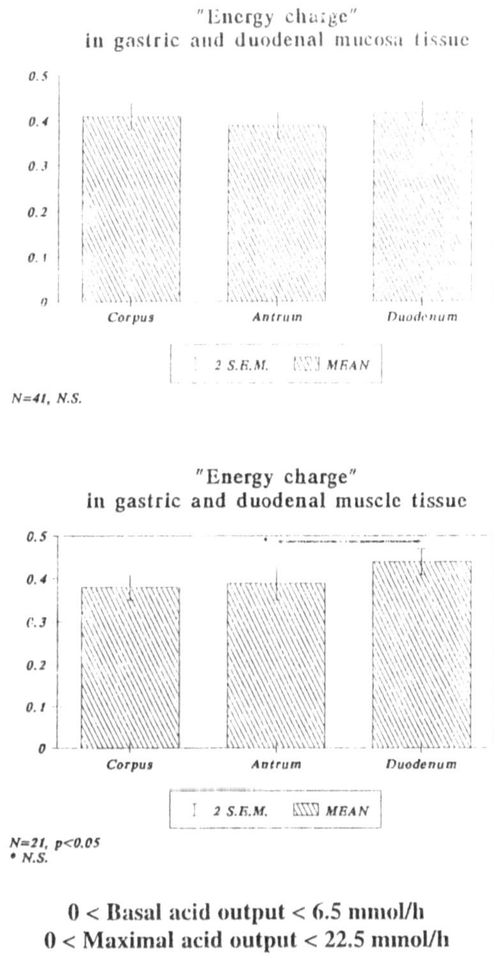

Figure 14. 'Energy charge' in gastric (corpus and antral) and duodenal mucosal and muscle tissue of the corpus, antrum and duodenum in patients

2. By the evaluation of the biochemical build up in the GI mucosal tissue specimens of patients with different basal (BAO) and maximal (MAO) secretory responses;

3. By the molecular–pharmacological approach to the membrane-bound ATP-dependent energy systems.

Before making these observations, similar experiments were performed on animals [7–9]. Of course, the conclusions drawn from the animal experiments were transformed to match the human problems, a process which was started at the end of the 1970s.

The biochemical measurements were made on the different tissue specimens of one

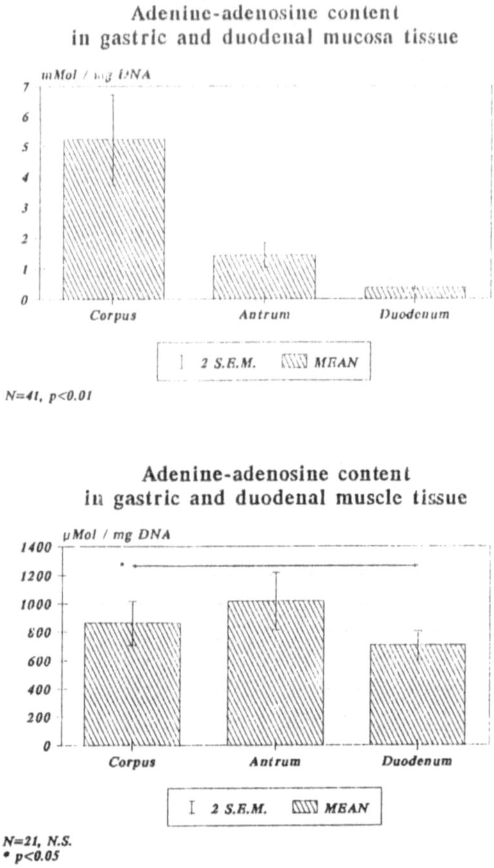

0 < Basal acid output < 6.5 mmol/h
0 < Maximal acid output < 22.5 mmol/h

Figure 15. Adenine–adenosine content in gastric (corpus and antral) and duodenal mucosal and muscle tissue of the corpus, antrum and duodenum in patients

patient in parallel so that possible technical errors would appear in the same manner. Furthermore, the measured contents were related to 1.0 mg of DNA, which represents the same number of cells in all cases.

A general biochemical approach to tissue biochemistry was used, involving the measurement of different biochemical parameters, such as adenosine compounds.

Cellular ATP is a storage molecule in animal cells. The actual level of ATP, in the different tissues, is determined by the equilibrium between ATP breakdown and its synthesis [10]. ATP is split in two ways, namely ATP–ADP transformation (by membrane ATPase) and ATP–cAMP transformation (by adenylate cyclase); ATP resynthesis occurs by intact oxidative phosphorylation. Intact oxidative phosphorylation can occur by two pathways:

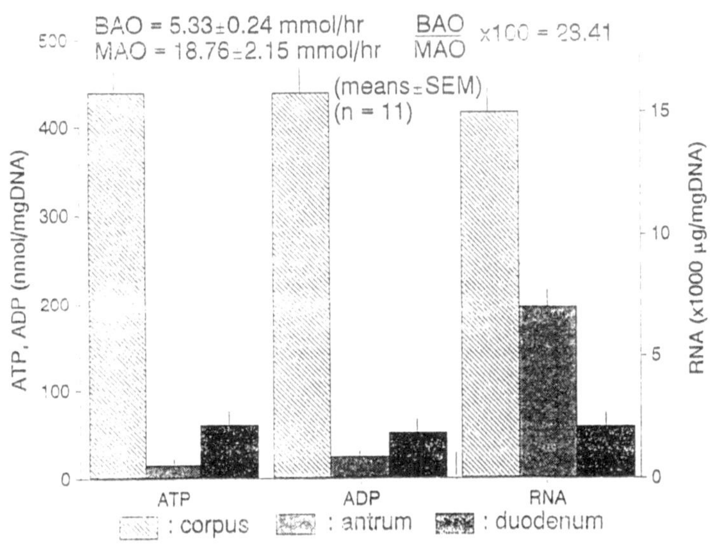

Figure 16. Absolute values of ATP, ADP, and RNA in the corpus, antrum and duodenum in hyperacid patients

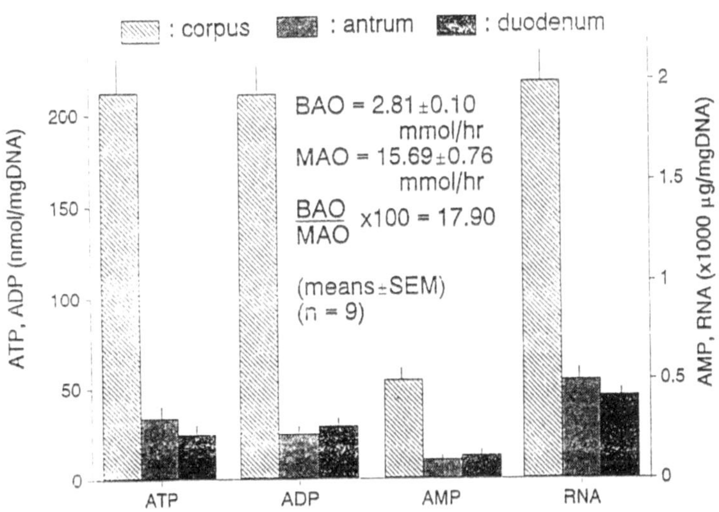

Figure 17. Absolute values of ATP, ADP, AMP and RNA in the corpus, antrum and duodenum in normacid patients

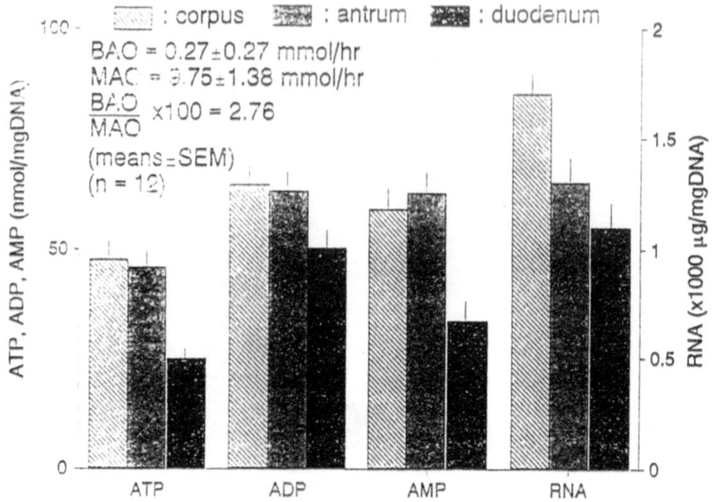

Figure 18. Absolute values of ATP, ADP, AMP and RNA in the corpus, antrum and duodenum in hypoacid patients with intact mucosa in the same places

1. In which the tissue lactate level does not change; and
2. In which the changes in the membrane-splitting enzyme and its substrate indicate parallel tendencies.

In our present study, the ATP–ADP transformation was detailed in different clinical situations: in ulcerated vs. non-ulcerated antral, duodenal and jejunal ulcers; in gastric corpus, antral and duodenal mucosa, without any ulceration; and, by the pharmacological testing of membrane ATPase and adenylate cyclase, gastric corpus, antral, duodenal and jejunal mucosa. Furthermore, the ratio of ATP/ADP, values of adenylate pool (ATP+ADP+AMP) and 'energy charge' [(ATP+0.5ADP)/(ATP+ADP+AMP)] were calculated based on biochemical results of observations.

The splitting of ATP to ADP by membrane ATPase provides a biochemical background of active movement of cations across the cell membrane. About 60–70% of total energy production of the cells is consumed by active transport of cations across the cell membranes.

The analysis of the biochemical results – in ulcerated vs. non-ulcerated mucosa of the antrum, duodenum and the jejunum – excludes hypoxaemic damage to mucosal tissues around antral, duodenal and jejunal mucosa in patients with 'genuine' ulcers. These statements are based on:

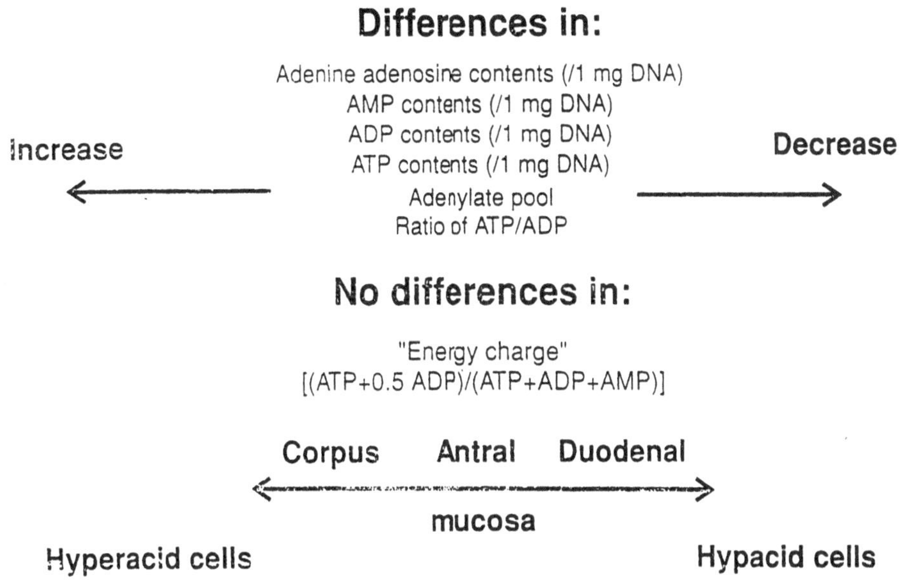

Figure 19. Schematic conclusions representing the comparison of corpus, antral and duodenum mucosal biochemistry in hyperacid and hypoacid patients

1. Increased tissue levels of ATP and ADP, in association with increased membrane ATPase activity in all types (antral, duodenal and jejunal) of mucosa around the ulcers. Interestingly, the value of 'energy charge' is unchanged;

2. The biochemical make-up of ulcerated antral, duodenal and jejunal mucosa is similar to that obtained from the gastric fundic mucosa of hyperacid patients. These patients showed gastric hypersecretion (the biochemical results were calculated per 1.0 mg DNA; membrane ATPase activity was calculated per 1.0 mg membrane protein).

These results demonstrate that increased energy metabolism exists in the ulcerated antral, duodenal and jejunal mucosa of patients with 'genuine' ulcers. These results are in contrast with suggested hypoxaemic damage of mucosal tissues in proven forms of ulcers. The biochemical observations give a cross-section of tissue energy metabolism. The changes in blood-flow can be obtained under physiological circumstances or massive bleeding.

Similar results were obtained in animal experiments under different experimental conditions [7–9]. If the tissue level of ATP decreases rapidly (without increase in tissue lactate), this indicates an enormous ATP breakdown (so that ATP breakdown and resynthesis can be separated under experimental conditions) [10].

The appearance of 'genuine' ulcer represents the insufficient metabolic adaptation to stimuli reaching the upper part of the GI tract (primarily HCl). The extent of positive metabolic adaptation depends on the original biochemical build up (reserves) of mucosal tissue in the stomach as well as in the proximal part of the small intestine (in the duodenum when there has been no previous surgery and in the jejunum after partial gastrectomy according to the Billroth II method). There are energy and biochemical gradients between corpus vs. antrum and antrum vs. duodenum in patients with gastric hyperacidity; similar gradients exist between corpus vs. antrum and smaller gradient between antrum vs. duodenum in patients with normal gastric secretions. Interestingly, no biochemical and energy gradient exists between corpus vs. antrum or between antrum vs. duodenum in patients with decreased gastric acid secretion (Figure 19).

The endogenous HCl produced by parietal cells located in the gastric corpus mucosa suggests a high energy production. The HCl reaches the antral and duodenal mucosa, in contrast with the jejunal mucosa after Billroth II resection. The gastric or small intestinal mucosa responds by increasing metabolic adaptation (theoretically only a positive or a negative metabolic adaptation due to the different endogenous or exogenous stimuli). The mucosal injury can be produced by an extremely increased metabolism (as in acute pancreatitis) or by an extremely decreased metabolism (as in massive bleeding). Of course, ulcer disease is a multifactorial process in the initial phase of the disease; however, a few factors will dominate in the tissues around the ulcer. There is no question that the biochemical structure (in terms of adenosine metabolism) is exactly the same in ulcerated gastric antral, duodenal and jejunal mucosa as in corpus mucosa (without ulcer). Furthermore, significant energy and biochemical gradients exist between corpus vs. antral and antral vs. duodenal (or jejunal) mucosa in patients with different gastric acid secretion rates (without ulcer); also, significant energy and biochemical gradients exist between non-ulcerated vs. ulcerated mucosa in the antrum, duodenum and jejunum. The capacity of mucosal tissues for positive metabolic adaptation is limited by the original energy and biochemical background of normal mucosal tissues. The duodenal mucosa is a more vulnerable tissue, in terms of metabolic adaptation, than the antral mucosa in hyperacid patients. A similar situation can be found in the jejunal mucosa vs. corpus (or antral) mucosa in patients after Billroth II gastric resection. This could be due to a positive metabolic adaptation caused by the endogenously produced HCl. In patients with normal or decreased gastric acidity, the HCl usually reaches the antral mucosa (and not the duodenum) so this situation may explain the location of 'genuine' ulcer in the duodenum. The 'genuine' ulcer (with typical histological features) without any HCl production is a rarity in clincial practice.

The mediators, hormones and drugs regulate adenosine metabolism in gastric and small intestinal mucosa at the level of the cell membrane (involving the membrane ATPase and adenylate cyclase) and intracellularly (involving the different products of ATP breakdown) [17]. The existence of a very complex feedback system has been proven between membrane-bound ATP-dependent energy systems in different experimental [10] and clinical [10] circumstances.

The effects of drug actions and surgical vagotomy await detailed description in terms of this biochemical explanation of 'genuine' gastric (antral), duodenal and jejunal ulcers.

ACKNOWLEDGEMENTS

This study was supported by grants from the Hungarian Welfare Ministry (ETT-03 660/93) and the Hungarian Research Fund (OTKA T 020098).

The authors acknowledge thanks to Margaret Jermás and Rosalie Nagy for their excellent help.

REFERENCES

1. Mózsik Gy, Jávor T, eds. Progress in Peptic Ulcer. Budapest: Akadémiai Kiadó; 1976.
2. Mózsik Gy, Hanninen O, Jávor T, eds. Gastrointestinal Defense Mechanisms. Advances in Physiological Sciences. Vol. 29. Oxford: Pergamon Press – Budapest: Akadémiai Kiadó; 1981.
3. Mózsik Gy, Pár A, Bertelli A, eds. Recent Advances of Gastrointestinal Cytoprotection. Budapest: Akadémiai Kiadó; 1984.
4. Mózsik Gy, Jávor T, Kitajama M et al., eds. Advances in gastrointestinal cytoprotection: Topics 1987. Acta Physiol Hung. 1989;72:111–391.
5. Mózsik Gy, Pár A, Csomós G et al., eds. Cell Injury and Protection in the Gastrointestinal Tract: From Basic Sciences to Clinical Perspectives. Budapest: Akadémiai Kiadó; 1993.
6. Rainsford KD, Mózsik Gy, Nagy L, Pár A, eds. Cell Injury and Protection in Gastrointestinal Tract: From Basic Sciences to Clinical Perspectives. Lancaster, UK: Kluwer Academic Publishers; 1986.
7. Mózsik Gy, Jávor T. A biochemical and pharmacological approach to the genesis of ulcer disease: I. A model study of ethanol-induced injury to gastric mucosa in rats. Dig Dis Sci. 1988;33:92–105.
8. Mózsik Gy, Garamszegi M, Jávor T et al. A biochemical and pharmacological approach to the genesis of ulcer disease: II. A model study of stress induced injury to gastric mucosa in rats. Ann NY Acad Sci. 1990;517:264–81.
9. Mózsik Gy, Pfeiffer CJ. A biochemical and pharmacological approach to the genesis of ulcer disease: III. A model study of epinephrine-induced injury to gastric mucosa in rats. Exp Clin Gastroenterol. 1992;2:196–200.
10. Mózsik Gy, Király Á, Sütő G, Vincze Á. ATP breakdown and resynthesis in the development of gastrointestinal mucosal damage and its prevention in animals and humans. Acta Physiol Hung. 1992;80:39–80.
11. Rainsford KD, Gaginella T, Mózsik Gy, eds. Biochemical Pharmacology as an Approach to Gastrointestinal Diseases: From Basic Science to Clinical Perspectives. Dordrecht: Kluwer Academic Publishers; 1997.
12. Mózsik Gy, Debreceni A, Juricskay I, Nagy L. Biochemical energetical backgrounds and their regulation in the gastric corpus mucosa in patients with different gastric secretory responses. In: Rainsford KD, Gaginella T, Mózsik Gy, eds. Biochemical Pharmacology as an Approach to Gastrointestinal Diseases: From Basic Science to Clinical Perspectives. Dordrecht: Kluwer Academic Publishers; 1997: 199–223.
13. Atkinson DE. The energy charge of the adenylate pool as a regulatory parameter. Interaction with feedback mediators. Biochemistry. 1968;7:4030–4.
14. Mózsik Gy, Figler M, Nagy L, Patty I, Tárnok F. Gastric and small intestinal energy metabolism in mucosal damage. In: Mózsik Gy, Hanninen O, Jávor T, eds. Advances in Physiological Sciences. Vol. 20. Gastrointestinal Defense Mechanisms. Oxford: Pergamon Press – Budapest: Akadémiai Kiadó; 1981:213–76.
15. Mózsik Gy, Figler M, Morón F, Nagy L, Patty I, Tárnok F. Molecular biochemistry and pharmacology of peptic ulcer treatment (review). Acta Med Hung. 1987;44:2–29.
16. Schmidt G, Tannhauser SJ. Method for determination of deoxyribonucleic acid, ribonucleic acid and phosphoproteins in animal tissues. J Biol Chem. 1945;161:83–9.
17. Mózsik Gy. Some feedback mechanisms by drugs in the interrelationship between the active transport system and adenylate cyclase system localized in the cell membrane. Eur J Pharmacol. 1969;7:319–27.
18. Mózsik Gy, Nagy L, Kutas F, Tárnok F. Interaction of cholinergic function with Mg^{+}-Na^{+}-K^{+}-dependent ATPase system of cells in the human fundic gastric mucosa. Scand J Gastroenterol. 1974;9:741–5.

19. Lowry OH, Rosenbrough NJ, Farr AL, Randal RJ. Protein measurements with folin phenol reagent. J Biol Chem. 1951;193:265–75.
20. Kleinbaum D, Kupper L, eds. The correlation coefficient and its relationship to straight-line regression analysis. In: Applied Regression Analysis. Boston: Duxbury Press; 1981:78–81.

Manuscript received 5 Nov. 95.
Accepted for publication 29 Dec. 95.

Section VI

MOLECULAR MECHANISMS OF PREMALIGNANT AND MALIGNANT DISEASES IN GI TRACT

TS Gaginella et al. (eds.), Biochemical Pharmacology as an Approach to Gastrointestinal Disorders, 337–346

CURRENT PROBLEMS AND RESULTS OF TUMOUR IMMUNOLOGY: DIAGNOSTIC AND THERAPEUTIC RELEVANCE OF TUMOUR-ASSOCIATED ANTIGENS

P. NEMETH[1*], T. BERKI[1] AND B. MARKUS[2]
[1]Immunological and Biotechnological Laboratory, University Medical School of Pécs;
[2]Department of General Surgery, Markusovszky Hospital, Szombathely, Hungary
*Correspondence

ABSTRACT

Tumour immunology is one of the most intensively studied fields of the medical/biological sciences this century. However, the clinical problems of tumour patients have not yet been completely solved. Immunological control of tumour growth has been investigated thoroughly and different escape mechanisms for tumour cells have been discovered recently. In spite of promising results, no appropriate generally accepted strategy has been developed. Targeting the tumour-associated antigens seems to be advantageous for both diagnosis and therapy.

Various monoclonal antibodies for diagnostic use have already been developed at our institute. During a retrospective study, remarkable prognostic relevances were defined with transforming growth factor (TGFα) and tumour necrosis factor (TNFα) on 82 breast-cancer patients.

In another experimental series, a new photoimmunotargeting method was developed for selective destruction of unwanted cell populations including tumour cells in vitro and (experimentally) in vivo. Gastrointestinal adenocarcinomas transplanted into nude mice were targeted successfully by this technique.

The paper reviews the main aspects of current tumour immunology using some of our own new results.

Keywords: tumour immunology, tumour-associated antigens, TNFα, TGFα, cytokines, immunotargeting, photoimmunotargeting

INTRODUCTION

Tumour immunology is one of the most intensively studied fields of the medical/biological sciences this century. The first experiments on transplanted tumours of experimental animals began more than one hundred years ago. These early investigations resulted in one of the biggest discoveries of molecular immunology: Goerer and his co-workers described the major histocompatibility antigens (named MHC) and the heredity and genetic localization of these antigens. It is peculiar: the discovery of MHC (in human named HLA) due to the tumour immunology [1]. During this century other important theoretical and practical immunological results were developed as 'side-products' of tumour biology. However, the clinical problems of the tumour patients have not been completely solved so far. Immunological control of tumour growth has

This paper was presented at the Section of IUPHAR GI Pharmacology Symposium on 'Biochemical pharmacology as an approach to gastrointestinal disorders (basic science to clinical perspectives)', October 12–14, 1995, Pécs, Hungary.

been investigated well and different escape mechanisms for tumour cells have been discovered recently. In spite of promising results in detail, no appropriate generally accepted strategy has been established [2].

A hypothesis for a basic role in human tumour development of immunological responsiveness and insufficiency against tumours and the theory of tumour-specific antigens have been put forward occasionally but have never been confirmed. These misconceptions have led to new research activities for possible specific immunotherapy of tumours [3,4]. However, these investigations for tumour-specific antigens have resulted in the correct analysis of the differences between chemically induced, virus-induced and spontaneously occurring tumours. A further important result of the tumour–biological experiments in recent decades is the discovery of different oncofetal (e.g. AFP, CEA) and differentiation antigens (e.g. βhCG, EGF, TGF) expressed by different tumour tissues. These tumour-associated antigens probably play no major role in tumour genesis; however, they have significant practical importance both in the diagnosis and treatment of tumour patients [5].

Practical applications of monoclonal antibodies for diagnostic use were developed at our institute. During a retrospective study, remarkable prognostic relevance was found of transforming growth factor (TGFα) and tumour necrosis factor (TNFα) in breast-cancer patients [6,7]. Similar analysis of the malignant tumours of the gastrointestinal system is under investigation.

In another experimental series, a new photoimmunotargeting method was developed for selective destruction of unwanted cell populations, including tumour cells in vitro and (experimentally) in vivo. Different tumour models, including gastrointestinal adenocarcinomas, were transplanted into nude mice and were targeted successfully by this technique [8].

The main goal of the present paper is to suggest new applications of tumour-associated antigens in experimental and clinical oncology.

PROGNOSTIC RELEVANCE OF IMMUNOHISTOCHEMICAL DETECTION OF TGFα AND TNFα ON TUMOUR TISSUES

It has already been confirmed that different cancer cells are able to synthesize and secrete various tissue hormones, growth factors (e.g. EGF, TGFα) and their receptors [9,10]. These cytokines may stimulate tumour growth by autocrine and/or paracrine mechanisms [11,12]. According to another hypothesis, cytotoxic cytokines, e.g. tumour necrosis factor (TNF) are applicable in antineoplastic treatment based on experimental and clinical investigations [13,14]. Though direct antitumour action of TNFα was described in accordance with in vitro and in vivo experiments, in many patients with malignant tumours, elevated endogenous TNF production was found [15,16]. The detection and function of different cytokines in tumour-bearing patients may have prognostic relevance concerning the disease [17,18]. The local effect of these cytokines on tumour cells is significantly greater in importance than the general effect. Histological/immunohistochemical techniques for the analysis of cytokines in tumour tissues seems to be optimal.

Monoclonal antibodies against TGFα and TNFα have been developed in our department previously [6,7] and used in routine pathohistological specimens in a retrospective study. The prognostic role of these cytokines in breast-cancer cases was analysed statistically [6].

A retrospective study was performed on 82 primary-breast-cancer patients (age 34–79 years) treated between January 1, 1986 and December 31, 1988 at the Department of General Surgery of Markusovszky Hospital (Szombathely, Hungary). TNM stages of tumour patients were clinically classified, and tumour recurrence, lymph-node involvement, and survival time were regularly recorded for more than 5 years after surgical treatment. The recording of data from patients ended on 31 May, 1994. All the patients were treated by generally accepted protocols [7]. The surgically removed tumour tissues were examined using our monoclonal antibodies.

Synthetic peptide fragments of TGFα (sequence 34–43) and TNFα (sequence 115–130) were the original antigens for hybridoma production in the classic way [19]. The specificity of our antibodies was controlled by human recombinant TNFα (E. Duda, BRC Szeged, Hungary) and TGFα (Peninsula Labs, USA). Monoclonal antibodies were selected by simple binding and competition ELISA [20] examined by both synthetic and human recombinant antigens. The anti-TGFα and anti-TNFα monoclonal antibodies were characterized immunocytochemically as well. Clones were selected for immunoreactivity both in native (frozen) and formol-paraffin tissue sections [21]. Monoclonal antibodies were prepared by in vitro hybridoma fermentation using Harvestmouse (Serotec, UK) hollow-fibre fermentor and purified by protein G affinity chromatography (FPLC, Pharmacia, Sweden).

The surgically removed tumour tissues were fixed routinely in formaldehyde solution (4% v/v) and embedded in paraffin as usual. Tissue sections (4 μm) were stained for daily histopathological examination. The tumour-positive samples were analysed immunohistochemically by our anti-TGFα and anti-TNFα monoclonal antibodies by direct immunoperoxidase technique according to the standard protocols [20,23]. The immunoreactivity of anti-TNFα and anti-TGFα monoclonal antibodies was examined microscopically and scored visually.

The statistical correlation between TGFα and TNFα expressed in the tumours, and the clinical prognostic factors (TNM stage, lymph node involvement, survival time, tumour recurrence) were evaluated by chi-square probe.

Results and discussion of the immunohistochemical study of 82 breast cancers

The histological localization of TGFα and TNFα showed focal appearance in the tumour tissues. TGFα occurred mainly in the cytoplasm of tumour cells localized in scars. TNFα staining was found both in the cytoplasm and in the extracellular space around the tumour cells.

Distribution of the TGFα and TNFα expression in 82 breast cancers is shown in Table 1. The correlation between TGFα and TNFα expression and survival time and tumour recurrence can be seen in Table 2. Significant negative correlation ($p < 0.05$) was found between TGFα production in tumour cells and the recurrence of tumours

TABLE 1
The TGFα and TNFα expression of 82 primary breast cancer tissues detected immunohistochemically

	TNFα+	TNFα–	Total number
TGFα+	24	17	41
TGFα–	12	29	41
Total number	36	46	82

TABLE 2
Correlation between TGFα/TNFα expression and the survival time and tumour recurrence

	TNFα+	TGFα–	TGFα+	TNFα–
Survival <5 y	5	8	15	18
Recurrent tumour	7	4	4	1
Tumour free	24	29	22	27
Total number	36	41	41	46

TABLE 3
Correlation between the co-expression of TGFα and TNFα and the prognostic values

	TGFα– TNFα+	TGFα+ TNFα+	TGFα– TNFα–	TGFα+ TNFα–
Survival <5 y	1	4	6	11
Recurrent tumour	3	4	1	0
Tumour free	8	16	22	6
Total number	12	24	29	17

and/or survival time. Co-expression of both TGFα and TNFα, or exclusive expression of TNFα, indicates a relatively good prognosis ($p<0.05$; Table 3). The TGFα and TNFα expression were not significantly associated with TNM score or the pathohistological type in our preliminary study (data not shown) [6,7].

The technique of surgical treatment of malignant tumours has recently been changed from radical mastectomy to the partial quadrectomy or the simple mastectomy [24]. Finding new prognostic factors has great clinical importance. According to different in vivo and in vitro studies, TGFα has been described as an autocrine and paracrine mediator of tumour growth [11,23]. Several laboratories have described the expression of TGFα in different tumour tissues [24,25] but it was not associated with TNM score or lymph node status [24] corresponding to our results.

Some literature data suggests that TNFα might be an endogenous antineoplastic agent [26] but the role of increased TNF production in malignancy has remained unclear [14,27]. According to other experiments, TNFα increases the number of EGF receptors which may be related to the mitogenic activity of TNF [28,29]. On the other hand, TGFα and EGF interfere with the cytostatic activity of TNF on cervix carcinoma cell lines in vitro in a dose-dependent manner [30].

Our study was initiated to determine the TGFα and TNFα content of primary breast cancers, investigated by monoclonal antibodies immunohistochemically on a statistically homogeneous group of breast-cancer patients. We compared the levels of TGFα and TNFα in the tumour tissue to the progression and recurrence of disease after surgical treatment for more than five years. Our findings that TGFα occur in a proportion of breast cancers and that they can be detected by monoclonal antibodies corresponds to some other observations [16]. However, in our follow-up study, TGFα-positive patients had a significantly worse prognosis ($p<0.05$) than patients who were TNFα-positive, TGFα/TNFα co-expressing, or who expressed neither of them. The interaction of TGFα and other growth factors with TNFα in tumour proliferation is poorly understood [30]. Some results suggest that production of growth factors by certain tumour cells might account for their TNFα-resistant phenotype in vitro [30]. Further studies are necessary to investigate the biological effect of locally occurring TNFα and/or TGFα on the progression and recurrence of malignant tumours. It would be important both theoretically and clinically to learn more details about the in vivo effects of these cytokines.

According to our experiments, the immunohistological detection of TGFα and TNFα in breast-cancer tissues seems to be a simple technique suitable for routine pathohistology. A series of human tumours, including some of gastrointestinal origin, are under examination for anti-TGFα and anti-TNFα monoclonal antibodies in a multicentre study.

The conclusion of our current immunohistochemical investigations is that exclusive TGFα expression (without TNFα) can predict unfortunate biological behaviour of breast carcinomas in the early stages. TNFα expression suggests a beneficial clinical prognosis.

EXPERIMENTAL PHOTOIMMUNOTARGETING OF DIFFERENT CELL SURFACE ANTIGENS

The use of different photosensitizer dye molecules activated by visible or laser light has provided new possibilities in the treatment and diagnosis of different malignant tumours [31]. This so-called photodynamic therapy (PDT) [31,32] is based on the toxic effect of light-activated photosensitizer molecules, accumulated in the neoplastic tissue [33,34]. The haematoporphyrin (HP) molecules and their modified analogues (the so-called haematoporphyrin derivative, HPD) [33] are the most widespread photosensitizers. They become active and destructive to the living cells after light irradiation only [35]. Photon energy of visible light activates the molecule to its triplet energy state [36], which initiates a free-radical-generating chain reaction [37,38] finally causing peroxidation of lipid [39] and protein molecules present in the biological membranes [40–42] and thus leading to the destruction of different cellular components [32].

The specificity of the photosensitization can be enhanced by conjugating photosensitizer molecules to different carrier molecules, e.g. monoclonal antibodies (mAbs) recognizing surface markers of the targeted cell types [43]. In our previous study, an a-PNAr-I monoclonal antibody (IgG_1), reacting with human gastric cancer cells (and with the normal gastric mucosal chief cells as well) [8,43], was used as carrier for the photosensitizer haematoporphyrin (HP) molecules. The complex was used as immunotoxin in vivo in an animal model (human-gastric-cancer-bearing nude mice) [8]. The ability of the antibody–HP conjugate to kill the labelled tumour cells after irradiation was tested both macroscopically and microscopically.

Recently, we developed an in-vitro targeting model where mouse T lymphoid cell lines (EL4) and thymocytes (bearing the Thy-1. antigen) were used for testing the toxic effect of an HP–mAb conjugate (HP–a-Thy-1., produced in our laboratory) [50] after visible light irradiation. The selectivity of the method was detected by treating a mixed cell population consisting of a Thy-1.-positive (EL4) and a Thy-1.-antigen-negative cell line with the HP–Thy-1. conjugate. This procedure can serve as a preliminary experiment for the selective killing of unwanted cell populations (e.g. in bone marrow purging).

The a-Thy-1. monoclonal antibody was covalently crosslinked through EDC1 to HP molecules in our recent experiment [44]. The chemical coupling reaction had no destructive effect on the antigen-binding ability of the antibodies controlled by immunocytochemistry. Both the monoclonal antibody and its HP conjugate at equivalent concentrations selectively recognize Thy-1.-antigen-bearing cell types, e.g. mouse thymocyte and T cell lines (e.g. EL4), while all B cell types (Sp-2/0 Ag-14, hybridomas) showed a negative reaction.

The cytotoxic potential of the conjugate was pretested in vitro on the EL4 cell line and mouse thymocytes, with Sp-2/0 Ag-14 cells as a negative control. The cells were treated with the HP–anti-Thy-1. conjugate (for 1 h at 4°C in the dark). The HP content of the conjugate ranged from 0 to 15 μg/ml HP (0–11 μg/ml mAb) and its effects were compared with those following the administration of free HP alone at the same concentrations (also at 37°C), or with mAb added alone, or culture medium as negative controls. After removing the unbound agents with intensive washing, the cells were

TABLE 4
Landagren colorimetric cell proliferation assay of in-vitro cultured EL-4 cells 48 h after photosensitization

	0.00 J/cm^2	10.0 J/cm^2
HP–a-Thyl.2 conjugates		
1.26 μg/ml HP + 10.0 μg/ml mAb	2.625	0.038
0.63 μg/ml HP + 5.0 μg/ml mAb	2.497	0.145
0.31 μg/ml HP + 2.5 μg/ml mAb	2.614	0.274
Free HP (1.0 μg/ml)	2.627	2.291
Free mAb (10.0 μg/ml)	2.467	2.302
Untreated	2.639	2.547

Numbers indicate average OD values measured at 405 nm in triplicates. mAb: monoclonal antibody; HP: haematoporphyrin

plated and irradiated either with a low-power He-Ne laser at 1–200 J/cm^2 energy level on 632.8 nm wavelength, or with an Hg-lamp at a wavelength peak of 400 nm at 2–12 J/cm^2, while the control samples (labelled, unirradiated) were kept in the dark. The viability of the cells was tested 1, 24 and 48 h after irradiation using proliferation assays [51].

The HP–anti-Thy-1. conjugate at 0.75 μg/ml HP concentration (5 μg/ml mAb) caused 98% EL4 cell destruction and 95% thymocyte death (see Table 4), while the control samples remained intact and cell proliferation could be observed microscopically 24 h later. The a-insulin hybridoma cell line and Sp-2/0 myeloma cells did not show any sign of photosensitization after the same treatment of the conjugate.

The selectivity of the method was measured in mixed cell populations, where EL4 cells and hybridoma cells were mixed at 1:1 ratio, treated with the conjugate at the above mentioned concentrations and/or HP alone, or mAb alone and irradiated with the Hg-lamp at 400 nm wavelength peak. Twenty-four hours later the cell viability was measured by trypan blue dye exclusion test and the cells were examined by immunocytochemistry for Thy-1. expression and antibody production, respectively. The photosensitization following treatment with the conjugate induced the selective disappearance of the Thy-1.-positive cells (data not shown).

A new phototargeting method has been developed, which can be used effectively both in vitro and in vivo for selective cell destruction. The photochemical treatment of malignant tumours has already been extensively investigated in animal models and human diseases [31,44,46]. The light-activated haematoporphyrin has been shown to be effective in the treatment of different malignant carcinomas, sarcomas and melanomas [36,45]. Unfortunately, the sensitizer molecules at the concentrations used in the protocols sometimes cause severe side-reactions in normal tissue, and the molecules cannot be used for in-vitro selective cell destruction [49].

The use of different protein carriers, specific for a cell surface antigen, as tools for selective cell destruction is another possibility for tumour treatment [46]. Monoclonal antibody technology has made it possible to produce antibodies with high antigen specificity, which, however, does not mean the same selectivity in the living material, since the epitope recognized by the antibody might be expressed on different components of living organism [47]. Using non-selective cytotoxic agents (e.g. ricin alpha chain, or bacterial toxins, e.g. diphtheria toxin A fragment) [47–49], toxic side-reactions in normal tissue, and unwanted cells frequently occur [48]. The combination of different, by themselves non-toxic, agents together with cytotoxic reagents, could decrease the non-specific side-reactions and increase the selectivity of the targeting methods. Our method combines a selective cell-labelling method with a local physical influence (light irradiation) to activate the cytotoxic HP molecules carried by a monoclonal antibody.

The amount of HP in the conjugate necessary for cell destruction was determined [50,51]. Compared with the free HP necessary for target cell destruction, a ten-fold lower amount of HP in the conjugate has proved effective. No side-effects at this low concentration of mAb, both in free and conjugated form, without irradiation have been observed. The mAbs permit concentration of the drug in the target cell type where the light activates the HP molecules to their excited free-radical-producing state, destroying cells.

ACKNOWLEDGEMENTS

The development of anti-TGFα and anti-TNFα monoclonal antibodies was supported by the National Council of Technical Development of Hungary (OMFB) (Project G-3, Grant No 13583/90). The retrospective study of the 82 breast-cancer patients was supported by the National Committee of Health Sciences (ETT) (Grant No. 187/94KO). The photoimmunotargeting experiments were supported by the National Scientific Foundation of the Hungarian Academy of Sciences (OTKA) (Grant No. 6215).

REFERENCES

1. Klein J. Natural History of the Major Histocompatibility Complex. New York: Wiley; 1986.
2. Siegel BV. Immunology and oncology. Int Rev Cytol. 1985;96:89–120.
3. Reisfeld RA, Cheresh DA. Human tumor antigens. Adv Immunol. 1987;40:323–77.
4. Zákány J, Jánossy T, Németh P, Chihara G, Fachet J, Petri G. Mechanism of the A/Ph.Mc.S1 tumor graft rejection in syngeneic mice. Gann (Jpn J Cancer Res). 1983;74:712–22.
5. Sulitzeanu D. Human cancer-associated antigens: present status and implications for immunodiagnosis. Adv Cancer Res. 1985;44:1–42.
6. Bêbok Zs, Márkus B, Brittig F, Németh P. Emlorákok szöveti TGF-α és TND-α tartalmának immunhisztokémiai vizsgálata és prognosztikai elemzése. Lege Artis Med. 1993;3:142–6.

7. Bebôk Zs, Márkus B, Németh P. Prognostic relevance of transforming growth factor alpha (TGF-α) and tumor necrosis factor alpha (TNF-α) detected in breast cancer tissues by immunohistochemistry. Breast Cancer Res Treat. 1994;29:229–35.
8. Berki T, Németh P. Photo-immune-targeting with low-power He-Ne laser activated hematoporphyrin conjugates. Cancer Immunol Immunother. 1992;35:69–74.
9. Sinkovics JG. Oncogenes and growth factors. Crit Rev Immunol. 1988;8:217–98.
10. McGuire WL, Dickson RB, Osborne CK, Salomon D. The role of growth factors in breast cancer (A panel discussion). Breast Cancer Res Treat. 1988;12:159–66.
11. Osborne CK, Arteaga CL. Autocrine and paracrine growth regulation of breast cancer: Clinical implications. Breast Cancer Res Treat. 1990;15:3–11.
12. Kurachi H, Morishige K, Amemiya K et al. Importance of transforming growth factor-α/epidermal growth factor receptor autocrine growth mechanism in an ovarian cancer cell line in vivo. Cancer Res. 1991;51:5956–9.
13. Sohmura Y, Nakata K, Yoshida H, Kashimoto S, Matsui Y, Furuichi H. Recombinant human tumor necrosis factor. II. Antitumor effect on murine and human tumors planted in mice. Int J Immunopharmacol. 1989;8:357–63.
14. Jakubowski A, Casper ES, Gabrilove JL, Templeton MA, Shervin SA, Oettgen HF. Phase I trial of intramuscularly administered tumor necrosis factor in patients with advanced cancer. J Clin Oncol. 1989;7:298–303.
15. Selby PJ, Hobbs S, Viner C, Jackson E, Smith IE, McElvain TJ. Endogenous tumor necrosis factor in cancer patients (Letter). Lancet. 1988;1:483.
16. Saarinen UM, Koskelo EK, Teppo AM, Siimes MA. Tumor necrosis factor in children with malignancies. Cancer Res. 1990;50:592–5.
17. Derynck R. Transforming growth factor-α: structure and biological activities. J Cell Biochem. 1986;32:203–4.
18. Old LJ. Tumor necrosis factor. In: Bonavida B, Granger G, eds. Tumor Necrosis Factor: Structure, Mechanisms of Action, Role in Disease and Therapy. Basel: Karger; 1990:1–30.
19. Köhler G, Milstein C. Continuous cultures of fused cells secreting antibody of predefined specificity. Nature (London). 1975;256:495–7.
20. Engvall E, Perlmann P. Enzyme-linked immunosorbent assay, ELISA. 3. Quantitation of specific antibodies by enzyme-labelled anti-immunoglobulin in antigen coated tubes. J Immunol. 1972;109:129–35.
21. Bebôk Zsuzsa, Szekeres Gy, Horváth Gy, Duda E, Németh P. Development and characterization of anti-TNFα and anti-TGFα monoclonal antibodies (In Hungarian). Orv Hetilap. 1993;134:1303–7.
22. Johnstone A, Thorpe R. Immunocytochemistry. In: Johnstone A, Thorpe R, eds. Immunochemistry in Practice. Oxford: Blackwell Scientific Publ; 1987:272.
23. Morishige K, Kurachi H, Amemiya K et al. Involvement of transforming growth factor α/epidermal growth factor receptor autocrine growth mechanisms in an ovarian cancer cell line *in vitro*. Cancer Res. 1991;51:5951–5.
24. Umekita Y, Enokizono N, Sagara Y et al. Immunohistochemical studies on oncogene products (EGF-R, c-erbB-2) and growth factors (EGF, TGF-α) in human breast cancer: their relationship to oestrogen receptor status, histological grade, mitotic index and nodal status. Virchows Archiv A Pathol Anat. 1992;420:345–51.
25. Finzi E, Ho T, Anhalt G, Hawkins W, Harkins R, Horn T. Localization of transforming growth factor-α in human appendageal tumors. Am J Path. 1992;141:643–53.
26. Carswell EA, Old LJ, Kassel RL, Green S, Fiore N, Williamson B. An endotoxin-induced serum factor that causes necrosis of tumors. Proc Natl Acad Sci USA. 1975;72:3666–70.
27. Cerami A. Inflammatory cytokines. Clin Immunol Immunopath. 1992;62:S3–10.
28. Baglioni C. Mechanisms of cytotoxicity, cytolysis, and growth stimulation by TNF. In: Beutler B, ed. Tumor Necrosis Factors: The Molecules and their Emerging Role in Medicine. New York: Raven Press Ltd; 1992:425–38.
29. Palombella V, Yamashiro JD, Maxfield FR, Decker SJ, Vilcek J. Tumor necrosis factor increases the number of epidermal growth factor receptors on human fibroblasts. J Biol Chem. 1987;262:1950–4.
30. Sugarman BJ, Lewis GD, Eessalu TE, Aggarwal B, Shepard HM. Effects of growth factors on the antiproliferative activity of tumor necrosis factor. Cancer Res. 1987;47:780–6.
31. Dougherty TJ. Hematoporphyrin derivative for detection and treatment of cancer. J Surg Oncol. 1980;15:209–12.
32. Allison AC, Magnus IA, Young MR. Role of lysosomes and cell membranes in photosensitization. Nature (London). 1966;209/5026:874.

33. Bugelsky PJ, Porter CW, Dougherty TJ. Autoradiographic distribution of HPD in normal and tumor tissue of mouse. Cancer Res. 1981;41:4606–13.
34. Tennant JR. Evaluation of trypan blue technic for determination of cell viability. Transplant. 1964;2:685–7.
35. Cowled PA, Grace JR, Forbes IJ. Comparison of the efficiency of pulsed and continuous-wave red laser light in induction of phototoxicity by HPD. Photochem Photobiol. 1984;39:115–19.
36. Bodaness RS, Heller DF, Krasinsky J, King DS. The two-photon laser induced fluorescence of the tumor-localizing photosensitizer hematoporphyrin derivative. J Biol Chem. 1986;261/26:12098–104.
37. Kimel S, Tromberg BJ, Roberts WG, Berns MW. Singlet oxygen generation of porphyrins, chlorines, and phthalocyanines. Photochem Photobiol. 1989;50:175–9.
38. Pótó L, Berki T. Investigation on the free radical producing effect of hematoporphyrin (a spin trapping study). Acta Physiol Hung. 1989;74:285–92.
39. Lakos Zs, Berki T. Effect ofhematoporphyrin-induced photosensitization on lipid membranes. J Photochem Photobiol B. 1995;29:185–91.
40. Berki T, Németh P, Pótó L, Németh Å. Effects of photosensitization and low-power He-Ne laser irradiation on liposomes and cell membranes. Scanning Microsc. 1991;5:1157–64.
41. Das M, Mukhtar H, Greenspan ER, Bickers DR. Photoenhancement of lipid peroxidation associated with the generation of reactive oxygen species in hepatic microsomes of hematoporphyrin derivative-treated rats. Cancer Res. 1985;45:6328–33.
42. Moan J, Vistnes AI. Porphyrin photosensitization of proteins in cell membranes as studied by spin-labelling and by quantification of DTNB-reactive SH-groups. Photochem Photobiol. 1986;44:15–18.
43. Németh P, Fischer J, Berki T. Differentiation of PNA-binding glycoprotein antigens by monoclonal antibodies. Acta Physiol Hung. 1988;71:122.
44. Mew D, Chi Kit Wat, Towers GH, Levy JG. Photoimmunotherapy: treatment of animal tumors with tumor-specific monoclonal antibody–hematoporphyrin conjugates. J Immunol. 1983;130:1473–7.
45. Gulliya KS, Pervaiz Sh. Elimination of clonogenic tumor cells from HL-60, Daudi, and U-937 cell lines by laser photoradiation therapy: implication for autologous bone marrow purging. Blood. 1989;73:1059–62.
46. Blythman HE, Casellas P, Gros O et al. Immunotoxins: Hybrid molecules of monoclonal antibodies and a toxin subunit specifically kill tumor cells. Nature (London). 1981;290:145–6.
47. Bernhard MJ, Foon KA, Oeltmann TN et al. Guinea pig line 10 hepatocarcinoma model: Characterization of monoclonal antibody and in vivo effect of unconjugated antibody and antibody conjugated to diphtheria toxin A chain. Cancer Res. 1983;43:4420–9.
48. Kishida K, Masuho Y, Saito M, Hara T, Fuji H. Ricin A-chain conjugated with monoclonal anti-L1210 antibody. In vitro and in vivo anti-tumor activity. Cancer Immunol Immunother. 1983;16:93–8.
49. Vitetta ES, Thorpe PE. Immunotoxins: In: New Avenues in Developmental Cancer Chemotherapy. New York: Academic Press; 1987:265.
50. Balogh P, Bebôk Zs, Németh P. Cellular enzyme-linked immunocircle assay. A rapid assay of hybridomas produced against cell surface antigens. J Immunol Meth. 1992;153:141–9.
51. Landegren U. Measurement of cell numbers by means of the endogenous enzyme hexosaminidase. Applications to detection of lymphokines and cell surface antigens. J Immunol Meth. 1984;67:379–88.

Manuscript received 6 Jan. 96.
Accepted for publication 18 Jan. 96.

Section VII

USE OF ISOLATED CELLS AND CELL CULTURES IN BIOCHEMICAL PHARMACOLOGICAL STUDIES TO APPROACH GI DISEASES

TS Gaginella et al. (eds.), Biochemical Pharmacology as an Approach to Gastrointestinal Disorders, 349–359

DOES OMEPRAZOLE-INDUCED HYPERGASTRINAEMIA CONTRIBUTE TO THE ENHANCED HEALING OF ACETIC ACID-INDUCED GASTRIC ULCERS IN RATS?

S. OKABE AND Y. TSUKIMI
Department of Applied Pharmacology, Kyoto Pharmaceutical University, Misasagi, Yamashina, Kyoto 607, Japan

This paper was first published in: Inflammopharmacology. 1996;4:267–277.

ABSTRACT

We examined the effects of omeprazole and SDZ CO-611 (an orally active somatostatin analogue) alone and in combination, on ulcer healing, gastric acid secretion and the serum gastrin level in rats. Two or 4-weeks' treatment with oral omeprazole significantly enhanced spontaneous healing and/or prevented delayed healing (caused by indomethacin) of acetic acid ulcers, with the inhibition of gastric acid secretion and hypergastrinaemia. While oral SDZ CO-611 had no effect on spontaneous ulcer healing, it significantly prevented delayed ulcer healing. On SDZ CO-611 treatment, gastric acid secretion was significantly inhibited but basal gastrin level remained unchanged. Hypergastrinaemia induced by a single treatment with oral omeprazole was markedly suppressed by SDZ CO-611 for >12 h. SDZ CO-611, administered together with omeprazole for 2 or 4 weeks, did not affect the enhanced ulcer healing or the antisecretory effect of omeprazole, despite a greater than 60% decrease. We conclude that omeprazole-induced hypergastrinaemia does not contribute to the mechanism by which omeprazole enhances ulcer healing.

Keywords: omeprazole, SDZ CO-611, somatostatin analogue, hypergastrinaemia, acetic acid ulcer

INTRODUCTION

The acid pump inhibitor, omeprazole, is a potent treatment for patients with Zollinger–Ellison syndrome, gastroduodenal ulcers, and reflux oesophagitis [1,2]. Even in animal studies, it apparently enhances the healing of chronic gastric ulcers [3–5]. Since omeprazole has potent and persistent antisecretory activity, long-term treatment with the drug invariably induces mild to profound hypergastrinaemia in both man and animals [6–9]. Gastrin has a trophic action on the oxyntic mucosa in the stomach, including on enterochromaffin-like cells (ECL-cells) [10–12]. Ryberg et al. [7] reported the increased incorporation of [^{3}H]thymidine in the oxyntic mucosa of rats with hypergastrinaemia caused by a 1-week treatment with omeprazole. Therefore, these results suggest that hypergastrinaemia caused by omeprazole is involved in the mechanism underlying the enhanced healing of experimental ulcers. Somatostatin inhibits gastrin release from G-cells in both in-vivo and in-vitro experiments [13–15]. Of interest, Cadiot et al. [16] reported that SMS 201-995, a somatostatin analogue,

This paper was presented at the Section of IUPHAR GI Pharmacology Symposium on 'Biochemical pharmacology as an approach to gastrointestinal disorders (basic science to clinical perspectives)', October 12–14, 1995, Pécs, Hungary.

significantly prevented the hypergastrinaemia caused by omeprazole and the trophic effect of hypergastrinaemia on the oxyntic mucosa in rats.

To elucidate the role of hypergastrinaemia in ulcer healing, we examined the effect of a new long-lasting, orally active somatostatin analogue, SDZ CO-611, on hypergastrinaemia and ulcer healing caused by omeprazole.

MATERIALS AND METHODS

Animals

Male Donryu rats (Nihon SLC, Shizuoka, Japan), weighing 240–260 g, were used in all experiments. The animals were not fasted prior to ulcer production to facilitate injection of the acetic acid solution into the gastric wall. Before the autopsy and secretory studies, they were fasted for 18 h in raised-mesh-bottom cages with free access to tap water. Between 8 and 21 rats were used for each study.

Induction of gastric ulcers

Gastric ulcers were induced by the previously reported method [17]. Briefly, under ether anaesthesia, the abdomen was incised and the anterior portion of the stomach exposed. Then, 0.03 ml of 20% acetic acid (v/v) was injected into the submucosal layer at the junction of the fundus and antrum, i.e. about 1 cm proximal to the pylorus. Postoperatively, the animals were maintained on rat chow and water ad libitum. Since well-defined and deep ulcers were observed 5 days later, we defined the 5th day as the day of ulceration. Two experiments were performed:

1. The effects of test compounds or the vehicle on the spontaneous healing of ulcers were determined with oral administration by gastric intubation once (9.30 am) daily for 2 weeks after ulceration; and

2. Since indomethacin delays the healing of acetic-acid-induced ulcers [18,19], the effects of the test compounds on this delayed ulcer healing were also studied. Indomethacin (1 mg/kg, Sigma, St Louis, MO) suspended in saline with a minimal amount of Tween 80 (0.02% v/v), was administered subcutaneously once daily (9.00 am) for 4 weeks after ulceration. The test compounds or the vehicle were administered orally once daily for 4 weeks after ulceration together with indomethacin. The animals were killed 24 h after the final administration of the test compounds and the stomachs removed. Then the stomach was inflated with 8 ml of 2% formalin and immersed in the same solution for 15 min. The stomach was then opened along its greater curvature and the ulcerated area was determined under a dissecting microscope (× 10, Olympus, Tokyo). The person (S.O.) who determined the ulcerated area did not know which treatment the animals had been given.

Gastric secretory studies

The effects of the test compounds or a combination of them on basal gastric acid secretion were determined in normal rats or rats with ulcers, using pylorus ligation. In the normal rats, omeprazole or SDZ CO-611 was administered orally 30 or 60 min before pylorus ligation. Combined administration of them was performed according to the same time schedule. The control animals received the vehicle alone. In the rats with ulcers, secretory studies were performed after the final administration of omeprazole or SDZ CO-611 for 2 or 4 weeks. One hour or 30 min before pylorus ligation, the animals received an additional dose of the drugs. Under ether anaesthesia, the pylorus was ligated. Four hours later, the gastric contents were collected and analysed as to volume and acidity. Total acidity was determined by titration of the gastric contents against 0.1 N NaOH to pH 7.0, using an automatic titrator (Comtite 5; Hiranuma, Tokyo, Japan). Total acid output (AOP: volume × acidity) was expressed as μEq/h.

Determination of the serum gastrin level

Before collecting the gastric contents, about 5 ml blood was collected from the aorta and left for 1 h. Each sample was then centrifuged at 3500 rpm for 20 min. The serum was stored frozen until analysis of the gastrin level. The gastrin concentration was determined by ^{125}I-radioimmunoassay (Sanyoh-Kasei, Kyoto, Japan). The results were expressed as pg gastrin per ml of serum.

Drugs

Omeprazole (Fujisawa Astra, Osaka, Japan) or SDZ CO-611 (*N*-[α-D-glucopyranosyl (1→4)-1-desoxy-D-fructosyl]-D-phenylalanyl-L-hemicystyl-L-phenylalanyl-D-tryptophyl-L-lysyl-L-threonyl-L-hemicystyl-L-threoninol cyclic (2→7)disulphide acetate; Sandoz, Basel, Switzerland) was either suspended in 0.5% carboxymethylcellulose or dissolved in saline, respectively. The test drugs were given in the volume of 0.5 ml/100 g of body weight.

Analysis of data

All data are presented as means ± SEM. Statistical analysis was performed using two-tailed Dunnett's multiple comparison test, values of $p < 0.05$ being regarded as significant.

RESULTS

Effects of omeprazole on ulcer healing, gastric acid output and the serum gastrin level

When the acetic acid solution was injected into the submucosal layer, deep round gastric ulcers developed, with a 100% incidence. The ulcerated area was about 30 mm^2 on the day of ulceration. The ulcers healed with time, the area after 2 weeks being 6.6 ± 1.0 mm^2 ($n = 11$). When omeprazole was administered for 2 weeks, it accelerated spontaneous ulcer healing in a dose-dependent manner (Figure 1). With 30 and 60 $mg\,kg^{-1}\,day^{-1}$, the healing rates were 59.1% and 83.3%, respectively. Gastric acid output in these rats was almost completely inhibited. The serum gastrin concentration was significantly increased (about 5-fold at 30 and 60 $mg\,kg^{-1}\,day^{-1}$). After 4-weeks' treatment with indomethacin, the ulcerated area was 8.5 ± 0.9 mm^2 ($n = 21$). Omeprazole (60 $mg\,kg^{-1}\,day^{-1}$) also significantly prevented the delay in ulcer healing, the healing rate being 60.0% (Figure 2). Similar to the 2-weeks' treatment, the acid output was completely inhibited and the serum gastrin level apparently increased (about 4–5-fold) with 30 or 60 $mg\,kg^{-1}\,day^{-1}$.

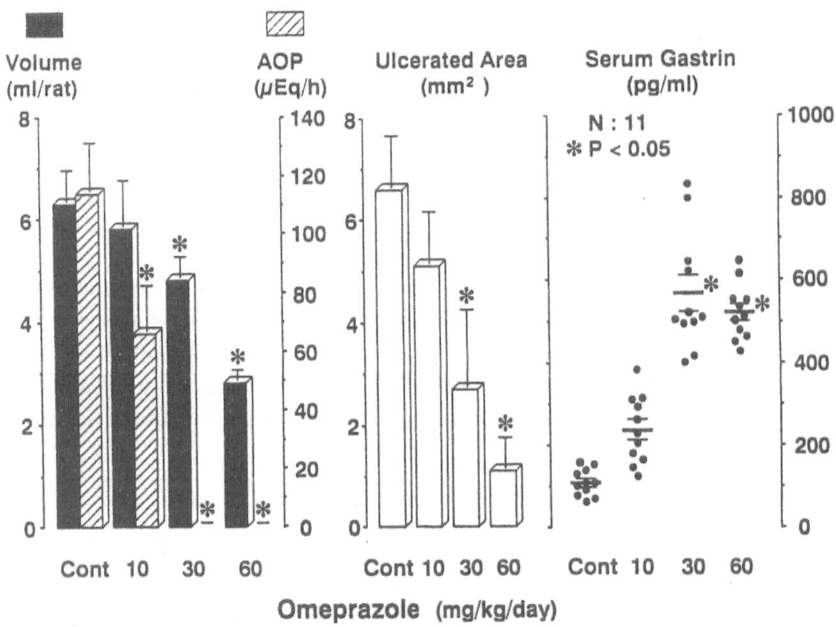

Figure 1. Dose–response relationship of omeprazole: spontaneous healing of acetic acid ulcers, serum gastrin levels and gastric basal acid output in rats. Omeprazole was administered orally once daily for 2 weeks after ulceration. Data are means ± SEM. *Significantly different from the corresponding control groups at $p < 0.05$

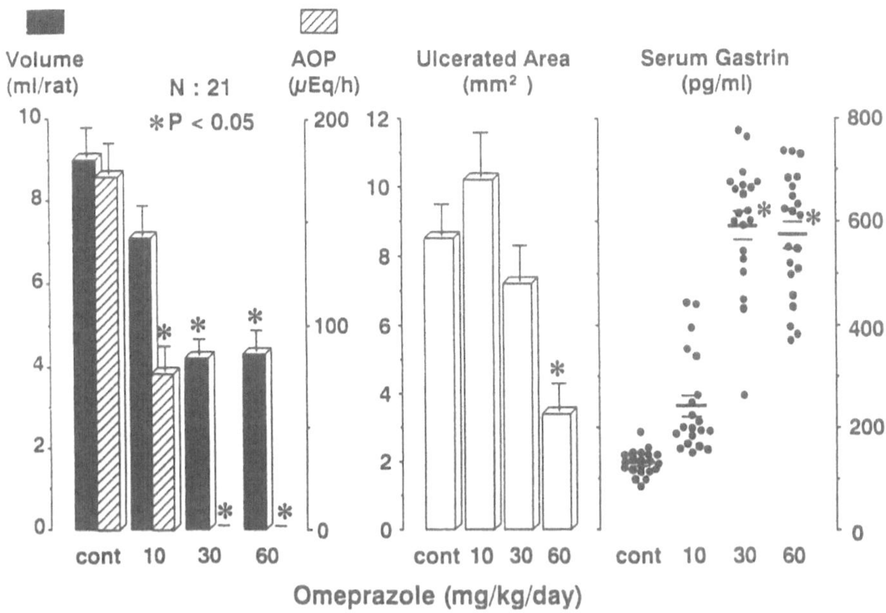

Figure 2. Dose–response relationship of omeprazole: delayed healing of acetic acid ulcers, serum gastrin levels and gastric basal acid secretion in rats. Omeprazole was administered orally once daily for 4 weeks. Delayed ulcer healing was caused by daily subcutaneous administration of indomethacin (1 mg/kg) for 4 weeks. Data are means ± SEM. *Significantly different from the corresponding control groups at $p < 0.05$

Effects of omeprazole, SDZ CO-611 or a combination thereof on acid output and serum gastrin levels in normal rats

Omeprazole (30 or 60 mg/kg) alone markedly inhibited acid output and increased the serum gastrin level (Figure 3). SDZ CO-611 also significantly inhibited acid output in a dose-dependent manner, the inhibition being 66.4% and 72.9% at 1 and 3 mg/kg, respectively. With these doses, the serum gastrin level was 135.8 ± 23.9 and 84.0 ± 6.7 pg/ml vs. 101.1 ± 8.5 pg/ml ($n = 8$) in the control groups, respectively. On the combined treatment, SDZ CO-611 had no appreciable effect on acid output inhibition by omeprazole. However, at 3 mg/kg, it significantly reduced the increased serum gastrin level due to omeprazole (30 and 60 mg/kg), the reduction being 75.6% and 76.1%, respectively.

The increase in the serum gastrin level in response to a single administration of omeprazole (60 mg/kg) reached a maximum 6 h later, and then returned to the basal value by 24 h (Figure 4). However, pretreatment with SDZ CO-611 (3 mg/kg) significantly reduced the increase in the serum gastrin level caused by omeprazole for

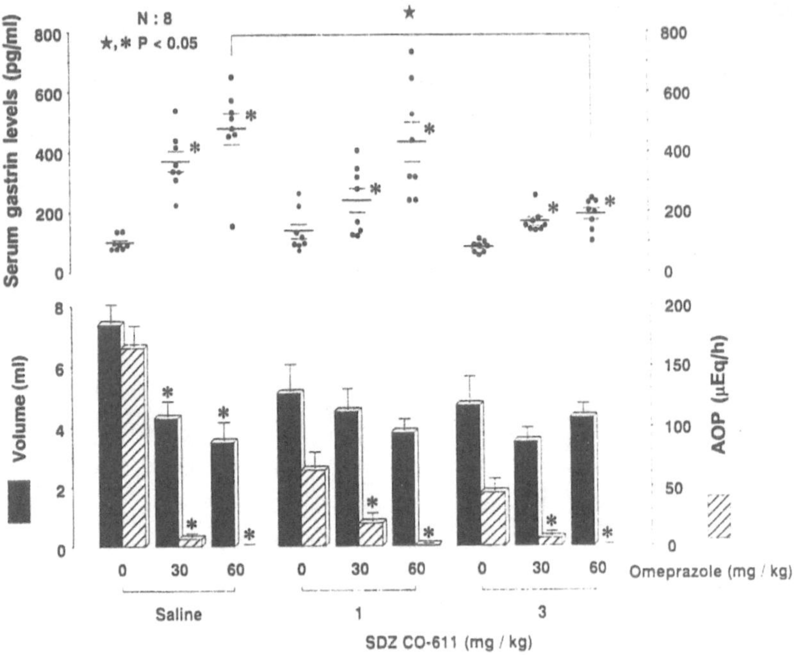

Figure 3. Effects of omeprazole, SDZ CO-611 and a combination of both on serum gastrin level or gastric basal acid output in normal rats. Data are means ± SEM. Note that SDZ CO-611 alone significantly inhibited gastric acid secretion without affecting the serum gastrin level. ✱,★ Significantly different from the corresponding control groups or from the omeprazole-treated groups at $p<0.05$

>12 h. However, the reduction did not increase when the dose of SDZ CO-611 was increased to 6 mg/kg. Indeed, the serum gastrin level was 334.4 ± 37.5 pg/ml vs. 526.2 ± 53.8 pg/ml in the omeprazole-treated control group 6 h later. At that time, diarrhoea was observed in all animals which had received the drug.

Effect of omeprazole, SDZ CO-611 and the combination of them on ulcer healing, acid output and serum gastrin level

Omeprazole (60 $mg\,kg^{-1}\,day^{-1}$) administered for 2 weeks apparently enhanced the spontaneous healing of acetic acid ulcers, the healing rate being 77.4% (Figure 5). Acid secretion was nearly completely inhibited after the treatment. SDZ CO-611 (3 $mg\,kg^{-1}\,day^{-1}$) administered for 2 weeks had no effect on ulcer healing or on serum gastrin levels but it did significantly inhibit acid output by 84.5%. SDZ CO-611 had little or no effect on the inhibition of acid output or the enhancement of ulcer healing caused by omeprazole. However, it significantly reduced the increased serum gastrin level due to

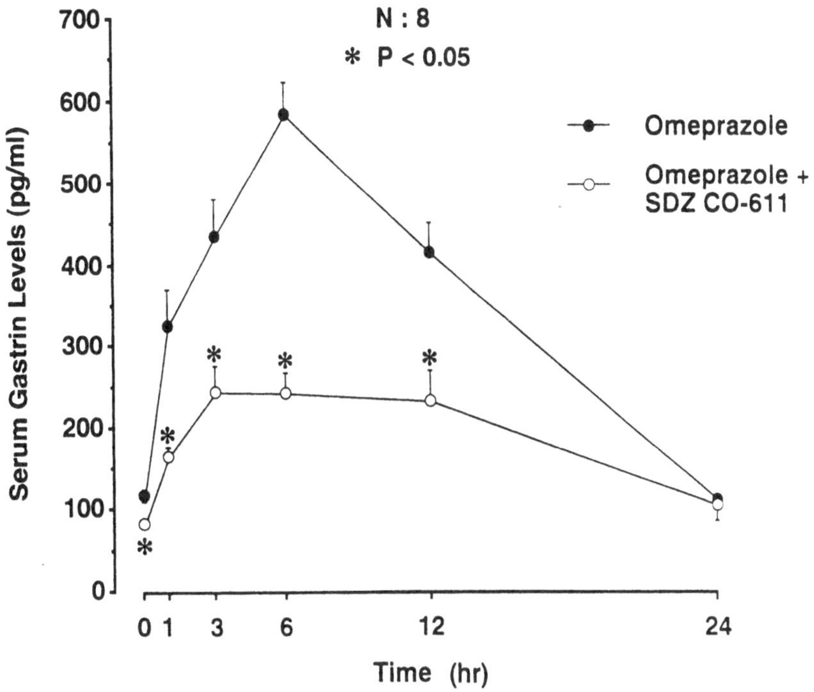

Figure 4. Time course changes in the serum gastrin level in rats treated with omeprazole alone or omeprazole + SDZ CO-611. Note that the increased serum gastrin level was apparently suppressed by SDZ CO-611 for >12 h. Data are means ± SEM. *Significantly different from the omeprazole-treated groups at $p<0.05$

omeprazole (248.8 ± 26.1 pg/ml vs. 511.4 ± 28.6 pg/ml, $n = 17$).

Four weeks' administration of omeprazole (60 mg kg^{-1} day^{-1}) gave results similar to those of the 2-week experiments: the delay in ulcer healing was significantly prevented by 85.0% and acid output was completely inhibited (Figure 6). SDZ CO-611 (3 mg kg^{-1} day^{-1}) administered for 4 weeks also significantly prevented the delay in ulcer healing by 33.6% and acid secretion by 89.9%. On the combined treatment, the serum gastrin level was significantly lower than that observed with omeprazole alone (263.1 ± 20.5 pg/ml vs. 605.1 ± 30.3 pg/ml, $n = 17$).

DISCUSSION

In these studies, we confirmed our previous findings [3,5] that omeprazole could enhance the spontaneous healing of acetic acid ulcers and prevent the delayed ulcer healing caused by indomethacin in rats. In addition, we confirmed the development of hypergastrinaemia in response to single or repeated treatment with omeprazole [4,6–

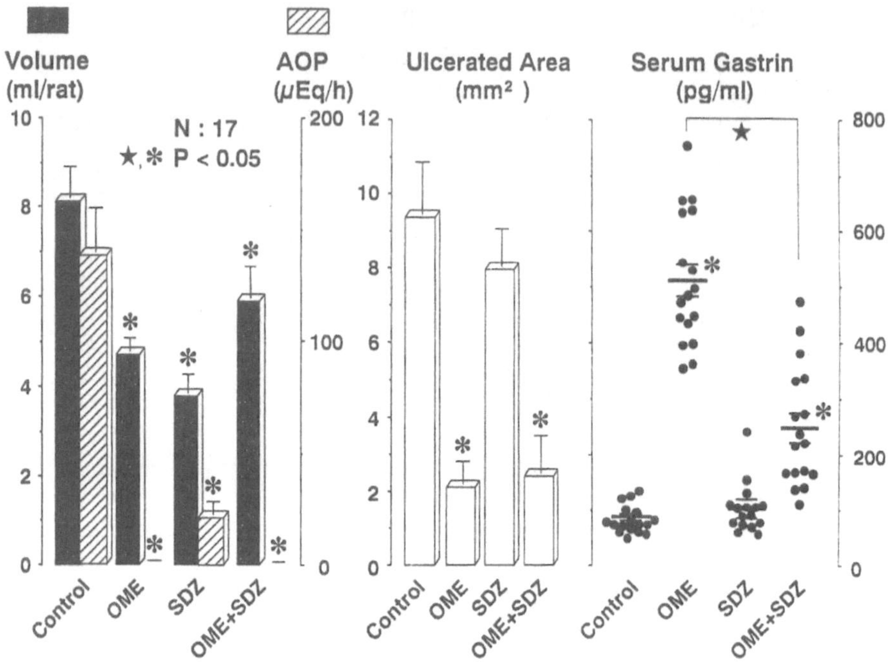

Figure 5. Effects of omeprazole, SDZ CO-611 (SDZ) and a combination of both on spontaneous healing of acetic acid ulcers, the serum gastrin level and gastric basal acid output in rats. The drugs were administered once daily for 2 weeks. Data are means ± SEM. *, ★Significantly different from the corresponding control groups or from the omeprazole-treated groups at $p < 0.05$

9,20]. Such elevation of the serum gastrin level seems to be caused by the increased intragastric pH due to the profound inhibition of gastric acid secretion by omeprazole.

As expected, we found that, while the somatostatin analogue, SDZ CO-611, had little or no effect on the basal gastrin level, it could prevent the hypergastrinaemia caused by omeprazole for >12 h. These effects of SDZ CO-611 were observed even after 2 or 4 weeks' treatment, i.e. the increased serum gastrin level was reduced by >60%. Interestingly, we found that, despite the reduced gastrin level, the healing promoting effect of omeprazole was not affected at all by SDZ CO-611. These results suggest that omeprazole-induced hypergastrinaemia is not involved in the mechanism by which omeprazole enhances ulcer healing. Certainly, the inhibition of hypergastrinaemia by SDZ CO-611 was not complete with the dose we used. Since mild or severe diarrhoea was observed in most of the animals which received 3 or 6 mg/kg SDZ CO-611, a further increase in the dose of the drug was not investigated. Accordingly, we could not rule out the possibility that the increased serum gastrin output, about 120 pg/ml, which was not suppressed by SDZ CO-611, contributes to

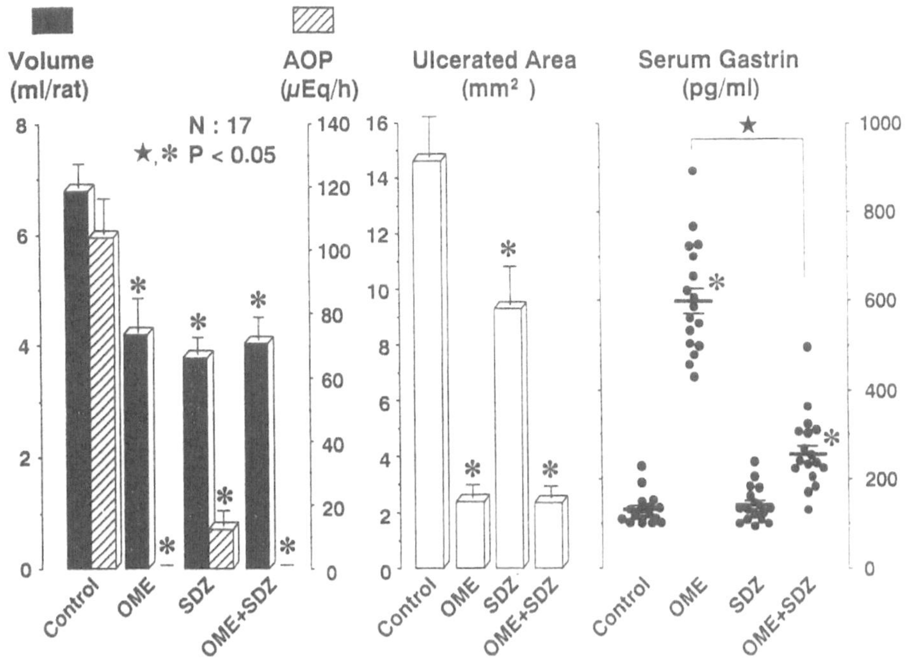

Figure 6. Effects of omeprazole, SDZ CO-611 (SDZ) and a combination of both on delayed healing of acetic acid ulcers, the serum gastrin level and gastric basal acid output in rats. The drugs were administered once daily for 4 weeks. Data are means ± SEM. *, ★Significantly different from the corresponding control groups or from the omeprazole-treated groups at $p<0.05$

enhanced healing. However, this is not possible because omeprazole administered for 2 or 4 weeks at 10 mg/kg had no effect on ulcer healing despite an increase in serum gastrin level to about 110–130 pg/ml.

Konturek et al. [21] found that growth-hormone-releasing factor (GRF) induced hypergastrinaemia and enhanced the healing of acetic-acid-induced gastroduodenal ulcers in rats, and that these effects were completely inhibited by somatostatin. They suggested that the increased gastrin level is involved in the mechanism by which GRF enhances ulcer healing. Our results are apparently different from those of Konturek et al. [21] who reported the abolition of the ulcer healing effect of GRF by somatostatin. The reason for the difference in results between these two groups appears to be the different location of the ulcers induced. They produced ulcers in the fundus while our ulcers were located in the border area between the antrum and fundus. Ulcers in the fundus may be much more sensitive to gastrin. Inauen et al. [4] reported that while omeprazole caused hypergastrinaemia and enhanced ulcer healing in rats, there was no increase in the proliferative index in the ulcer margin. Such results seem to support our postulation, that is, hypergastrinaemia is not involved in ulcer healing.

Takeuchi and Johnson [22] reported that, in rats fed with a liquid diet alone, circulating gastrin levels were reduced and healing of acetic-acid-induced gastric ulcers was significantly delayed. However, this delayed ulcer healing rate was apparently reversed in chow-fed rats after repeated treatment with pentagastrin. Accordingly, they suggested that basal gastrin plays an important role in ulcer healing. At this moment, it is unknown whether basal gastrin level contributes to the enhanced healing by omeprazole. It would be of interest to study whether or not omeprazole could enhance the ulcers in rats fed with a liquid diet alone.

In the present study, we found that SDZ CO-611 alone was less effective for promoting spontaneous ulcer healing. The reason seems to be the short duration of its antisecretory activity (<5 h) on rat basal gastric acid secretion compared with that of omeprazole (unpublished data). However, it significantly prevented the delay in ulcer healing. It is possible that SDZ CO-611 might interfere with the action of indomethacin to delay ulcer healing.

Long-term treatment with omeprazole or ranitidine induces hyperplasia of ECL cells and development of carcinoids, most probably through persistent hypergastrinaemia [6,11,12]. Meijer et al. [23] reported that subcutaneously administered SMS 201-995, a long-lasting somatostatin analogue, for 5 days significantly prevented basal and meal-stimulated increases in serum gastrin during omeprazole therapy in man. They suggested that concurrent treatment with omeprazole and SMS 201-995 might reduce the possible development of ECL cell hyperplasia through omeprazole-induced hypergastrinaemia. Accordingly, the inhibition of hypergastrinaemia induced by omeprazole by combined treatment with somatostatin analogues, such as SDZ CO-611 and SMS 201-995, might be beneficial for prevention of the possible mucosal hyperplasia during omeprazole therapy in man, without affecting its ulcer-healing effect.

We conclude that omeprazole-induced hypergastrinaemia does not contribute to the mechanism by which omeprazole enhances ulcer healing.

ACKNOWLEDGEMENTS

We wish to thank N.J. Halewood for critical reading of the manuscript. We are also grateful to Sandoz Inc. for the supply of SDZ CO-611, and Fujisawa Astra Inc. for the supply of omeprazole.

REFERENCES

1. Holt S, Howden CW. Omeprazole: overview and opinion. Dig Dis Sci. 1991;36:385–93.
2. Freston JW. Emerging strategies for managing peptic ulcer disease. Scand J Gastroenterol. 1993;29(Suppl 201):49–54.
3. Yamamoto O, Okada Y, Okabe S. Effects of a proton pump inhibitor, omeprazole, on gastric secretion and gastric and duodenal ulcers or erosions in rats. Dig Dis Sci. 1984;29:394–401.
4. Inauen W, Wyss PA, Kayser S et al. Influence of prostaglandins, omeprazole, and indomethacin on healing of experimental gastric ulcers in the rat. Gastroenterology. 1988;95:636–41.

5. Wang JY, Nagai H, Okabe S. Effect of omeprazole on delayed healing of acetic acid-induced gastric ulcers in rats. Jpn J Pharmacol. 1990;54:82–5.
6. Sundler F, Carlsson E, Hakanson R, Larsson H, Mattsson H. Inhibition of gastric acid secretion by omeprazole and ranitidine, effects on plasma gastrin and gastric histamine, histidine decarboxylase activity and ECL cell density in normal and antrectomized rats. Scand J Gastroenterol. 1986;21(Suppl 118):39–45.
7. Ryberg B, Mattsson H, Carlsson E. Effects of omeprazole and ranitidine on gastric acid secretion, blood gastrin levels and [^{3}H]-thymidine incorporation in the oxyntic mucosa from dogs and rats. Digestion. 1988;39:91–9.
8. Decktor DL, Pendleton RG, Kellner AT, Davis MA. Acute effects of ranitidine, famotidine and omeprazole on plasma gastrin in the rat. J Pharmacol Exp Ther. 1989;249:1–5.
9. Olbe L, Cederbberg C, Lind T, Olausson M. Effect of omeprazole on gastric acid secretion and plasma gastrin in man. Scand J Gastroenterol. 1989;24(Suppl 166):27–32.
10. Johnson LR. Regulation of gastrointestinal growth. In: Johnson LR, ed. Physiology of the Gastrointestinal Tract, Vol 1, 2nd ed. New York: Raven Press; 1987:307–15.
11. Axelson J, Hakanson R, Rosengren E, Sundler F. Hypergastrinemia induced by acid blockade evokes enterochromaffin-like (ECL) cell hyperplasia in chicken, hamster and guinea-pig stomach. Cell Tissue Res. 1988;254:511–16.
12. Hakanson R, Tielemans, Y, Chen D, Andersson K, Mattsson H, Sundler F. Time-dependent changes in enterochromaffin-like cell kinetics in stomach of hypergastrinemic rats. Gastroenterology. 1993;105:15–21.
13. Bloom SR, Mortimer RH, Thorner MO et al. Inhibition of gastrin and gastric acid secretion by growth-hormone release-inhibiting hormone. Lancet. 1974;2:1106–9.
14. Hayes JR, Johnson DG, Koerker D, Williams RH. Inhibition of gastrin release by somatostatin in vitro. Endocrinology. 1975;96:1374–6.
15. Koop H, Bothe E, Eissele R. Somatostatin–gastrin interaction in the rat stomach. Res Exp Med. 1988;188:115–21.
16. Cadiot G, Lehy T, Bonfils S. Action of somatostatin analogue (SMS 201-995) on the growth-promoting effect resulting from sustained achlorhydria in rat gastric mucosa, with special reference to endocrine cell behaviour. Eur J Clin Invest. 1988;18:360–8.
17. Takagi K, Okabe S, Saziki R. A new method for the production of chronic gastric ulcer in rats and the effect of several drugs on its healing. Jpn J Pharmacol. 1969;19:418–26.
18. Wang JY, Yamasaki S, Takeuchi K, Okabe S. Delayed healing of acetic acid induced gastric ulcers in rats by indomethacin. Gastroenterology. 1989;96:393–402.
19. Tarnawski A, Stachura J, Douglass TG, Kause WJ, Gergely H, Sarfeh IJ. Indomethacin impairs quality of experimental gastric ulcer healing: A quantitative histological and ultrastructural analysis. In: Garner A, O'Brien PE, eds. Mechanism of Injury, Protection and Repair of the Upper Gastrointestinal Tract. New York: Wiley; 1991:521–31.
20. Brenna E, Hakanson R, Sundler F, Sandvik AK, Waldum HL. The effect of omeprazole-induced hypergastrinemia on the oxyntic mucosa of mastomys. Scand J Gastroenterol. 1991;26:667–72.
21. Konturek SJ, Brzozowski T, Dembinski A, Warzecha Z, Konturek PK, Yanaihara N. Interaction of growth hormone releasing factor and somatostatin on healing and mucosal growth in rats: Role of gastrin and epidermal growth factor. Digestion. 1988;41:121–8.
22. Takeuchi K, Johnson LR. Effect of cell proliferation on healing of gastric and duodenal ulcers in rats. Digestion. 1986;33:92–100.
23. Meijer JL, Jansen JBMJ, Crobach LFSJ, Biemond I, Lamers CBHW. Inhibition of omeprazole induced hypergastrinemia by SMS 201-995, a long acting somatostatin analogue in man. Gut. 1993;34:1186–90.

Manuscript received 7 Nov. 95.
Accepted for publication 10 Nov. 95

TS Gaginella et al. (eds.), Biochemical Pharmacology as an Approach to Gastrointestinal Disorders, 361–371

MODIFICATION OF PATHOBIOLOGICAL EVENTS BY POTENTIAL HEPATOPHARMACOLOGICAL AGENTS

A. JENEY*, I. KOVALSZKY, F. TIMÁR, Zs. SCHAFF, A. ZALATNAI, K. LAPIS, J. OLÁH, A. DIVALD AND B. SZENDE
Semmelweis University of Medicine, I. Institute of Pathology and Experimental Cancer Research, Budapest, Hungary
*Correspondence

This paper was first published in: Inflammopharmacology. 1997;5:93–103.

ABSTRACT

The elucidation of the pathobiological events in chronic liver diseases – such as cellular injury, cell proliferation, remodelling of extracellular matrix – has considerable importance for establishing the rational bases of hepatopharmacology. To follow this concept, the molecular–pathological features of chemically induced liver damage in rats were characterized and modulated by potential hepatopharmacological compounds. Among the 55 chemical compounds tested, acute liver damage could be most effectively abolished by prostacyclin (PGI_2). In addition, prostacyclins were also able to prevent cirrhosis in experimental animals. The modes of action of the prostacyclins were investigated in short-term hepatocyte culture. The hepatotoxin-induced metabolic alterations (reduced gluconeogenesis and protein synthesis, lipid peroxidation, etc.) could be restored by prostacyclin. It was shown that PGI_2 could circumvent the augmented catabolic rate of 4,5-phosphatidyl inositol-diphosphate (PIP_2) in CCl_4-induced hepatocyte injury. In addition, the increased intracellular calcium concentration in the injured cells was also normalized by PGI_2. Thus, PIP_2 metabolism appears to be a critical process in the mechanism of hepatocyte damage and its protection. Interestingly, PGI_2 was effective at an advanced stage of liver injury, whereas thiazolidines were only active when administered before the application of the hepatotoxic agent. The formation of collagen could be reduced by amino-imidazolcarboxamide and silymarin. The increase in glycosaminoglycans could be abolished by the application of 5-hexyl-2-deoxyuridine. The presented data provide further evidence that compounds with various targets are required in hepatopharmacology.

hepatopharmacological agents, prostacyclin

INTRODUCTION

As it is well documented that chronic liver diseases represent an ever increasing concern for contemporary health services, it is surprising that there is still a lack of guidelines for the design and testing of hepatopharmacological agents.

This may be explained by the strategy for pharmacological studies which requires an appropriate experimental model system, including a characteristic feature of the relevant human disease, to test the efficacy of the selected chemicals. Clearly, drug-development programmes prefer to target aetiological agents of a biological nature

This paper was presented at the Section of IUPHAR GI Pharmacology Symposium on 'Biochemical pharmacology as an approach to gastrointestinal disorders (basic science to clinical perspectives)', October 12–14, 1995, Pécs, Hungary.

because the differences between the biochemical features of microbes and mammalian cells are great enough to obtain selective toxicity. Certainly, the elimination of the pathogenic microbes from the human organism by chemotherapeutic agents has resulted in dramatic recovery from many infectious diseases. In these instances, the success of targeting aetiological factors may be due to the disease being dependent on the presence of microbes. Since infectious diseases are maintained by the production of toxic substances and no lesions remain after the disappearance of the causative agent, the 'magic bullet' idea of Ehrlich is applicable in drug design. Thus, the elective destruction of pathogenic microbes without affecting the macro-organism has been an effective strategy to combat the major infectious diseases. However, in many other diseases, the causative agents induce permanent lesions in the host organism, i.e. lasting after their elimination, and frequently trigger alterations in the regulatory mechanisms between various cell populations, leading to a chronic pathological entity. The pattern of pathogenesis characterized by the progression of acute cellular damage to the chronic state is well illustrated in liver disease in which various pathobiological events are implicated [1]. In the highly industrialized countries, besides the hepatotoxins and viral agents from the environment, certain harmless chemicals (at low concentrations and by themselves) may also contribute to the development of liver disease, acting as sensitizers or sometimes promoters. Although acute liver damage can be lethal in some cases, the major problem is the transition from acute liver damage to the chronic state.

Thus, hepatopharmacological investigation of liver diseases must be viewed as a series of pathological alterations closely linked to each other. Consequently, for effective therapy, drugs with various molecular targets are required.

In order to outline a rational basis of hepatopharmacology, recognition of the critical pathobiological events and their underlying molecular mechanisms has paramount importance because these data would offer appropriate means of selecting potentially hepatoprotective chemicals. This concept was used in our laboratory when the molecular–pathological features of acute and chronic liver damage induced by hepatoxins were characterized in both in-vitro and in-vivo experimental model systems. In these studies, those metabolic alterations which may be associated with hepatocyte injury or with the remodelling of the extracellular liver matrix were utilized to determine the potential hepatopharmacological values of more than sixty chemical compounds over the last two decades [2–5].

MATERIALS AND METHODS

Hepatotoxins

Carbon tetrachloride (CCl_4) from Reanal (Budapest, Hungary) and thioacetamide from P.P.H. Polskie Odczynniki Chemiczne (Gliwice, Poland) were purchased in analytical pure form.

Hepatoprotective substances

Prostacyclin (PGI_2) was synthesized by Dr G. Galambos, Dr I. Tömösközi, Dr I. Székely and Dr G. Kovács [6]. The 1-phosphate-4-amino-5-carboxamido-imidazole (AICA-P) was a product of Chinoin Pharmaceutical Works (Budapest, Hungary). [+]Cyanidanol, silymarin and 4-carboxy-5,5-dimethyl-2[5-nitro-2-furyl]-thiazolidine were obtained from Biogal Pharmaceutical Works (Debrecen, Hungary).

Assay systems

Hepatocyte cultures

Rat liver hepatocytes were isolated by the method of Seglen [7] using female Fisher 344 rats of 220–240 g weight after an 18-h fast period. Hepatocyte suspensions of viability higher than 90%, as determined by the trypan blue exclusion test, were plated in collagen-coated Petri dishes at a density of 8×10^4 cell/cm^2 [8]. Hanks-MEM culture medium (Flow Laboratories Ltd., Irvine, UK) supplemented with 5% fetal calf serum (Flow Laboratories Ltd), 0.1% glucose, 10^{-6} mol/L insulin, 10^{-6} mol/L dexamethasone (Richter Pharmacy Works, Budapest, Hungary) and 0.05 mg/ml gentamycin (Serva, Heidelberg, Germany) was used for seeding (3 h in CO_2:O_2:N_2; 4.8:21:74.2 by volume atmosphere). Subsequently, the medium was changed for fresh medium without the additives and the hepatocytes cultured for a further 18 h.

Animal experiments

In-vivo acute liver damage was induced by the administration of CCl_4 (1.5 ml/kg in CFY and 1.0 ml/kg in F344 male rats per os). Treatment with test compounds was performed before or after poisoning at the time indicated.

For the induction of cirrhosis, either CCl_4 or thioacetamide was administered for the time indicated. The test compounds were administered either simultaneously with the hepatotoxin or after the development of cirrhosis.

Biochemical measurements

In the experiments with isolated hepatocytes, gluconeogenesis was investigated by measuring the formation of glucose from lactate [3]. For the study of protein synthesis, hepatocytes were labelled with 400 kBq/ml [^{14}C]amino acid mixture (CB59, UVVVR, Prague, Czech Republic) [9].

Fatty acid catabolism was estimated in hepatocytes prelabelled with 1 MBq [U-^{14}C]palmitate (40 MBq/mmol) as reported previously [10]. Phospholipid biosynthesis was measured after 1 h labelling with 1.6 MBq/ml $^{32}P_i$ (Izinta, Budapest, Hungary). The phospholipids were isolated and separated as described previously [9].

In the in-vivo experiments, serum glutamine oxalate transaminase (SGOT) activity, serum glutamate pyruvate transaminase (SGPT) activity, triglyceride, glycogen and collagen-associated hydroxyproline were measured as described by Reitmann and Frankel [11], Biggs et al. [12], Morris [13], Divald et al. [14] and Ujhelyi et al. [15]. The glycosaminoglycan concentration in the cirrhotic liver was determined by measuring the amount of uronic acid in the cetylpyridinium chloride precipitates of the trichloroacetic acid extracts as described previously by Kovalszky et al. [16].

RESULTS

Modification of acute liver damage

CCl_4 administration per os gave rise to a substantial increase in liver triglycerides in CFY male rats. Forty-eight hours after ip treatment with PGI_2 at 10, 30 and 100 μg/kg applied 24 h after CCl_4 poisoning, a time when both pathomorphological and pathobiological alterations were already pronounced, a remarkable hepatoprotective action could be observed (Figure 1). It is worth noting that PGI_2 applied shortly (1 h) before CCl_4 administration was much less effective. PGI_2 was also able to mitigate the

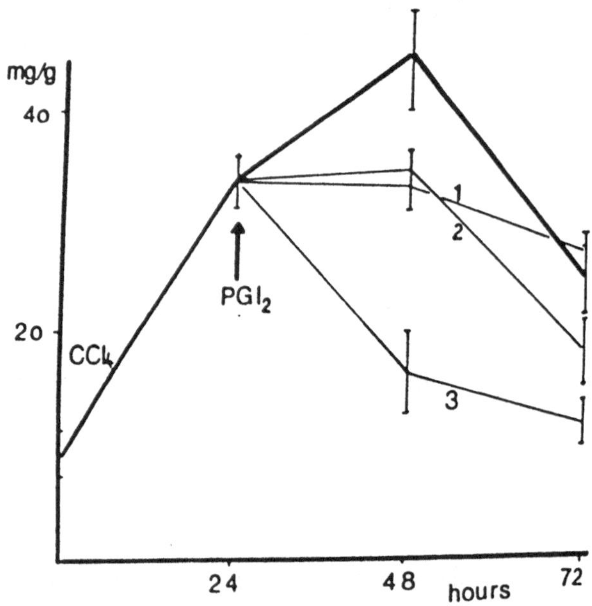

Figure 1. The dose–response relationship of prostacyclin action on fatty liver. Male CFY rats (180–200 g) received CCl_4 intragastrically 1.6 ml/kg after a 16-h starvation period and the animals were refed 1 h later. Prostacyclin (PGI_2) was administered 24 h after hepatotoxin administration at doses of 10 (line 1), 30 (line 2) and 100 (line 3) mg/kg ip. The bold line shows the control response. Triglyceride concentration in the liver was quantified as reported previously [14]

TABLE 1
Modulation of acute liver damage by PGI_2 and thiazolidine* in CFY rats

Treatment†	SGOT (U/L)	Triglyceride (mg/g wet weight)	Glycogen (mg/g wet weight)
No treatment	87 ± 9	6.9 ± 1.3	46.3 ± 6.4
CCl_4	415 ± 45	39.0 ± 4.4	3.9 ± 1.3
Prostacyclin + CCl_4	391 ± 92	19.4 ± 2.6	5.6 ± 2.6
CCl_4 + prostacyclin	127 ± 53	11.8 ± 5.8	39.0 ± 2.5
Thiazolidine + CCl_4	275 ± 47	14.2 ± 2.8	32.5 ± 2.1

*Thiazolidine = 2-(5-nitro-2-furyl)-4-carboxy-5,5-dimethyl thiazolidine

†Test substances were administered either 3 h before or 24 h after carbon tetrachloride (CCl_4, 1.6 ml/kg) administration as indicated. Glutamine oxalate transaminase in serum (SGOT), triglyceride and glycogen in liver were measured 48 h after poisoning

elevation of serum glutamate oxalate transaminase and the reduction in glycogen concentration, both induced by CCl_4. By contrast, thiazolidine was effective only if it was given before and not after CCl_4 poisoning (Table 1).

Protection against CCl_4-induced liver cell injury was also demonstrated in vitro, using isolated liver cells or primary hepatocyte cultures. In these studies, measurements of dye exclusion and release of intracellular enzymes are normally used as parameters to detect the extent of cell injury. We completed our arsenal of test systems by including measurements of protein synthesis, gluconeogenesis, fatty acid oxidation and also the phosphatidylinositol cycle.

Table 2 shows that PGI_2 enhances triglyceride catabolism and gluconeogenesis in CCl_4-injured hepatocytes. The CCl_4 reduces the transition of the radioactivity from that [^{14}C]palmitate prelabelled triglyceride to that released as carbon dioxide. In the presence of PGI_2 this reduction was not only cancelled, but in fact more radioactivity appeared in the CO_2 than in the case of normal untreated hepatocytes. At the same time, the CCl_4-induced reduction of gluconeogenesis was also mitigated by PGI_2.

Membrane integrity was studied by metabolic labelling of phospholipids both before and after the induction of injury, and a highly sensitive response to CCl_4 was observed in the metabolism of PIP_2. The labelling of PIP_2 in $^{32}P_i$ preincubated cells substantially declined after 60 min treatment with CCl_4, while the major phospholipid components (PC, PE or PI) showed no marked differences from controls up to this time. The elevation of the production of labelled inositol phosphates after CCl_4 treatment in [^{3}H-*myo*]inositol prelabelled cells may indicate that a phosphatidylinositol diphosphate-specific phospholipase C was simultaneously activated, i.e. a pathway by which PIP_2 can be metabolized (Table 3). The decreased labelling of PIP_2 may be interpreted in terms of either an increased catabolism or a decreased synthesis rate, but the lack of accumulation of radioactivity in PIP, the metabolic precursor of PIP_2, argues for the former possibility. The fact that, upon CCl_4 administration, a change in the

TABLE 2
Modification of hepatocyte injury by prostacyclin and catergen (in % of intact hepatocytes)

	CCl_4 3 mm	CCl_4 + PGI_2 0.1 μmol/L	CCl_4 + catergen** 10 μmol/L
Protein synthesis[a]	34±4%	73±5%*	46±6%
Gluconeogenesis[b]	10±4%	54±4%*	82±5%
Fatty acid oxidation[c]	308±8%	150±17%*	–
Lipid peroxidation[d]	372±16%	227±20%	–
Membrane fragmentation[e]	252±13%	228±14%*	189±10%

Hepatocytes were treated with CCl_4 for 1 h followed by treatment with the test substance and reincubation in the absence of CCl_4

[a] [^{14}C]amino acid incorporation (cpm (mg protein)$^{-1}$ h^{-1});

[b] Glucose formation from 2 mmol/L pyruvate (nmol (mg protein)$^{-1}$ min^{-1});

[c] $^{14}CO_2$ production from [^{14}C]palmitate (cpm (mg protein)$^{-1}$ h^{-1});

[d] nmol malondialdehyde per g liver, in-vivo experiment CCl_4 0.1 mg/kg, 24 h, PGI_2 0.1 mg/kg 3 h after CCl_4;

[e] GPT release (mU (mg protein)$^{-1}$ h^{-1});

*Significantly different ($p<0.05$) from CCl_4-treated cells

** = cyanidanol

TABLE 3
Prostacyclin modulation of phosphatidylinositol cycle (in % of control values)

	PI	→	PIP	→	PIP_2	→	$[IP+IP_2+IP_3]$*	Calcium
CCl_4 (3 mmol/L)	80%		50%		10%		180%	300%
PGI_2 (0.1 μmol/L)	120%		120%		100%		100%	100%
CCl_4 + PGI_2	150%		80%		100%		115%	160%

*Hepatocytes treated with CCl_4 for 1 h. After CCl_4 removal, the cells were further incubated in the presence or absence of PGI_2 and labelled with $^{32}P_i$ for 4 h

metabolism of PIP_2 precedes the reduction in the labelling of major phospholipids and also dominates at later stages of injury suggests that PIP_2 catabolism may represent a critical event in CCl_4-induced cell injury. It was concluded by Lamb and Schwertz [17] that both ischaemia and CCl_4 exposure cause increases in hepatic phospholipase C. The present observation that this metabolic shift may be effectively controlled by PGI_2 seems to indicate that the key mechanism for cytoprotection in this experimental system may also operate at this level.

Modification of chronic liver damage

It has been found that PGI_2 and thiazolidine compound partially prevent the development of collagen accumulation. Morphological examinations as reported by Lapis et al. [5] revealed that characteristic features of cirrhosis, such as abortive regeneration, parenchymal nodules encircled by fibrous tissue, were markedly decreased. Measurements of the amount of collagen are in agreement with the morphological observations (Table 4).

TABLE 4
Prevention of collagen accumulation by drug treatment induced by carbon tetrachloride or thioacetamide in F344 rat livers

	Liver collagen (μg/mg DNA)
Control	854 ± 77
CCl_4	2562 ± 357
CCl_4 + 7-oxo-PGI_2 0.01 mg/kg	1267 ± 658*
CCl_4 + 7-oxo-PGI_2 0.1 mg/kg	1064 ± 420*
CCl_4 + thiazolidine 100 mg/kg	1932 ± 266
CCl_4 + thiazolidine 10 mg/kg	2135 ± 448
Thioacetamide	1638 ± 84*
Thioacetamide + 7-oxo-PGI_2 0.1 mg/kg	1288 ± 182*
Thioacetamide + thiazolidine 100 mg/kg	1204 ± 511

F344 male rats (5-5 in each experimental group) received 0.3 ml/kg CCl_4 po and 5 h later either 7-oxo-PGI_2 or thiazolidine (ip)

Thioacetamide was administered as 0.1% solution in the drinking water.

*Significantly different from the CCl_4 group ($p < 0.05$)

Another series of investigations addressed the question of whether pre-existing cirrhosis could be affected or not. To test this possibility, cirrhotic rat livers were produced by repeated administration of hepatotoxin, and, after the development of cirrhosis, administration of the test compounds was begun. In this type of experimental layout, neither PGI_2 nor the thiazolidine compound showed any sign of hepatopharmacological activity. However, AICA-P and silymarin showed remarkable effects in reducing the amount of collagen in the liver (Table 5). This observation was confirmed by morphometric examination in cirrhosis, the ratio between connective tissue and parenchyma was 24 μm^2 per 1000 μm^2, whereas after AICA-P or silymarin treatment, this value was reduced to 16.3 and 11.1 μm^2, respectively.

In the next series of experiments, the importance of changes of glycosaminoglycans in cirrhotic liver was studied by applying 5-hexyl-2′-deoxyuridine (HUdR), an agent

TABLE 5
Reduction of collagen in cirrhotic liver by drug treatment in CFY rats

Induction of cirrhosis	Treatment with drug	Liver collagen (μg/mg DNA)
Control	Normal liver	1400 ± 360
CCl_4	No treatment	5866 ± 860
CCl_4	Legalon	4200 ± 720
CCl_4	Silymarin	3642 ± 500
CCl_4	AICA-P	3607 ± 428
TAA	No treatment	5500 ± 2170
TAA	Legalon	2380 ± 1720
TAA	Silimarin	4911 ± 1597
TAA	AICA-P	2044 ± 883

Induction of cirrhosis: carbon tetrachloride (1 ml/kg po) was administered three times per week for 2 months; or thioacetamide (150 mg/kg im) was given every 2 days for 6 months

Drug treatment: (given after the end of CCl_4 or thioacetamide poisoning) three times per week for 1 month: silimarin (Biogal, Hungary) 4 mg/kg po, Legalon (silymarin) (Madaus, Germany) 4 mg/kg po, AICA-P (Chinoin, Hungary) 100 mg/kg po

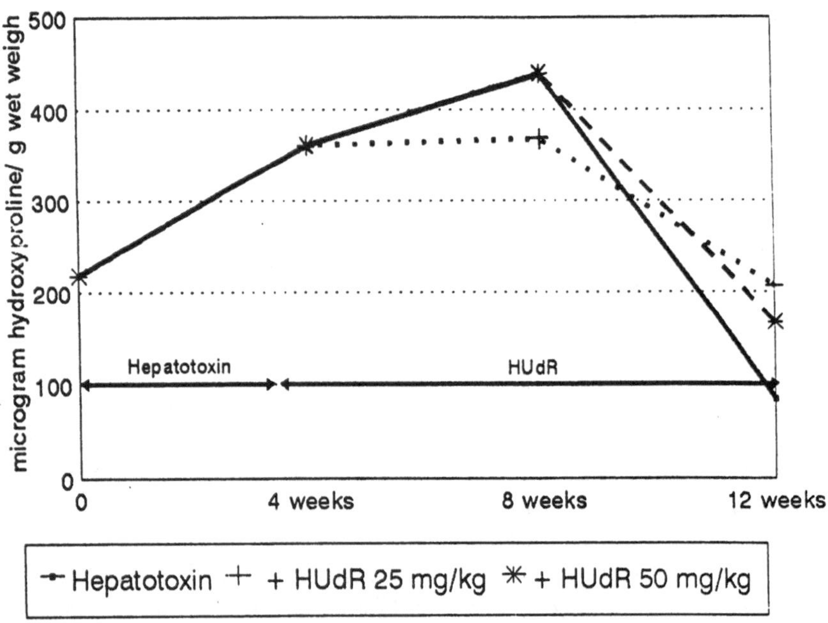

Figure 2. The effect of 5-hexyl-2′-deoxyuridine on collagen concentrations in cirrhotic liver. Fischer 344 male rats (150–180 g body weight) received 0.2 ml/kg carbon tetrachloride intragastrically twice a week for 1 month and also phenobarbital (0.2 g/L) in drinking water. 5-Hexyl-2′-deoxyuridine at the indicated dose was administered after hepatotoxin administration

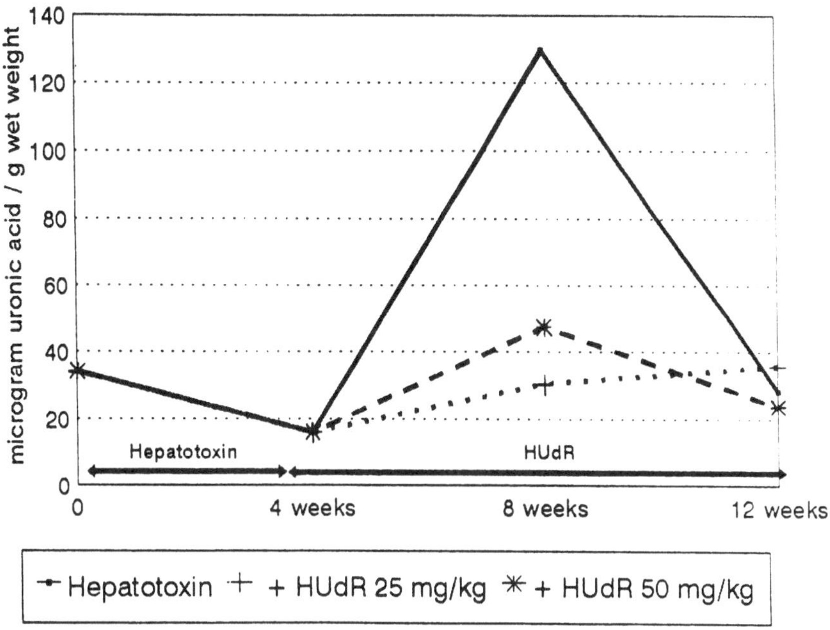

Figure 3. The effect of 5-hexyl-2′-deoxyuridine on glycosaminoglycan concentrations in cirrhotic liver. Fischer 344 male rats (150–180 g body weight) received 0.2 ml/kg carbon tetrachloride intragastrically twice a week for 1 month and also phenobarbital (0.2 g/L) in drinking water. 5-Hexyl-2′-deoxyuridine at the indicated dose was administered after hepatotoxin administration

which inhibits the biosynthesis of certain glycosaminoglycans. Figure 2 shows that the amount of collagen increases even after the end of hepatotoxin administration and HUdR has no effect at all. However, in the same animals, the hepatotoxin maintained the glycosaminoglycan concentration below normal levels, but, after the cessation of CCl_4 administration, there was a remarkable elevation of glycosaminoglycan concentration, which was abolished by HUdR treatment (Figure 3).

DISCUSSION

Although diseases are well defined by their morphological appearances, there is an increasing need to elucidate those biological and underlying molecular–biological alterations that contribute to the development and maintenance of a pathological condition. The knowledge of at least some of these critical events is essential for establishing pharmaceutical assays and for designing drugs which can interfere with the progression of a particular disease. Methodological progress has led to the molecular–pathological characterization of several diseases and made it possible to learn more about the basic elements involved in pathogenesis.

It is now widely accepted that cell injury has great importance, not only in eliciting a pathogenetic process, but also in the self-perpetuation of pathobiological events, such as accumulation of various cell products, proliferation, disorder in intercellular contacts, etc. It is likely that the injured cells play a major role in the progression of the disease. This is well illustrated by the transition from the acute to the chronic stage of a disease, when the cells start to produce abnormal amounts of extracellular substances. Therefore, to develop powerful therapeutic approaches in a particular disease, the involved injured cells must be considered the main target. To this end, several drugs, capable of modifying various types of alteration in cell metabolism, must be developed since there is no general pattern of cell injury. The appearance of cell injury shows great variation in different organs and at different stages during the progression of a disease. This implies that, beside determining the cytoprotective behaviour of a chemical structure, data must also be collected concerning the molecular mechanism of its action. Information, both about the subcellular target of a cytoprotective drug and the molecular pattern of the cell injury, makes it possible to select the most appropriate drug for treatment of a disease; e.g. fatty liver could be treated effectively with drugs which reduce the triglyceride content of the liver. To develop potent drugs for hepatopharmacology, the cytoprotective actions of various chemical agents and their modes of action were investigated at our institute.

As far as hepatocyte injury is concerned, it is conceivable that some of the numerous alterations related to various metabolic pathways, e.g. reduced gluconeogenesis and protein synthesis, ATP depletion etc., are elicited by the uncontrolled and higher rate of PIP_2 conversion. Since it has been well documented that changes in phosphatidyl inositol metabolism have a variety of consequences for cell metabolism, the data presented here, showing that PGI_2 acts at this level, may elucidate the mechanism by which PGI_2 modifies various metabolic changes in the injured cell.

Important differences were recorded between the anticirrhotic activities of the four compounds, i.e. PGI_2, thiazolidine compound, AICA-P and silymarin. AICA-P does not prevent the development of cirrhosis, but is highly effective for alleviating cirrhosis which has already developed. By contrast, PGI_2 and thiazolidine compounds are effective in preventing the development of cirrhosis, but cannot modify the cirrhotic state.

Our results demonstrate that the hepatoprotective compounds examined have different effects on the various types of liver damage. This suggests that complex studies are required in hepatopharmacology for the development of drugs which act on the different forms of human liver disease.

REFERENCES

1. Perrisond D, Testa B. Hepatic pharmacology mechanism of action and classification of antinecrotic hepatoprotective agents. Trends Pharmacol Sci. 1982;3:365–7.
2. Szepesházy K, Lapis K, Jeney A et al. Morphological and biochemical studies on the effect of agents with liver protecting properties. Exp Pathol. 1978;15:271–87.
3. Ujhelyi E, Divald A, Vajta G, Jeney A, Lapis K. Effect of PGI_2 in carbon tetrachloride induced liver injury. Acta Physiol Hung. 1984;64:425–30.

4. Jeney A, Divald A, Szende B et al. Hepatoprotective action of prostacyclin and its possible mechanisms. In: Kecskeméti V, Gyires K, Kovács G. Proceedings of the 4th Congress of Hungarian Pharmacology Society, Budapest, 1985:503–59.
5. Lapis K, Jeney A, Divald A, Vajta G, Zalatnai A, Schaff Zs. Experimental studies on the effect of hepatoprotective compounds. Tokai J Exp Clin Med. 1986;14(Suppl.):135–45.
6. Kovács G, Simonidesz V, Tömösközi P et al. A new stable prostacyclin mimic, 7-oxoprostaglandin I_2. J Med Chem. 1982;25:105–7.
7. Seglen PO. Preparation of isolated rat liver cells. Meth Cell Biol. 1976;13:29–83.
8. Vajta G, Divald A, Elek J, Paku S, Lapis K. Fatty degeneration in cultured hepatocytes – a new experimental model. Virchows Arch B Cell Pathol. 1986;52:177–84.
9. Divald A, Jeney A, O-Nagy J, Timáer F, Lapis K. Modification of the inhibitory effects of CCl_4 on phospholipid and protein biosynthesis by prostacyclin. Biochem Pharmacol. 1990;40:1477–83.
10. Divald A, Vajta G, Oláh J, Jeney A, Lapis K. Effect of prostacyclin on the triglyceride catabolism in CCl_4 poisoned hepatocytes. IRCS Med Sci (Biochem). 1985;13:1117–18.
11. Reitman S, Frankel S. A colorimetric method for the determination of serum oxalacetic and glutamic pyruvic transaminases. Am J Clin Pathol. 1977;28:56–63.
12. Biggs HG, Erikson JM, Moorehead WR. A manual colorimetric assay of triglycerides in serum. Clin Chem. 1975;21:437–41.
13. Morris DL. Quantitative determination of carbohydrates with Dreywood's anthron reagent. Science. 1948;107:254.
14. Divald A, Ujhelyi E, Jeney A, Lapis K, Institoris L. Hepatoprotective effects of prostacyclin on CCl_4-induced liver injury in rats. Exp Mol Pathol. 1985;42:163–6.
15. Ujhelyi E, Kovács L, Szepesházi K, Jeney A, Lapis K. Morphological and biochemical study of the hepatoprotective effect of AICA phosphate. Acta Med Acad Sci Hung. 1980;37:99–103.
16. Kovalszky I, Pogány G, Molnár G et al. Altered glycosaminoglycan composition in reactive and neoplastic human liver. Biochem Biophys Res Commun. 1990;167:883–90.
17. Lamb RG, Schwertz DW. The effect of bromobenzene and carbon tetrachloride exposure in vitro on phospholipase C activity of rat liver cells. Toxicol Appl Pharmacol. 1982;65:216–29.

Manuscript received 14 Oct. 95.
Accepted for publication 10 Nov. 95.

4. Jancsó A, Hávári A, [illegible] et al. Hepatoprotective action of prostacyclin and its possible mechanisms. In: [illegible] Gyires K, [illegible] Proceedings of the 4th Congress of Hungarian Pharmacology Society, Budapest, 1985, [illegible]
5. Lapis K, Jeney A, [illegible] Experimental studies on the effect of [illegible] hepatoprotective compounds. [illegible] 1988; [illegible]
6. Kovács G, [illegible] et al. A [illegible] Med Chem 199[illegible]
7. [illegible]
8. [illegible]
9. [illegible]
10. [illegible]
11. [illegible]
12. [illegible]
13. [illegible]

TS Gaginella et al. (eds.), Biochemical Pharmacology as an Approach to Gastrointestinal Disorders, 373–385

ORGANOPROTECTION AND CYTOPROTECTION OF HISTAMINE DIFFER IN RATS

B. BÓDIS, O. KARÁDI, O.M.E. ABDEL-SALAM, R. FALUDI, L. NAGY AND Gy. MÓZSIK*
First Department of Medicine, Medical University School of Pécs, Pécs, Hungary
*Correspondence

This paper was first published in: Inflammopharmacology. 1997;5:29–41.

ABSTRACT

Aims
The aim of the present study was to compare the organoprotective (in vivo) and cytoprotective (in vitro) effects of histamine.

Methods
In vivo, gastric mucosal damage was produced by intragastric (ig) administration of 1 ml 96% ethanol (EtOH) in Sprague–Dawley rats. The animals were sacrificed 1 h after EtOH administration, when the gastric mucosal damage was measured. Histamine was given subcutaneously (sc) 30 min before administration of EtOH with and without PGI_2Na (5 μg/kg sc). Gastric acid secretion was also measured 1 h after pylorus ligation in control (saline-), histamine- and PGI_2-treated animals. The affinity, intrinsic activity curves and the values of pD_2 and pA_2 were determined in EtOH-treated and in PGI_2-treated animals.

For the in-vitro studies, a mixed population of rat gastric mucosal cells was isolated by pronase digestion. Cells were preincubated for 60 min with histamine (10^{-8}–10^{-6} mol/L) with or without PGI_2Na (10^{-4} mol/L). At the end of this incubation period, cells were treated with 15% EtOH with or without 10^{-6}–10^{-3} mol/L indomethacin (IND) for 5 min. Cell viability was tested by trypan blue exclusion test and succinic dehydrogenase activity.

Results
1. Histamine (20 mg/kg) stimulated, while PGI_2 (5 μg/kg) had no effect on gastric acid secretion in rats;
2. Histamine inhibited the development of EtOH-induced gastric mucosal damage (pD_2=4.0, pA_2=3.75);
3. Histamine stimulated the PGI_2-induced gastric cytoprotection in vivo (pD_2=4.7, pA_2=3.75);
4. There was no measurable acid secretion by our method in isolated cells after incubation with 10^{-8}–10^{-6} mol/L histamine;
5. Histamine preincubation did not prevent the EtOH- or IND-induced cell injury.

Conclusions
1. Histamine has a protective effect in a non-acid-dependent model in vivo;
2. This organoprotection has a metabolic component;
3. The cytoprotective effect of histamine failed in vitro;
4. The mechanisms of histamine-induced organo- and cytoprotection seem to be different in rats.

Keywords: gastric organoprotection, gastric cytoprotection, histamine, isolated gastric mucosal cells

---

This paper was presented at the Section of IUPHAR GI Pharmacology Symposium on 'Biochemical pharmacology as an approach to gastrointestinal disorders (basic science to clinical perspectives)', October 12–14, 1995, Pécs, Hungary.

INTRODUCTION

The phenomenon of gastric cytoprotection was described by Chaudhury and Jacobson in 1978 [1] and was generally accepted after the publication of Robert et al. in 1979 [2]. Its essential point is the protection of gastric mucosa by exogenous prostaglandins against different necrotizing agents, such as 0.6 mol/L HCl, 0.2 mol/L NaOH, 25% NaCl and 96% ethanol, without any inhibition of gastric acid secretion.

The terminology 'gastric cytoprotection' underwent several critical evaluations. Szabo used earlier the term 'organoprotection' [3]. Later, Gyires demonstrated that not all general cytoprotective agent(s) can be used for the stomach [4]. The title of the 'International Symposium on Gastrointestinal Cytoprotection' was changed to 'Cell Injury and Protection in the Gastrointestinal Tract' owing to the previously obtained results [5,6].

Questions remain open about the similarities and differences between the phenomena of 'organoprotection' and 'cytoprotection'. Observations are needed in living animals (organoprotection) and in separated or cultured cells (cytoprotection) to provide data necessary to answer these questions.

The cellular mechanisms involved in the gastric acid secretion of rats in ethanol-induced mucosal damage and prostacyclin (PGI_2)-induced gastric cytoprotection have been studied: atropine, adrenalin, cimetidine, prostacyclin, actinomycin D and Degranol (mannomustine) inhibited gastric acid secretion and ethanol-induced mucosal damage [7] while surprisingly histamine, pentagastrin and 2,4-dinitrophenol (which enhanced gastric acid secretion over a short time period) stimulated the PGI_2-induced gastric cytoprotection [8]. So, drugs stimulating the aggressive side (HCl) of the stomach, could enhance the PGI_2-induced gastric cytoprotection. Furthermore, it was proved that an intact vagus is necessary for gastric cytoprotection and mucosal protection from atropine, cimetidine, PGI_2 and β-carotene [9].

The aims of our present study were:

1. To determine the stimulating effect of histamine on (a) gastric acid secretion and (b) ethanol-induced mucosal damage and PGI_2-induced gastric cytoprotection;

2. To evaluate the stimulating effects of histamine and pentagastrin (drugs acting at the receptor level) on PGI_2-induced gastric cytoprotection;

3. To identify the affinity and intrinsic activity curves (including the determination of pD_2 and pA_2 values) for these drugs on PGI_2-induced gastric cytoprotection; and

4. To study the direct cellular effect of histamine on the viability of freshly isolated rat gastric mucosal cells in the ethanol- and indomethacin-induced cell injury model [10].

MATERIALS AND METHODS

In-vivo studies

Observations were carried out on both sexes of Sprague–Dawley rats weighing 180–210 g. The animals were fasted for 24 h before experiments but received water ad libitum.

Gastric mucosal injury was produced by ig administration of 1 ml 96% ethanol (EtOH; Reanal, Hungary). The animals were killed 60 min after administration of necrotizing agents. The number and severity of gastric mucosal lesions were determined on a semiquantitative scale [7], and they were expressed as the average ± SEM for one rat stomach.

Gastric secretory responses

Pylorus ligation was carried out under light ether anaesthesia [11]. Immediately after surgery, each rat received 1 ml saline solution ig. Histamine (Peremin, Chinoin, Hungary), PGI_2 (Chinoin, Hungary) or saline were given sc 30 min before pylorus ligation. The animals were killed 60 min after surgery and the gastric juice of each rat was collected for measurements of acid output (μmol H^+). The results were expressed as μEq/rat.

Determination of affinity and intrinsic activity curves for drugs inhibiting EtOH-induced gastric mucosal damage

Histamine and PGI_2 were given sc 30 min before EtOH administration. The gastric mucosal damage was measured, and the intrinsic activity, pD_2 and pA_2 were calculated from affinity and intrinsic activity curves according to Csáky [12]. The value of the intrinsic activity of atropine was taken to be equal to 1.00. The results were calculated in percent values (means ± SEM) of the inhibition of EtOH-induced gastric mucosal damage.

Determination of PGI_2-induced gastric cytoprotection

Prostacyclin (PGI_2; Chinoin, Hungary) was given sc at doses of 5 and 50 μg/kg 30 min before EtOH injury; the control groups were treated with saline solution. The changes in the number and severity of EtOH-induced gastric mucosal damage were studied as described above.

Determination of affinity and intrinsic activity curves for drugs stimulating the PGI_2-induced gastric cytoprotection

Histamine and pentagastrin (Peptavlon, ICI, England) were given sc to modify the PGI_2-induced gastric cytoprotection. The gastric mucosal damage was measured, the intrinsic activity, pD_2 and pA_2 were calculated from affinity and intrinsic activity curves [11]. The intrinsic activity of pentagastrin was taken to be equal to 1.00. The results were calculated as percent values (means $\pm$ SEM) of 5 µg/kg PGI_2-induced gastric cytoprotection.

In-vitro studies

Preparation of mixed gastric mucosal cells (GMCs)

Gastric mucosal cells from 1–2 unfasted Sprague–Dawley rats were isolated by the method of Nagy et al. [13]. Briefly, the segments of glandular stomach without blood vessels or surrounding connective tissue were sequentially incubated in a physiological solution containing 0.5 mg/ml pronase E (type XXV, Sigma Chemical Co.) and 10^{-3} mol/L EGTA. After several washings cells were resuspended and kept in a shaking water bath at 37°C in a solution (0.157 mol/L, pH 7.4) produced freshly with the following ingredients: 98.0 mmol/L NaCl, 5.8 mmol/L KCl, 2.5 mmol/L NaH_2PO_4, 5.1 mmol/L Na pyruvate, 6.9 mmol/L Na fumarate, 2.0 mmol/L glutamine, 24.5 mmol/L HEPES Na, 1.0 mmol/L Trizma base, 11.1 mmol/L D-glucose, 1.0 mmol/L $CaCl_2$, 1.0 $MgCl_2$ and 2.0 mg/ml (w/v) bovine serum albumin. Also, all examinations were carried out in this solution. The mixed population of isolated rat GMCs contained at least three types of cell: parietal (20–25%), chief (40%) and epithelial (40–45%) cells. An initial viability of the isolated cells of 85–95% was maintained for 6–7 h.

Histamine

The isolated rat gastric mucosal cells were incubated with 10^{-8}–10^{-6} mol/L histamine (Peremin, Chinoin, Hungary) for 60 min with or without 10^{-4} mol/L prostacyclin (PGI_2Na, Chinoin, Hungary). Acid secretion was observed by measurements of pH in the incubating medium (Radelkis, Hungary).

Toxicological studies

After the histamine preincubation, GMCs were treated with ethanol (EtOH, EC_{50}=15%; Reanal, Hungary) alone, or in cotreatment with indomethacin (IND, ED_{50}=10^{-3} mol/L; Chinoin, Hungary) for 5 min. After this process, cells were treated as described above.

Examinations of cell viability

1. Trypan blue exclusion test:

   Trypan blue is excluded by viable cells but is taken up by damaged cells, staining the cytoplasm blue [14]. Trypan blue (0.14%; Sigma Chemical Co.) was mixed with the same volume of cell suspension and, 5 min later, the proportions of stained (dead) and unstained (viable) cells were calculated as a percentage after counting 100 cells in a haemocytometer.

2. Succinic dehydrogenase (SDH) assay

   The mitochondrial integrity was tested in 2×10^6 previously treated and redispersed cells [15]. The colour formazan product was quantified by Hitachi 124 spectrophotometer at 500 nm and calculated as nmol min^{-1} $(2 \times 10^6 \text{ cells})^{-1}$.

Statistics

Values in figures and text are expressed as means ± SEM. Comparisons were performed by unpaired Student's *t*-test. Results were considered significant at $p < 0.05$.

RESULTS

In-vivo studies

Acid secretory response

The acid output of the control group was 70.5 ± 6 μEq/rat 1 h after pylorus ligation. Addition of 20 mg/kg histamine significantly increased acid output to 304 ± 24 μEq/rat (n=6, $p < 0.01$). PGI_2 (5 μg/kg) had no detectable effect on gastric acid secretion of 1-h pylorus-ligated rats.

Effect of histamine on EtOH-induced gastric mucosal damage

Histamine dose-dependently reduced the number and severity of gastric mucosal lesions produced by ethanol. The values of pA_2 (doses required to produce 50% inhibition) for histamine were found to be 4.1 for the number, and 4.0 for the severity, of the mucosal lesions (Figures 1 and 2). The pD_2 for histamine ($\alpha_{atropine}$ was regarded as 1.00) was 3.75 for both number and severity of gastric lesions (Table 1).

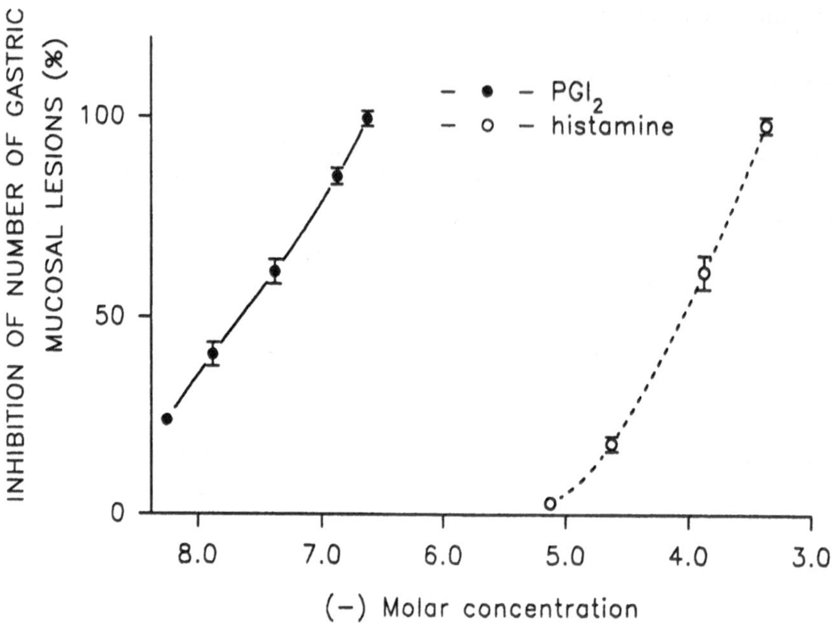

Figure 1. Affinity curves for PGI_2 and histamine inhibiting the extent of ethanol-induced gastric mucosal damage (number of lesions) in rats ($n = 12$)

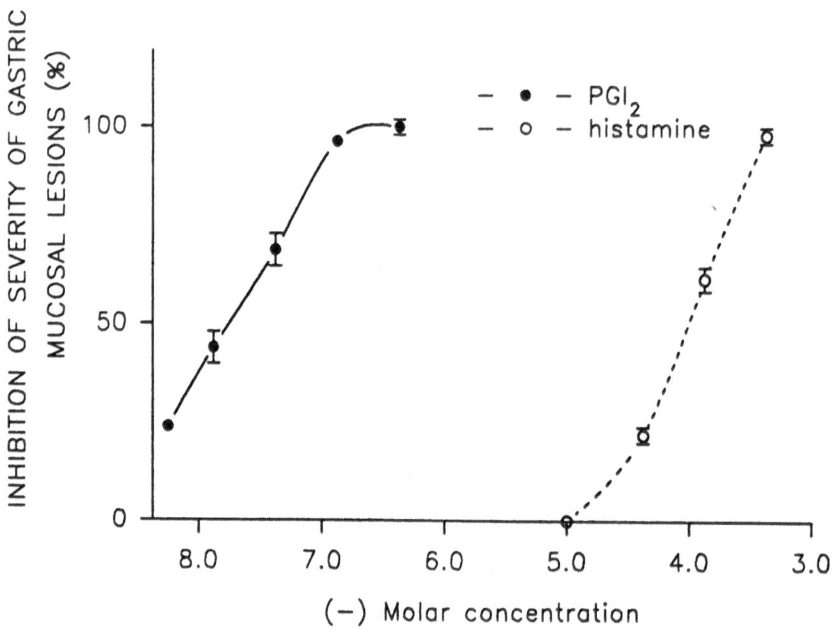

Figure 2. Affinity curves for PGI_2 and histamine inhibiting the severity of ethanol-induced gastric mucosal damage in rats ($n = 12$)

TABLE 1
Values of pD_2, α and pA_2 for histamine and PGI_2 inhibiting EtOH-induced gastric mucosal damage on the number (A) and severity (B) of mucosal lesions produced by intragastric administration of 96% ethanol ($\alpha_{atropine}$=1.00)

	Affinity		Intrinsic activity			
	pD_2		α		pA_2	
	A	B	A	B	A	B
Histamine	3.75	3.75	0.72	0.75	4.10	4.00
PGI_2	7.66	6.60	0.81	0.81	7.63	7.72

TABLE 2
PGI_2-induced gastric cytoprotection on 96% ethanol-induced gastric mucosal damage. The values are expressed as means ± SEM ($n = 12$)

	Control	5 μg/kg PGI_2	50 μg/kg PGI_2
Number	14±1	9±1	5±0.5
Severity	52±3	18±2	9±1

Effect of PGI_2 on EtOH-induced gastric mucosal damage

PGI_2 (5 and 50 μg/kg) significantly decreased both the number and severity of 96% EtOH-induced gastric mucosal injury. The cytoprotective effect of 5 μg/kg PGI_2 was regarded as 100% (Table 2). The values of pA_2 were 7.63 for the number and 7.72 for the severity of mucosal lesions (Figures 1 and 2). The pD_2 values of PGI_2 ($\alpha_{atropine} = 1.00$) were 7.66 for the number and 6.60 for the severity of gastric lesions (Table 1).

Effect of histamine on PGI_2-induced cytoprotection

Histamine stimulated PGI_2-induced gastric cytoprotection. The value of pA_2 was 3.75 for both the number and the severity of mucosal lesions; pD_2 values for histamine ($\alpha_{pentagastrin}$ was regarded as 1.00) were 3.7 for both number and severity of gastric mucosal damage (Figures 3 and 4, Table 3).

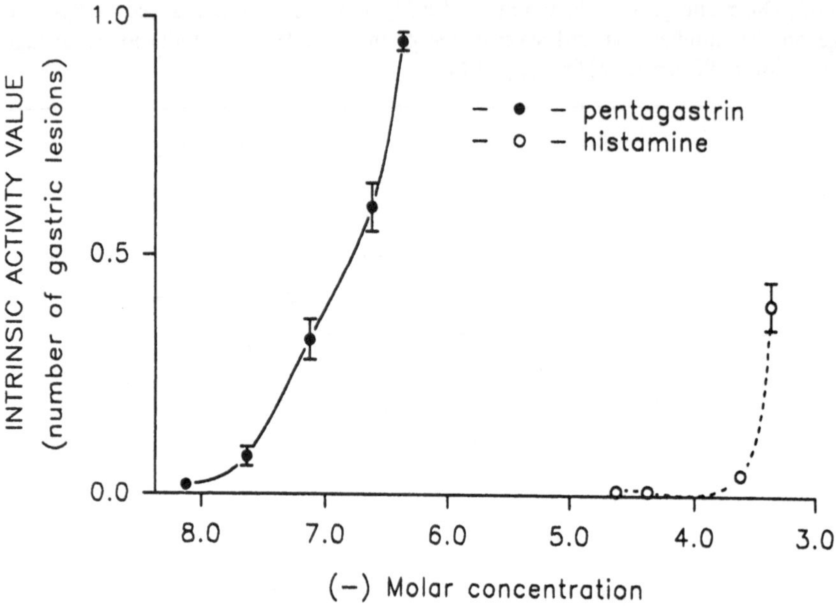

Figure 3. Intrinsic activity curves for histamine and pentagastrin stimulating PGI_2-induced gastric cytoprotection after administration of 96% ethanol on the number of gastric lesions ($\alpha_{pentagastrin}$=1.00) ($n = 12$)

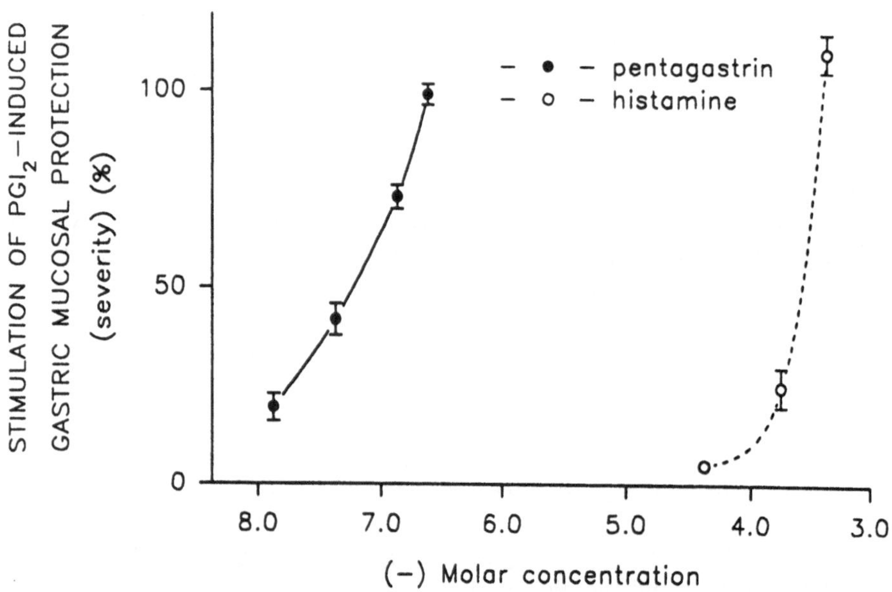

Figure 4. Affinity curves for histamine and pentagastrin stimulating PGI_2-induced gastric cytoprotection after administration of 96% ethanol on the severity of gastric mucosal lesions ($n = 12$)

TABLE 3
Values of pD_2, α and pA_2 for histamine and pentagastrin stimulating PGI_2-induced gastric cytoprotection on the number (A) and severity (B) of gastric mucosal damage produced by intragastric administration of 96% ethanol ($\alpha_{pentagastrin}$=1.00)

	Affinity		Intrinsic activity			
	pD_2		α		pA_2	
	A	B	A	B	A	B
Histamine	3.70	3.70	0.40	0.05	3.75	3.75
Pentagastrin	7.12	7.12	1.00	1.00	7.00	7.25

In-vitro studies

Effect of histamine

Preincubation with 10^{-8}–10^{-6} mol/L histamine, alone or in combination with 10^{-4} mol/L PGI_2, for 60 min did not cause any changes in the viability of GMCs, detected by trypan blue exclusion test or SDH activity (Figures 5–8). There was no measurable acid secretion in this incubation system caused by histamine, PGI_2 or their combination.

Effect of EtOH

After 5 min incubation with 15% EtOH, we could not observe any protective effect of histamine alone or in combination with 10^{-4} mol/L PGI_2 (Figures 5–8).

Combined effect of EtOH and IND

After 5 min incubation with 15% EtOH, alone or in combination with 10^{-3} mol/L IND treatment, there was no detectable cytoprotective effect of histamine, alone or in combination with 10^{-4} mol/L PGI_2 (Figures 5–8).

DISCUSSION

In this study, the organoprotective and cytoprotective effects of histamine were analysed in rats and on isolated rat gastric mucosal cells.

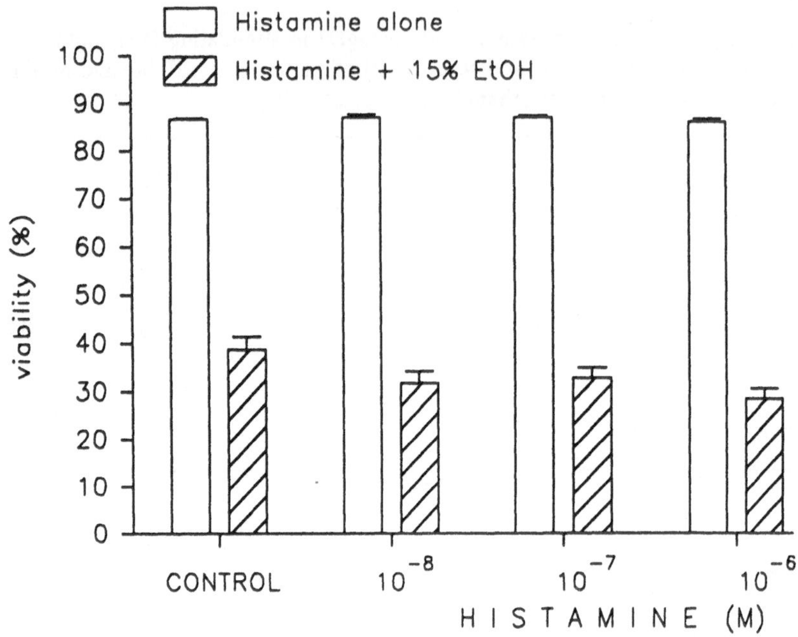

Figure 5. Effect of 60 min incubation of 10^{-8}–10^{-6} mol/L histamine on the viability of freshly isolated rat gastric mucosal cells detected by trypan blue exclusion test with or without 5 min 15% ethanol (EtOH) treatment ($n = 4$)

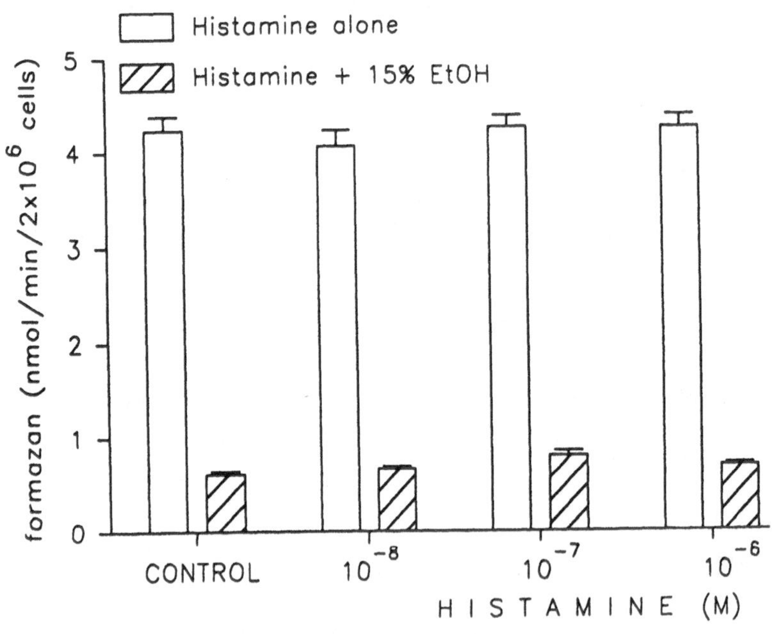

Figure 6. Changes in succinic dehydrogenase activity of freshly isolated rat gastric mucosal cells after 60 min incubation by 10^{-8}–10^{-6} mol/L histamine with or without 5 min 15% ethanol (EtOH) treatment ($n = 4$)

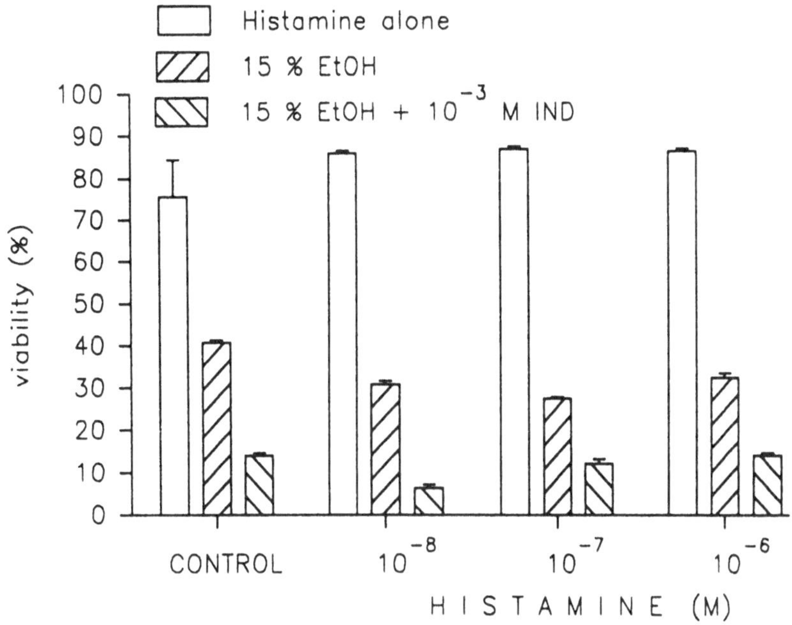

Figure 7. Effect of 60 min incubation of 10^{-8}–10^{-6} mol/L histamine and 10^{-4} mol/L PGI_2 on the viability of freshly isolated rat gastric mucosal cells detected by trypan blue exclusion test with or without 5 min 15% ethanol (EtOH) and 10^{-3} mol/L indomethacin (IND) treatment ($n = 4$)

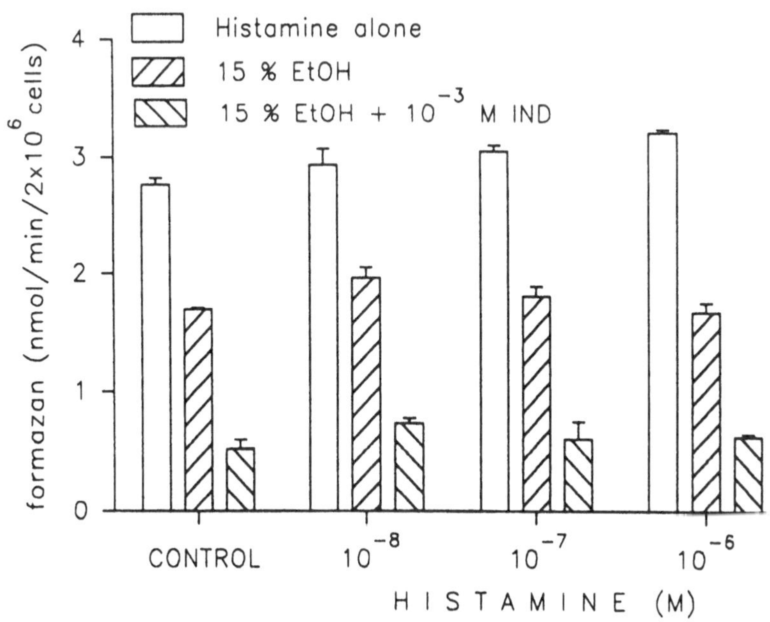

Figure 8. Changes in succinic dehydrogenase activity of freshly isolated rat gastric mucosal cells after 60 min incubation of 10^{-8}–10^{-6} mol/L histamine and 10^{-4} mol/L PGI_2 with or without 5 min 15% ethanol (EtOH) and 10^{-3} mol/L indomethacin (IND) treatment ($n = 4$)

Our results indicate that:

1. Histamine increases the short-term acid output in rats, while PGI_2 has no effect on gastric acid secretion;

2. Despite being itself aggressive, histamine has a protective effect (so-called cytoprotection) on the development of gastric mucosal lesions in a non-acid-dependent model;

3. Histamine stimulates PGI_2-induced gastric cytoprotection;

4. In vitro, there is no detectable cytoprotective effect of histamine.

We provided further evidence that PGI_2 has no influence on gastric acid secretion and that it can protect the mucosa against EtOH without any inhibition of aggressive factors (HCl). On the other hand, histamine (as histamine dihydrochloride, $C_5H_9N_3 \times 2$ HCl) increases acid secretion at a dose of 20 mg/kg (1.08×10^{-4} mol/L). This dose is within the range which provides a protective effect, both alone or by stimulating PGI_2-induced gastric cytoprotection in the EtOH-model. Thus, the secretory and organoprotective effects of histamine are linked at the same doses.

What could be the biochemical background to the in-vivo cytoprotective effect of this aggressive drug? It is known that, surprisingly, both gastric acid secretion inhibiting and stimulating drugs can prevent EtOH-induced mucosal damage [16]. The inhibitory drugs, such as cimetidine and atropine, decrease the cell metabolism, while pentagastrin, histamine and 2,4-dinitrophenol (for a short time) increase it. PGI_2-induced gastric cytoprotection is decreased by gastric acid inhibitory drugs; however, histamine, pentagastrin and 2,4-dinitrophenol can stimulate it. This effect can be partly explained at the level of the receptors due to reduction of ATP–ADP transformation and increase in the cellular cAMP content (in the case of histamine and pentagastrin) [16] but the mechanism of 2,4-dinitrophenol is quite different (inhibition of the respiratory chain). It seems that metabolic components must play a role in the protection of gastric mucosal damage.

In in-vitro circumstances, we could not detect any cytoprotective effect of histamine alone or in combination with PGI_2. One of the possible explanations of this negative result is that the surface receptors of the cells were damaged during pronase digestion. Freshly isolated GMCs can be stimulated by high levels of carbachol and histamine [13] but, in this study, we used physiological doses.

In respect of these in-vivo and in-vitro studies, the organoprotective and cytoprotective effects of histamine seem to be different in rats.

REFERENCES

1. Chaudhury TK, Jacobson ED. Prostaglandin cytoprotection of gastric mucosa. Gastroenterology. 1978;74:59.

2. Robert A, Nezamis JE, Lancaster C, Hanchar AJ. Cytoprotection by prostaglandins in rats. Prevention of gastric mucosal necrosis by alcohol, HCl, hypertonic NaCl, and thermal injury. Gastroenterology. 1979;77:433–43.
3. Szabó S. Critical and timely review of the concept of gastric cytoprotection. Acta Physiol Hung. 1989;73:115–27.
4. Gyires K. Are all 'cytoprotective' drugs gastroprotective? Acta Physiol Hung. 1992;80:247–55.
5. Mózsik Gy, Jávor T, Kitajima M, Pfeiffer CJ, Rainsford KD, Simon L, Szabó S, eds. Advances in Gastrointestinal Cytoprotection: Topics 1987. Budapest: Akadémiai Kiadó; 1989.
6. Mózsik Gy, Pár A, Csomós G, Kitajima M, Kondo M, Pfeiffer CJ, Rainsford KD, Sikiric P, Szabó S, eds. Cell Injury and Protection in the Gastrointestinal Tract: From Basic Sciences to Clinical Perspectives. Budapest: Akadémiai Kiadó; 1993.
7. Mózsik Gy, Morón F, Jávor T. Cellular mechanisms of the development of gastric mucosal damage and of gastroprotection induced by prostacyclin in rats. A pharmacological study. Prostagl Leukotr Med. 1982;9:71–84.
8. Mózsik Gy, Süto G, Király A, Vincze Á, Abdel-Salam OME, Karádi O. Cholinergic, gastrinergic, histaminergic and metabolic pathways of PGI_2-induced gastric cytoprotection in ethanol-induced mucosal damage in rats. Gastroenterology. 1995;108(Suppl.):A171.
9. Mózsik Gy, Bódis B, Garamszegi M et al. Role of vagal nerve in the development of gastric mucosal injury and its prevention by atropine, cimetidine, β-carotene and prostacyclin in rats. In: Szabo S, Taché Y, eds. Neuroendocrinology of Gastrointestinal Ulceration. New York: Plenum Press; 1995:175–90.
10. Bódis B, Karádi O, Nagy L, Mózsik Gy. Effect of ethanol, indomethacin and their combination on mixed gastric mucosal and Sp2 cells in vitro. Can J Physiol Pharmacol. 1994;72(Suppl 1):605.
11. Shay H, Sun DCH, Gruenstein M. A quantitative method for measuring spontaneous gastric secretion in the rat. Gastroenterology. 1954;26:906–13.
12. Csáky TZ. Introduction to General Pharmacology. New York: Appleton–Century–Crofts Educational Division, Meredith Corporation; 1969:17–34.
13. Nagy L, Szabo S, Morales RE, Plebani M, Jenkins JM. Identification of subcellular targets and sensitive tests of ethanol-induced damage in isolated gastric mucosal cells. Gastroenterology. 1994;107:907–14.
14. Baur H, Kasperek S, Pfaff E. Criteria of viability of isolated liver cells. Z Physiol Chem. 1975;356:827–38.
15. Mosmann T. Rapid colorimetric assay for cellular growth and survival: application to proliferation and cytotoxicity assays. J Immunol Meth. 1983;65:55–63.
16. Mózsik Gy, Jávor T. Biochemical and pharmacological approach to the genesis of ulcer disease. I. A model study of ethanol-induced injury to gastric mucosa in rats. Dig Dis Sci. 1988;33:92–105.

Manuscript received 31 Oct. 95.
Accepted for publication 18 Dec. 95.

TS Gaginella et al. (eds.), Biochemical Pharmacology as an Approach to Gastrointestinal Disorders, 387–394

COMPARATIVE VIABILITY STUDIES ON ISOLATED GASTRIC MUCOSAL MIXED CELLS AND HEPATOMA AND MYELOMA CELL LINES WITH ETHANOL, INDOMETHACIN AND THEIR COMBINATION

I. SZABÓ[1], B. BÓDIS[1], P. NÉMETH[2] AND Gy. MÓZSIK[1*]
[1]First Department of Medicine, [2]Immunological and Biotechnological Laboratory, University Medical School of Pécs, Pécs, Hungary
*Correspondence

This paper was first published in: Inflammopharmacology. 1997;5:21–28.

ABSTRACT

The toxic effects of ethanol (EtOH), indomethacin (IND) and their combination were studied in vitro. The experiments were performed on freshly isolated gastric mucosal mixed cells and two types of stable cultured cells: Sp2/0-Ag14, which is a non-secreting mouse myeloma cell line, and Hep G2, which is a human hepatocellular carcinoma cell line. EtOH decreased the viability of all types of cells in a concentration-dependent manner. At all concentrations, the EtOH caused a greater decrease in the viability of gastric mucosal cells than in the viability of Sp2/0-Ag14 cells. IND had no effect on the viability of the cultured cells, when this was employed without any other aggressive factor, such as EtOH. When used in combination, IND aggravated the EtOH-induced cell injury. These results show that the endogenous prostaglandins may play a role in the maintenance of cell integrity in all three types of cells.

Keywords: isolated rat gastric mucosal cells, Sp2/0-Ag14 cell line, Hep G2 cell line, ethanol, indomethacin

INTRODUCTION

The meaning of the original term 'gastric cytoprotection', which was described by Robert in 1979 [1,2], is limited at the level of the cell, and new concepts have been defined, such as organoprotection and gastroprotection, which are widely accepted and have been studied recently in in-vivo experiments. In these investigations, many environmental factors, e.g. central nervous system [3], vagal nerve [4,5], blood flow [6,7], vascular permeability [6] and rapid epithelial restitution of neck cell [8] have been studied as defence mechanisms of gastric mucosa.

The in-vivo and in-vitro experiments essentially differ from each other. Investigations on isolated cells have many advantages: all the effects originating from other organs or tissues can be eliminated, so the behaviour of a single cell can be examined. Unfortunately, these kinds of studies might have harmful consequences. Acutely

This paper was presented at the Section of IUPHAR GI Pharmacology Symposium on 'Biochemical pharmacology as an approach to gastrointestinal disorders (basic science to clinical perspectives)', October 12–14, 1995, Pécs, Hungary.

isolated cells are less suitable for pharmacological studies of the gastric mucosa because of their isolation procedure [9]. Stress may reduce the cell responsiveness, and surface receptors are damaged during the digestive stages of the isolation procedure. These effects may be eliminated by using stable cultured cells in the experiment, though their number is small and some properties of the original tumour can be seen in their behaviour.

Ethanol (EtOH) is widely used as a toxic agent in gastric cytoprotection investigations in vivo [9]. Indomethacin (IND) is also generally used for experiments [10–12]. It inhibits prostaglandin synthesis, which is responsible for the maintenance of gastric mucosal integrity due to stimulation of mucosal blood flow, preservation of cellular ion transport and protection of the mucosal proliferative zone [13]. These chemical agents have been studied widely in in-vivo experiments, but only a few experiments have been carried out in vitro on isolated cells with these toxic agents.

The aims of this study were:

1. To analyse the toxic effects of 5 min EtOH treatment in vitro on acutely isolated mixed gastric mucosal cells (GMC);

2. To compare the differences between the GMC and the stable cultured cells;

3. To evaluate the differences between the myeloma (Sp2/0-Ag14) and the hepatoma (Hep G2) cell lines;

4. To study the effect of IND on GMC and Sp2/0-Ag14 cells;

5. To examine the combined effect of EtOH and IND on these two types of cells.

MATERIALS AND METHODS

Preparation of mixed gastric mucosal cells

Gastric mucosal cells from Sprague–Dawley rats were isolated by the method of Nagy et al. [9]. The segments of the glandular stomach were separated from the blood vessels and the surrounding connective tissue and were incubated in a physiological solution containing 0.5 mg/ml pronase E (type XXV, Sigma Chemical Co.) and 10^{-3} mol/L EGTA. After several washings, the cells were resuspended in a solution (0.157 mol/L, pH 7.4) produced freshly with the following ingredients: 98.0 mmol/L NaCl, 5.8 mmol/L KCl, 2.5 mmol/L Na_2PO_4, 5.1 mmol/L sodium pyruvate, 6.9 mmol/L sodium fumarate, 2.0 mmol/L glutamine, 24.5 mmol/L HEPES Na, 1.0 mmol/L Trizma base, 11.1 mmol/L D-glucose, 1.0 mmol/L $CaCl_2$, 1.0 mmol/L $MgCl_2$, and 2.0 mg/ml (w/v) bovine serum albumin. All examinations were carried out in this solution.

Stable cultured cells

Sp2/0-Ag14 (CRL 1581) is a non-secreting mouse myeloma; Hep G2 is a human hepatocellular carcinoma cell line obtained from the American Type Culture Collection (ATCC). Cells were cultured and the examinations were carried out in Dulbecco's modified Eagle's medium containing 10% fetal calf serum in a humidified incubator containing 95% air and 5% CO_2 at 37°C.

Toxicological studies

The cells were incubated with different concentrations of EtOH (1, 5, 10, 15, 20 and 50% (v/v)), IND (10^{-8}–10^{-3} mol/L dissolved in 5% $NaHCO_3$, pH 7.4 with 5 N HCl) and their combination (15% EtOH and 10^{-3} mol/L IND) for 5 min in a shaking water bath at 37°C. Each study used 10^5 cells. After 5 min incubation the cells were separated from the supernatant by centrifugation (500*g*, 10 min), washed out (10 min water bath and centrifugation again) and resuspended in a toxic-free medium.

Trypan blue exclusion test

Trypan blue is taken up by damaged cells, staining the cytoplasm blue; viable cells can resist this staining. Trypan blue (0.2%) was mixed with the same volume of cell suspension and, after 5 min latency, the numbers of stained (dead) and unstained (viable) cells were calculated as percentages in a haemocytometer. In the comparison with stable cultured cells, we examined the viability over longer periods (5 min, 60 min, 4 h and 24 h) after the 5-min EtOH incubation.

Statistics

Values in figures and text are expressed as means ± SEM. Comparisons were performed using the unpaired Student's *t*-test and *p* values were considered significant at $p < 0.05$.

RESULTS

Effect of EtOH on GMC

EtOH (1, 5, 10, 15, 20 and 50%) concentration-dependently decreased the viability of GMC. The EC_{50} was 13.5% (Figure 1).

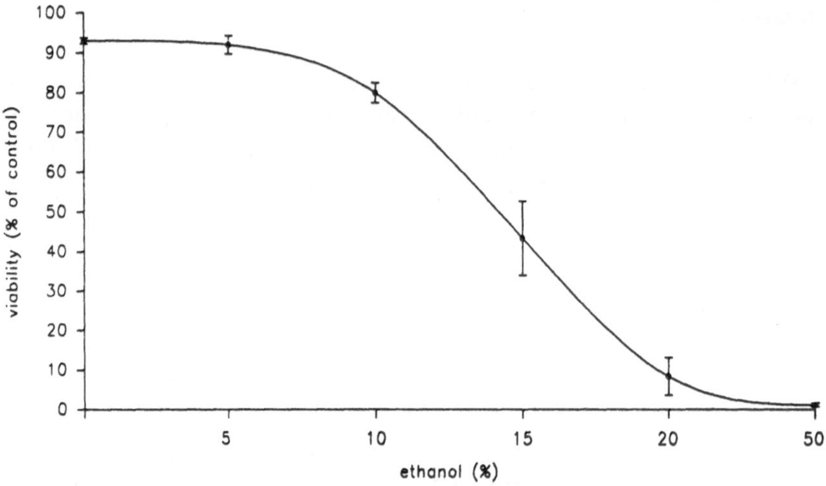

Figure 1. Changes in the viability of acutely isolated rat gastric mucosal cells (GMC) after 5 min incubation with 1–50% ethanol, detected by trypan blue exclusion test (% of control). The results are expressed as means ± SEM ($n = 5$)

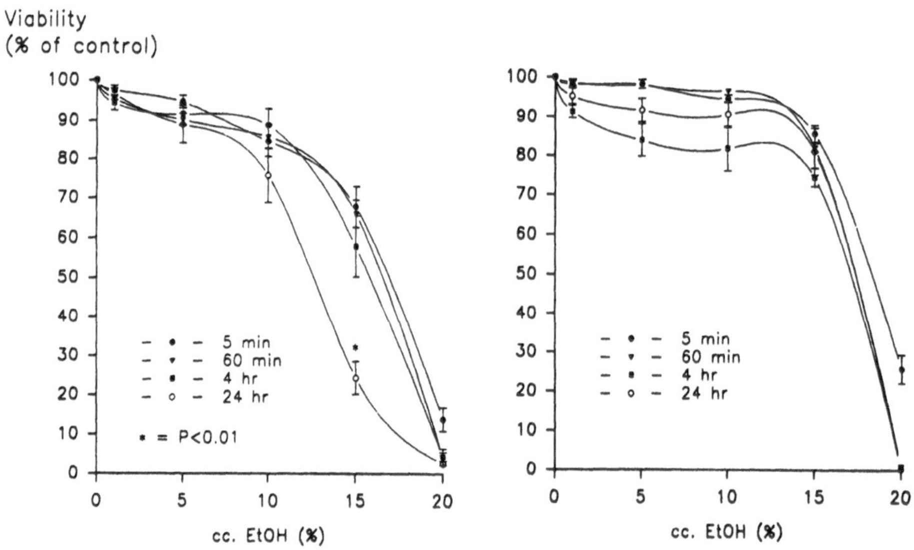

Figure 2. Changes in the viability of the Sp2/0-Ag14 (left) and Hep G2 (right) cell lines at various times (5 min, 60 min, 4 h and 24 h) after incubation with different concentrations of EtOH, detected by trypan blue exclusion test. The results are expressed as means ± SEM ($n = 5$). $^*p < 0.01$ compared with the 4-h value

Effect of EtOH on Sp2/0-Ag14 and Hep G2 cell lines

EtOH concentration-dependently decreased the viability of stable cultured cells. In the case of Sp2/0-Ag14 cells, there was no significant difference between the viability values counted at 5 and 60 min, but 4 h after incubation with 10% or 15% of EtOH, a significant level of cell destruction could be detected. In the case of the Hep G2 cell line, a greater level of resistance was found up to a concentration of 15% EtOH; above that concentration, a similar level of cell destruction occurred (Figure 2).

Comparing GMC and stable cultured cells

At all concentrations, the EtOH decreased the viability of GMC much more potently than the viability of the stable cultured cells. The EC_{50} for GMC was 13.5%; the EC_{50} for Sp2/0-Ag14 was 16% (Figures 1 and 2).

Effect of IND

Five minutes incubation with 10^{-8}–10^{-3} mol/L IND had no effect on the viability of Sp2/0-Ag14 cells. In the case of GMC, only the highest dose (10^{-3} mol/L) of IND decreased significantly ($p<0.02$) the number of viable cells (Figure 3).

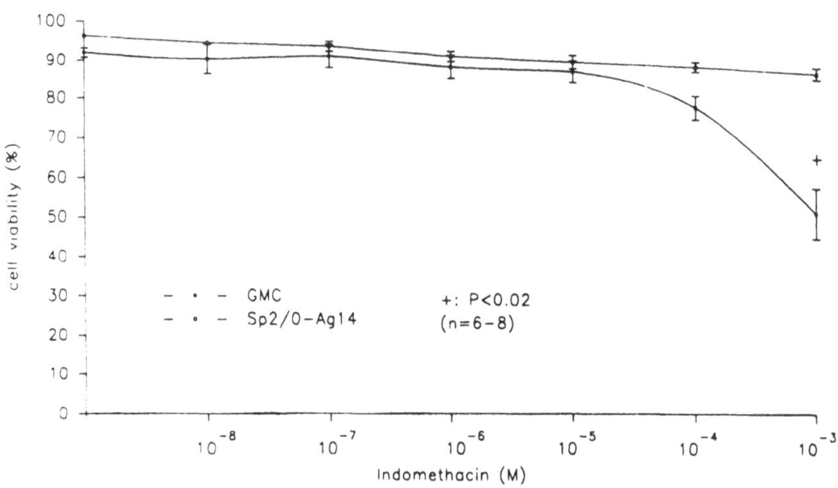

Figure 3. Changes in the viability of GMC and Sp2/0-Ag14 cells after 5-min incubation with 10^{-8}–10^{-3} mol/L indomethacin, detected by trypan blue exclusion test. The results are expressed as means ± SEM ($n=6$–8). $^{+}p<0.02$ compared with GMC

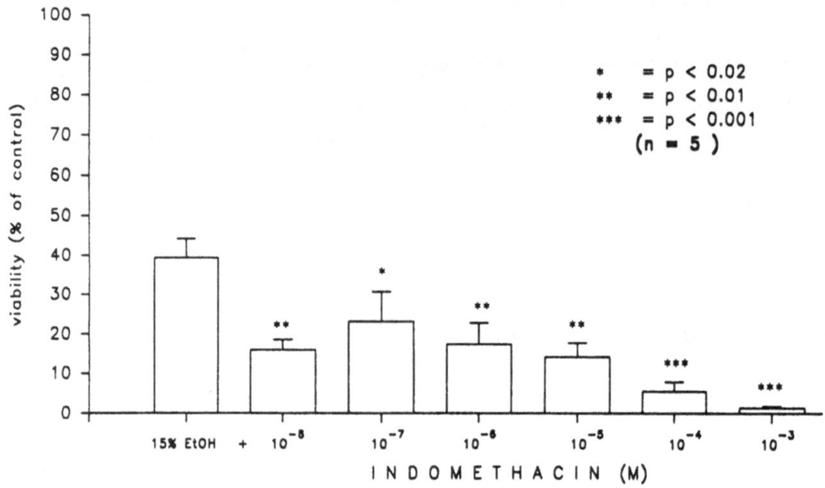

Figure 4. Changes in the viability of GMC after combined incubation with 15% ethanol and 10^{-8}–10^{-3} mol/L indomethacin, detected by trypan blue exclusion test. The results are expressed as means ± SEM ($n = 5$). $^{*}p<0.02$; $^{**}p<0.01$; $^{***}p<0.001$ compared with treatment with 15% EtOH alone

Combined effect of EtOH and IND

After the combined treatment a greater cell destruction could be detected. Using different concentrations, the 10^{-3} mol/L dose was the most aggressive; the amount of necrotic cell loss was concentration dependent (Figure 4). Comparing the response of the GMC with the myeloma cells, the GMC are much more vulnerable than Sp2/0-Ag14 cells after EtOH treatment, and after the combined treatment too (Figure 5).

DISCUSSION

In these studies freshly isolated rat gastric mucosal cells and two types of stable cultured cells were used to evaluate the effects of EtOH, IND and their combination in toxicological studies. The mixed population of isolated rat GMC contained at least three types of cells: parietal (20–25%), chief (40%), and epithelial (45%) cells. A viability of 80–95% could be maintained for 6–7 h. These cells do not have the potential for proliferation. Cultured cells were always kept in the same conditions, tests are reproducible and cells can survive for a longer time. During the calculation of viability, it must be remembered that the two cell lines have different proliferation rates. In particular, this should be borne in mind during the interpretation of the different viability values of longer incubation times.

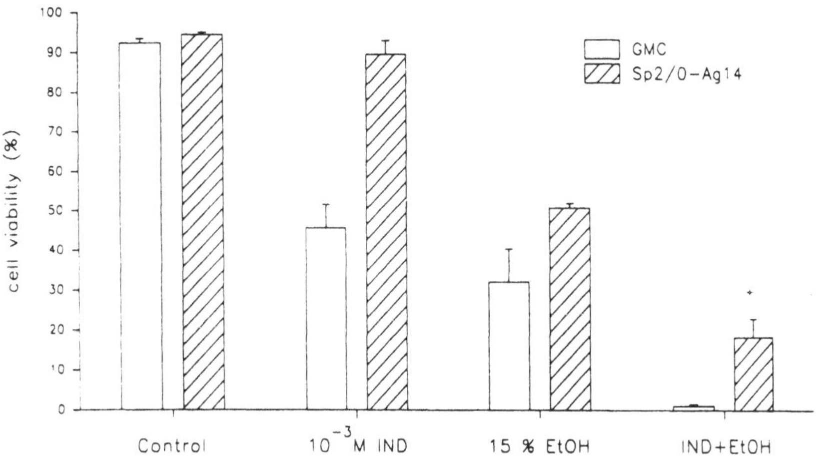

Figure 5. Changes in the viability of GMC and Sp2/0-Ag14 cells after 5-min incubation with 15% EtOH, with 10^{-3} mol/L IND and with 15% EtOH and 10^{-3} mol/L IND combined, detected by trypan blue exclusion test. The results are expressed as means ± SEM ($n = 6$–8). $^{+}p < 0.01$; $^{*}p < 0.05$ compared with 15% EtOH treatment

Our results indicate that the acutely isolated cells are more vulnerable than cultured cells. After EtOH treatment, in the case of Sp2/0-Ag14 cells, the EC_{50} was higher (16%) than that of GMC (13.5%). IND had no damaging effect on stable cultured cells. The combined treatment reduced the viability in both types of cells, but this effect was much smaller in Sp2/0-Ag14 cells; almost all the GMC were destroyed. These results show that cultured cells are more resistant to toxic agents than acutely isolated cells. Though different types of cells were used in this study, the differences in behaviour may derive from the differences in isolation procedure rather than from their differences in type. In-vivo experiments have shown that gastrointestinal ulceration can be produced by IND administration [9,10]. It is known that IND inhibits the activity of cyclooxygenase, producing less prostaglandins and excessive vasoconstrictor leukotrienes [14], and decreases the mucosal level of adenosine triphosphate [15]. These factors reduce the gastric mucosal resistance to acid. In the in-vitro study described here, IND was applied without any other aggressive factor, such as EtOH, and was not toxic for these cells. However, after the combination treatment, cell viability was considerably decreased compared with the effect of EtOH alone. It is likely that the decreased levels of endogenous prostaglandins might play a role in the enhanced toxic effect of EtOH. These results are in a good agreement with those of Tarnawski et al. [16] who observed a protective effect of exogenous prostaglandins on human isolated gastric glands against IND and EtOH injury.

ACKNOWLEDGEMENTS

This study was supported by the Hungarian National Research Fund (OTKA T020098) and the Ministry of Welfare and Health (ETT-03 660/93).

REFERENCES

1. Robert A, Nezamis JE, Lancaster C, Hancher AJ. Cytoprotection by prostaglandins in rats. Gastroenterology. 1979;77:433–43.
2. Robert A. Cytoprotection by prostaglandins. Gastroenterology. 1979;77:761–7.
3. Grijalva CV, Novin D. The role of the hypothalamus and dorsal vagal complex in the gastrointestinal function and pathophysiology. Ann NY Acad Sci. 1990;597:207–22.
4. Mózsik Gy, Karádi O, Király Á et al. Vagal nerve and the gastric mucosal defence. J Physiol (Paris). 1993;87:59–64.
5. Mózsik Gy, Király Á, Garamszegi M et al. Mechanism of vagal nerve in gastric mucosal defence: unchanged gastric emptying and increased vascular permeability. J Clin Gastroenterol. 1992;14(suppl 1):S140–4.
6. Szabo S, Trier JS, Broown A, Schoor J. Early vascular injury and increased vascular permeability in the gastric mucosal injury caused by ethanol in the rat. Gastroenterology. 1985;88:228–36.
7. Guth PH, Paulsen G, Nagata H. Histologic and microcirculatory changes in alcohol-induced gastric lesions in the rat: effects of prostaglandin cytoprotection. Gastroenterology. 1984;87:1083–90.
8. Lacy ER, Ito S. Rapid epithelial restitution of the rat gastric mucosa after ethanol injury. J Lab Invest. 1984;51:573–83.
9. Nagy L, Szabo S, Morales RE, Plebani M, Jenkins JM. Identification of subcellular targets and sensitive tests of ethanol-induced damage in isolated gastric mucosal cells. Gastroenterology. 1994;107:907–14.
10. Djahanguiri B. The production of acute gastric ulceration by indomethacin in the rat. Scand J Gastroenterol. 1969;17:265–7.
11. Brodie DA, Cook PG, Bauer BJ. Indomethacin-induced intestinal lesions in the rat. Toxicol Appl Pharmacol. 1970;17:615–24.
12. Karádi O, Bódis B, Király Á et al. Surgical vagotomy enhances the indomethacin-induced gastrointestinal mucosal damage in rats. Inflammopharmacology. 1994;2:389–99.
13. Lacy ER, Ito S. Microscopic analysis of ethanol damage to rat gastric mucosa after treatment with a prostaglandin. Gastroenterology. 1982;83:619–25.
14. Rainsford KD. Mechanism of NSAID-induced ulcerogenesis: structural properties of drugs, focus on the microvascular factors, and novel approaches for gastro-intestinal protection. Acta Physiol Hung. 1992;80:23–38
15. Rainsford KD. Prevention of indomethacin induced gastro-intestinal ulceration in the rat by glucose-citrate formulations: Role of ATP in mucosal defences. Br J Rheumatol. 1987;26(suppl):81.
16. Tarnawski A, Brzozowski T, Sarfeh IJ et al. Prostaglandin protection of human isolated gastric glands against indomethacin and ethanol injury. J Clin Invest. 1988;81:1081–9.

Manuscript received 31 Oct. 95.
Accepted for publication 5 Nov. 95.

INDEX